Handbook of Pediatric Drug Therapy and Immunization

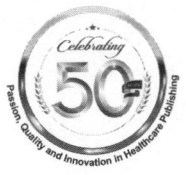

Handbook of Pediatric Drug Therapy and Immunization

Third Edition

RK Suneja MD DCH
Former Consultant and Head
Department of Pediatrics and
Medical Superintendent
Hindu Rao Hospital
New Delhi, India

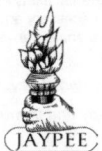

JAYPEE BROTHERS MEDICAL PUBLISHERS
The Health Sciences Publisher
New Delhi | London

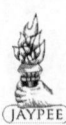

Jaypee Brothers Medical Publishers (P) Ltd

Headquarters

Jaypee Brothers Medical Publishers (P) Ltd
4838/24, Ansari Road, Daryaganj
New Delhi 110 002, India
Phone: +91-11-43574357
Fax: +91-11-43574314
E-mail: jaypee@jaypeebrothers.com

Overseas Office

JP Medical Ltd
83 Victoria Street, London
SW1H 0HW (UK)
Phone: +44 20 3170 8910
Fax: +44 (0)20 3008 6180
E-mail: info@jpmedpub.com

Website: www.jaypeebrothers.com
Website: www.jaypeedigital.com

© 2020, Jaypee Brothers Medical Publishers

The views and opinions expressed in this book are solely those of the original contributor(s)/author(s) and do not necessarily represent those of editor(s) of the book.

All rights reserved. No part of this publication may be reproduced, stored or transmitted in any form or by any means, electronic, mechanical, photocopying, recording or otherwise, without the prior permission in writing of the publishers.

All brand names and product names used in this book are trade names, service marks, trademarks or registered trademarks of their respective owners. The publisher is not associated with any product or vendor mentioned in this book.

Medical knowledge and practice change constantly. This book is designed to provide accurate, authoritative information about the subject matter in question. However, readers are advised to check the most current information available on procedures included and check information from the manufacturer of each product to be administered, to verify the recommended dose, formula, method and duration of administration, adverse effects and contraindications. It is the responsibility of the practitioner to take all appropriate safety precautions. Neither the publisher nor the author(s)/editor(s) assume any liability for any injury and/or damage to persons or property arising from or related to use of material in this book.

This book is sold on the understanding that the publisher is not engaged in providing professional medical services. If such advice or services are required, the services of a competent medical professional should be sought.

Every effort has been made where necessary to contact holders of copyright to obtain permission to reproduce copyright material. If any have been inadvertently overlooked, the publisher will be pleased to make the necessary arrangements at the first opportunity. The **CD/DVD-ROM** (if any) provided in the sealed envelope with this book is complimentary and free of cost. **Not meant for sale**.

Inquiries for bulk sales may be solicited at: jaypee@jaypeebrothers.com

Handbook of Pediatric Drug Therapy and Immunization

First Edition: **2004**

Second Edition: **2008**

Third Edition: 2020

ISBN: 978-93-88958-59-2

Printed at Rajkamal Electric Press, Plot No. 2, Phase-IV, Kundli, Haryana.

Preface to the Third Edition

Recent major advances in the field of Pediatric Drug Therapy and Immunization and the introduction of a large number of new drugs and vaccines have made the task of pediatricians, residents, postgraduate (PG) and undergraduate (UG) students, and general practitioners to stay abreast of them extremely difficult. The relevant information lies scattered among different textbooks and journals and cannot readily be accessed and utilized when required during management of patients in the clinic, wards, or in the intensive care unit (ICU).

To address this important issue, vital information about key aspects of drug therapy and immunization in neonates, infants, and children, derived from various authoritative sources has been presented in this concise manual in a simple, easy to access and apply format.

It covers treatment of a broad range of important pediatric disorders such as infections, asthma, epilepsy, congestive heart failure, diabetes, hereditary clotting disorders, blood component therapy, and management of emergencies such as shock, status asthmaticus, status epilepticus, diabetic ketoacidosis, anaphylaxis, hypertensive emergency, cardiac arrhythmias, and life support-requiring situations.

The spectrum of effectiveness of various antibiotics and their rational use in treatment of different types of infections have been set out.

The guidelines by Indian Academy of Pediatrics, World Health Organization (WHO), and other international authorities in respect of schedules of immunization, appropriate use of various vaccines, and measures for pre- and postexposure prophylaxis in children have been described.

A separate section provides information about drugs used in children—their indications, dosage, modes of use, precautions, and side effects along with trade names of some standard proprietary products. An alphabetical index of diseases and drugs has been provided for instant retrieval of the desired information.

The assistance and valuable suggestions by Dr Krishan Autar and Dr PR Oberoi are gratefully acknowledged.

RK Suneja

Preface to the First Edition

Clinicians engaged in the management of sick infants and children have to contend with some unique complexities. While the clinical manifestation of an infection may be the same, say pneumonia, in a neonate, infant or an older child, the causative organisms are generally quite different. Rational therapy requires proper knowledge about the diverse nature of aetiological agents and appropriate antimicrobial drugs suitable for their treatment in different age groups. The use of inappropriate antimicrobial drugs may result in ineffective therapy or contribute to the development of undesirable antibiotic resistance in the causative pathogens in the community.

There is no simple, appropriate age-based mathematical formula for calculation of drug dosage for children on the basis of their dose for adults. Without specific knowledge about correct pediatric dosage, based on body weight/surface area and other factors, such as gestational and post-natal age in neonates, a clinician is liable to prescribe the drug in an inappropriate suboptimal or excess dose with undesirable consequences.

Rapid advances in the field of pediatrics and steady introduction of a large number of new drugs have made the task of even experienced pediatricians of staying duly informed and capable of conducting rational drug therapy quite difficult. The difficulty is notably enhanced by the fact that the relevant information (especially in the context of conditions in South Asia and other neighboring countries) lies widely scattered among several textbooks, journals and monographs and busy clinicians frequently do not have sufficient time or resources to gather it. They feel particularly handicapped when they require quick information on some vital aspects of drug therapy during active management of a sick child in the clinic or hospital as no handy source of reliable information is available.

Keeping this in view, comprehensive information about important practical aspects of pediatric drug therapy (both during routine and emergency management) drawn from various authoritative sources has been compiled and presented in this manual in a simple, easy to access and apply format. The subjects covered include the choice and usage of appropriate drugs for therapy in different infections in neonates, infants and children, spectra and effectiveness of various antimicrobial agents, drug management of important cardiovascular, respiratory and other systemic disorders, emergency drugs, fluids, electrolytes and acid-base management in acute gastroenteritis, blood component transfusion therapy, vaccines and antidotes for common poisonings. A separate section provides information about drugs in pediatric use—their indications, dosage, mode of use, precautions and side effects along with trade names of some proprietary formulations. An alphabetical index of diseases and drugs has been incorporated for the convenience of the reader.

It is hoped that this concise, wide-ranging, ready reference handbook will be of immense help as a companion guide to residents, postgraduate students, pediatricians and other specialists as well as to the general practitioners involved in the care of neonates, infants and children.

RK Suneja

Acknowledgments

I am thankful to Shri Jitendar P Vij (Group Chairman), Mr Ankit Vij (Managing Director), Mr MS Mani (Group President), Ms Chetna Malhotra Vohra (Associate Director—Content Strategy), Ms Pooja Bhandari (Production Head) and Ms Prerna Bajaj (Development Editor) of M/s Jaypee Brothers Medical Publishers (P) Ltd, New Delhi, India, for giving a go-ahead at the very beginning and helping me in every way possible to bring out this book.

Contents

Section 1: Drug Therapy

1. Guidelines for Antimicrobial Therapy 3
2. Antibiotic Therapy in Neonatal Infections 31
3. Spectra and Effectiveness of Various Antimicrobial Agents 38
4. Preferred Antimicrobial Agents against Selected Bacteria 57
5. Antimicrobial Chemoprophylaxis in Patients/Contacts 70
6. Drug Therapy and Prevention in Childhood Tuberculosis 74
7. Malaria: Treatment and Chemoprophylaxis 80
8. Treatment of Helminthic, Protozoal, and Other Parasitic Infections 86
9. Drugs for Selected Viral Infections 90
10. Guidelines for HIV Treatment 92
11. Preferred Therapy for Selected Fungal Pathogens 96
12. Fluids, Electrolytes and Acid-base Management in Acute Gastroenteritis 99
13. Treatment of Acute Hyperkalemia and Hypokalemia 104
14. Management of Asthma 107
15. Drug Therapy in Epilepsy and Neonatal Seizures 115
16. Pharmacotherapy in Congestive Heart Failure 127
17. Pharmacotherapy in Hypertension and Hypertensive Emergencies 134

18. Guidelines for Management of Cardiac Arrhythmias 147
19. Pediatric Life Support Algorithms and Emergency Drugs 150
20. Understanding and Management of Shock 159
21. Management of Dengue 171
22. "Blue Spells" in Tetralogy of Fallot: Management and Prevention 177
23. Management of Childhood Type I Diabetes and Diabetic Ketoacidosis 179
24. Drug Therapy in Anaphylaxis 184
25. Management of Intracranial Hypertension 187
26. Management of Hemophilia 191
27. Blood Component Therapy 196

Section 2: Immunization and Immunoprophylaxis

28. Active Immunization 203
29. Pre- and Postexposure Prophylaxis 233

Section 3: Poisoning

30. Nontoxic Household Products and Pharmaceuticals 247
31. Antidotes for Common Poisoning 249
32. Medications Whose Single Dose may be Fatal for a Toddler 260

Section 4: Drugs in Pediatrics

33. Pediatric Drug Formulary 265
34. Dosage of Antimicrobial Agents in Neonates 467
35. Drugs in Renal Failure 470

Appendices *475-507*
Index *509*

Section 1

Drug Therapy

CHAPTER 1

Guidelines for Antimicrobial Therapy

It is crucial that antibiotics should be prescribed only when they are necessary for treatment following a clear diagnosis and that these be administered for the desirable, precise duration.

While choosing an antibiotic, the age of the child, his hepatic and renal status, history of allergy, comorbid condition; antibiotic sensitivity or resistance pattern of organisms in the local community or institution, culture sensitivity findings in the patients sample (if available) and the known effectiveness, limitations and potential adverse effects of the proposed antibiotic should be duly taken into account. As far as possible, a first-line simple antibiotic, which would suffice, should be chosen for treatment instead of the strong second-line one. In the event of hypersensitivity to the first-line antibiotic or lack of proper clinical response, suitable alternative second-line antibiotic may be employed.

Taking into consideration different important factors and the recommendations of various national and international regulatory bodies, guidelines for antimicrobial therapy in children have been described in this and following sections.

Note: For dosage, mode of use and other information regarding recommended drugs, see under the individual drug in "Pediatric Drug Formulary".

SKIN AND SOFT TISSUE INFECTIONS

Cellulitis and Erysipelas (Nonpurulent)

(Mainly Group A *Streptococcus*, *Staphylococcus aureus*; in immunocompromised—*Pseudomonas aeruginosa*, *Haemophilus influenzae* type b, and others).

Mild

Clindamycin or cephalosporin or cloxacillin per oral (PO).

Moderate

Ceftriaxone or cefazolin or clindamycin intravenous (IV).

Severe

Empirical: Vancomycin + piperacillin – tazobactam *IV*
Subsequently as per culture findings:
- Monomicrobial *Streptococcus pyogenes*; or clostridia species:
  - Penicillin + clindamycin
- Vibrio vulnificus
  - Doxycycline + ceftazidime
- Polymicrobial
  - Vancomycin + piperacillin – tazobactam.

Duration of treatment: 10 days

Cellulitis, Buccal

H. influenzae type b, Pneumococcus:
- *Initial*: Cefotaxime or ceftriaxone or cefuroxime IV/intramuscular (IM)
- *Alternative*: Chloramphenicol IV
- *Later*: Amoxicillin-clavulanate PO or a second or third generation cephalosporin PO
- *Duration of treatment*: 7–10 days.

BITES

Dog, Cat, Other Animals, and Human

[Streptococci, *S. aureus*, *S. epidermidis*, *Pasteurella multocida and canis* (in animal bites), and *Eikenella corrodens* (in human bites)]

Amoxicillin-clavulanate PO

For severe infection: Ampicillin-sulbactam or ticarcillin-clavulanate IV.

Alternative: Ampicillin + clindamycin IV.
For penicillin allergic patients: clindamycin + sulfamethoxazole.

Ludwig's Angina (Bilateral Submandibular Space Infection)

(Streptococcus species, anaerobes, *Eikenella corrodens*, and others)
- Clindamycin or ticarcillin-clavulanate IV or
- Piperacillin-tazobactam IV.

Pyoderma, Cervical Adenitis

(Streptococcal, *Staph. aureus*)
Cephalexin or cloxacillin PO × 5–10 days.
For serious infection: Cloxacillin or clindamycin IV.

Rat-bite Fever

(*Streptobacillus moniliformis* and *Spirillum minus*)
Penicillin G IV or procaine penicillin IM × 7–10 days, *alternatives*: Tetracycline, doxycycline, gentamicin, or streptomycin (in penicillin allergic patients).

Staphylococcal Scalded Skin Syndrome

- *Initial*: Cloxacillin or nafcillin; vancomycin [if methicillin-resistant *Staphylococcus aureus* (MRSA)] PO/IV
- *Later*: Add clindamycin.

OROPHARYNGEAL, NOSE, EAR, EYE, AND UPPER RESPIRATORY TRACT INFECTIONS

Pharyngitis, Tonsillopharyngitis

[(Group A β-hemolytic *Streptococcus* (GABHS)]
- *For patients who are not allergic to penicillin:*
  - Amoxicillin 50 mg/kg/day (max 1 g) div q 8–12 h PO × 10 days

- Penicillin V (i) wt <27 kg: 250 mg q BD; weight >27 kg: 500 mg div. in BD PO × 10 days.
- Benzathine penicillin (i) wt <27 kg: 600,000 units; >27 kg: 1.2 million units in single dose
- *For penicillin allergic patients:*
  - Erythromycin ethylsuccinate 40 mg/kg/day (max 1 g) div. in BID × 10 days PO
  - Azithromycin (12 mg/kg/day × 1 day; then 6 mg/kg/day div. in OD × 4 days PO
  - Clarithromycin 15 mg/kg/day (max 500 mg/day) div. in BID × 10 days PO.
- *For those with only type 1 allergy to patients:*
  - Cefaclor 20–40 mg/kg/day (max 1.8 g/day) div. in TID × 10 days PO
  - Cephalexin: 50 mg/kg/day div in q 6–8 hr PO × 10 days.
- *For recurrent GABHS culture positive pharyngitis and streptococcal carriers:*
  - Clindamycin 20 mg/kg/day div in TID PO × 10 days; (adults—150–450 mg/dose q TID PO)
  - *Alternative*: Amoxicillin-clavulanate @ amoxicillin 40 mg/kg/day up to 2000 mg/day div in TID × 10 days.

Retropharyngeal Cellulitis or Abscess

(Group A *Streptococcus*, oral anaerobes, staphylococci, *H. influenzae*, and *Klebsiella*)

Clindamycin or ampicillin-sulbactam + cefotaxime or ceftriaxone IV × several days; when improved PO (clindamycin + cefdinir or cefpodoxime).

Gingivostomatitis

(Herpetic)
Acyclovir × 7 days; for mild infection—PO; for severe cases—IV.

Diphtheria

- Erythromycin 40–50 mg/kg/day div. in q 6 h PO (max 2 g/day) × 14 days

- Or Procaine penicillin: <10 kg: 300,000 units/dose OD IM × 14 days
  >10 kg: 600,000 units/dose OD IM × 14 days
- Or Aqueous crystalline penicillin 100,000–150,000 U/kg/day. div q 6 hr IV/IM × 14 days.

  PLUS diphtheria antitoxin (*see* under "immunoglobulins and antitoxins" for dosage). *Antitoxin is the mainstay of therapy.*

Note: Parenteral penicillin is recommended till the patient is unable to swallow. It is followed by oral erythromycin (total duration 14 days).

Otitis Media (Acute)

Initial Treatment

- Amoxicillin 40–90 mg/kg/day div q BID × 7–10 days
- or amoxicillin clavulanate (amoxicillin 40–90 mg/kg/day) div q BID × 7–10 days
- or ceftriaxone 50 mg/kg IM/IV × 3 doses on alternate days

If patient allergic to penicillin:
- Cefdinir 14 mg/kg/day div in OD/BID × 7–10 days
- Or cefuroxime 30 mg/kg/day div in BID × 7–10 days
- Or cefpodoxime 10 mg/kg/day div in BID × 7–10 days
- Or ceftriaxone 50 mg/kg IM/IV × 3 doses on alternate days.

Antibiotic Treatment after 48–72 hours of Failure of Initial Treatment

Clindamycin 30–40 mg/kg/day div. in TID + cefuroxime or cefdinir.

Sinusitis (Acute)

(*Pneumococcus, H. influenzae, Moraxella catarrhalis, streptococci*)
- Uncomplicated mild/moderate acute bacterial sinusitis
  - *Initial:* Amoxicillin 45 mg/kg/day div in BID

- *For penicillin allergic cases:* Cefdinir or cefuroxime axetil or cefpodoxime or cefixime or levofloxacin (in an older child).
- *Severe sinusitis; no response to initial 3 days treatment; children age <2 years:*
  - Amoxicillin clavulanate high dose 80-90 mg/kg/day div in BID
  - Or ceftriaxone 75 mg/kg/day IV/IM initial followed by oral cefdinir or cefuroxime
  - *Duration of treatment:* Minimum 10 days or 7 days after resolution of symptoms

Note: Azithromycin and cotrimoxazole are not recommended (high microbial resistance)

Mastoiditis (Acute)

(Pneumococcus, group A *Streptococcus*, nontypable *H. influenzae, Pseudomonas aeruginosa*)
Obtain cultures and treat accordingly:
- *Initial:* Ceftriaxone 75 mg/kg/day + cloxacillin 75 mg/kg/day
- *Later*: As per culture and sensitivity findings.

Orbital Cellulitis

(*H. influenzae, S. aureus*, MRSA, *S. pneumoniae*, streptococci)
- Vancomycin + cefotaxime or ceftriaxone
- Add metronidazole if anaerobes suspected
- If no improvement, sinus drainage.

LOWER RESPIRATORY TRACT INFECTIONS

Epiglottitis

(*H. influenzae* type b in nonvaccinated children; streptococci, nontypable *H. influenzae, S. aureus*)
- *Initial:* Ceftriaxone or cefotaxime or meropenem IV × 10 days
- Later as per culture and sensitivity findings.

Tracheitis Bacterial

(*S. aureus, S. pneumoniae, S. pyogenes, Moraxella catarrhalis, H. influenzae*, anaerobes)
- Cloxacillin or clindamycin + cefotaxime or ceftriaxone IV
- If MRSA infection—use vancomycin in place of cloxacillin or clindamycin.

Bronchitis (Acute)

(Bacterial)
Same drugs as for acute otitis media.

Pneumonia

Community-acquired Pneumonia

- *Common causative organisms*:
  - Bacteria: *Strep. pneumoniae, H. influenzae, S. aureus*, Group A Streptococcus, *Klebsiella*, and *Escherichia coli*
  - Viruses: Respiratory syncytial virus (RSV), parainfluenza, rhinoviruses and adenoviruses
  - *Nonviral pathogens*: *Mycoplasma pneumoniae, Chlamydia pneumoniae*, and *Chlamydia trachomatis*
- *Age incidence:* Viral infections are common below 5 years of age; *S. pneumoniae, M. pneumoniae,* and *C. pneumoniae* are more common in above 5 year olds; gram-negative organisms (esp. *Klebsiella, E. coli,* and *C. trachomatis*) are common between 3 weeks and 3 months of age.
- *Guide to antibiotic therapy:* In view of the uncertain differentiation on clinical, radiologic, or laboratory findings between pneumonia caused by various bacterial, viral, and nonviral pathogens, antibiotic treatment is largely empirical. The choice of drugs is initially guided by the child's age and the likelihood of causative organisms in that age group, type of infection then prevalent in the community and its antibiotic sensitivity pattern, the child's immunity and nutritional status, the type

of infection likely to be present in association with the underlying illness* (Table 1.1) (if any) and the severity of illness.

- **Outpatient treatment for mild illness:**
  Initial: (i) Amoxicillin 40–50 mg/kg/day PO div q 8 h PO × 5 days
  - *If poor response to (i) or if high incidence of penicillin-resistant pneumococci in the community*: Amoxicillin high dose (80–90 mg/kg/day) PO
  - *Alternative*: Cefuroxime axetil or amoxicillin-clavulanate or cefdinir or cefpodoxime.
  - *Children >5 years, suspected M. pneumoniae, or C. pneumoniae infection*:
    - A macrolide (azithromycin 10 mg/kg/day OD × 5 days or clarithromycin 15 mg/kg/day div q BID × 10 days)
    - *Alternative in adolescents*: Levofloxacin or moxifloxacin.
- **Initial choice of antibiotics in severe pneumonia:**
  - *Under 2 months of age*:
    - Cefotaxime or ceftriaxone IV + gentamicin IV × 10 days
  - *Above 2 months of age*:
    - Ampicillin 200 mg/kg/day div q 6 h IV + gentamicin 7.5 mg/kg/day IV/IM OD × 7–10 days
    - If no response in 2 days, assess for complications, such as empyema;

Table 1.1: Illness and susceptibility to infection.	
*Underlying illness	Susceptibility to infection
Nephrotic syndrome, and hemoglobinopathies	Pneumococcal infection
Cystic fibrosis	*Staphylococcus, Haemophilus influenzae*, and *Pseudomonas*
HIV infection	Tuberculosis, gram-negative bacilli, *Pneumocystis carinii*, and fungi

HIV: Human immunodeficiency virus

- *If none:* Change ampicillin to cefotaxime 200 mg/kg/day div q 6 h IV or ceftriaxone 75–100 mg/kg/day div q 12 h IV + continue gentamicin.
  - *Above 5 years of age:*
    - Cefuroxime or ceftriaxone or cefotaxime IV + macrolide (macrolide to cover against *Mycoplasma* and *C. pneumoniae* infection instead of aminoglycoside)
  - Suspected *S. aureus* infection
    - Add cloxacillin or clindamycin to initial regime of cefotaxime or ceftriaxone + gentamicin
    - If suspected methicillin resistance, add vancomycin or teicoplanin or linezolid to initial regime
      - Vancomycin 25–30 mg/kg IV loading dose, followed by 15–20 mg/kg/day div q 8–12 h IV
      - or teicoplanin 10 mg/kg/dose q 12 h × 3 doses then 10 mg/kg/day IM or IV (bolus or slow infusion)
      - or linezolid 20 mg/kg/day div q 12 h IV
      - Total duration of treatment 3–4 weeks
  - Multidrug resistant *S. pneumoniae*
    - Vancomycin and linezolid
  - *Klebsiella pneumoniae*
    - Cefotaxime or ceftriaxone IV
- *Mode and duration of drug administration:* In patients with severe pneumonia, antibiotics should be given intravenously for first 7 days or so. Once the child improves, is stable and can take orally, treatment can be switched over to oral amoxicillin-clavulanate (in cases of infection by organisms sensitive to it). While some authorities consider this drug to be preferable to oral cephalosporins cefdinir, cefpodoxime, and cefuroxime-axetil, others consider them to be equally good. Alternatively, ceftriaxone IM can be given as a follow-up drug.

In general, antibiotics are administered for 10–14 days or till 5 days after subsidence of fever. Patients with pneumonia caused by staphylococci, gram-negative bacilli and *M. pneumoniae* and some cases of severe pneumonia of undiagnosed etiology need treatment for 2–3 weeks, while those due to *C. pneumoniae* need treatment for up to 6 weeks.

Hospital-acquired Pneumonia

Empirical therapy:

According to prevalence and sensitivity of causative organisms in hospital/ICU:

- Potential pathogens: *Pseudomonas aeruginosa*, *Klebsiella* pneumoniae (ESBL) or *Acinetobacter* species
  Antibiotics: Piperacillin-tazobactam PLUS
  a. Aminoglycoside (amikacin, gentamicin or tobramycin) or
  b. Antipseudomonal fluoroquinolone (ciprofloxacin or levofloxacin)
- Methicillin resistant staphylococci
  First-line antibiotics: Vancomycin or linezolid
  Second line: Daptomycin
- Anaerobes
  Antibiotic: Metronidazole or clindamycin
- Cytomegalovirus
  Antibiotic: Ganciclovir IV (+ IV immunoglobulin)
- *Pneumocystis carinii*
  Antibiotic: Trimethoprim–sulfamethoxazole
- *Legionella*
  Antibiotic: Erythromycin
- Herpes simplex
  Antibiotic: Acyclovir and foscarnet IV
- Respiratory syncytial virus
  Antibiotic: Ribavirin by aerosol.

Empyema

- *Initial*: Cloxacillin + cefotaxime or ceftriaxone
- Suspected staphylococcal infection: Vancomycin + cefotaxime or ceftriaxone
- *Suspected anaerobic infection*: IV clindamycin
- *Nosocomial empyema*: IV piperacillin-tazobactam or meropenem + vancomycin or linezolid

- *Subsequently*: As per in vitro sensitivity of the organisms grown on pus culture.

Lung Abscess or Necrotizing Pneumonia

Ceftriaxone or cefotaxime + cloxacillin or clindamycin.

Pertussis

- Erythromycin: 40–50 mg/kg div q 6 h × 14 days
- Age above 2 months: *Alternatives*—clarithromycin × 7 days or azithromycin × 5 days.

Tuberculosis

See in separate section on "Tuberculosis".

INFECTIONS OF CENTRAL NERVOUS SYSTEM

Meningitis (Bacterial)

0–2 months (>2 kg)
Initial empiric therapy
- *First-line therapy*
  i. Inj. cefotaxime 50 mg/kg/dose IV–age < 7 days: q 12 hr; age > 7 days: q 8 hr; for 2–3 weeks
  PLUS
  ii. Inj. gentamicin 5 mg/kg/dose IV age <7 days q 24 hr; × 2–3 weeks, age >7 days: 2.5 mg/kg/dose q 8 hr × 2–3 weeks
- *Second-line therapy*
  i. Meropenem 20 mg/kg/dose; age <7 days: 12 hrly; age > 7 days: 8 hrly × 2–3 weeks
  PLUS
  ii. Vancomycin 15 mg/kg/dose; age <7 days: 12 hrly and >7 days: 8 hrly × 2–3 weeks

Duration of treatment for gram–ve bacilli or *Staph* sp × at least 21 days

For 2 month and above
- First-line therapy

Inj ceftriaxone 100 mg/kg/day div. q 12 hr × 10–14 days

Note: If ceftriaxone not available, inj cefotaxime 200 mg/kg/day IV div q 8 hr/6 hr × 10–14 days

If clinically suspected staphylococcal infection, add inj. vancomycin; continue treatment for minimum 3 weeks
- Second-line therapy
  i. Inj. meropenem 120 mg/kg/day div q 8 hr × 10–14 days PLUS
  ii. Inj. vancomycin 60 mg/kg/day div q 6 hr × 10–14 days
- Subsequent drug therapy after isolation of organisms as per their antibiotic sensitivity.
- Meningococcal meningitis: Ceftriaxone × 7 days
- *Haemophilus influenzae type b (Hib) meningitis*: Ceftriaxone × 10 days
- *Streptococcus pneumoniae type b meningitis*: Ceftriaxone × 14 days.
- Other organisms: *See* Table 1.2.

Suspected Tuberculosis Infection

See under section "Drug Treatment of Childhood Tuberculosis".

Ventriculoperitoneal Shunt Infection

- *Initial*: Vancomycin + ceftriaxone or cefotaxime + metronidazole
- *Subsequently*: As per organisms grown on culture:
  - *For coagulase negative Staphylococcus:* Vancomycin + rifampicin 10–14 days
  - *For E. coli:* Cefotaxime or ceftriaxone × 21 days + gentamicin × 10 days or till cerebrospinal fluid (CSF) becomes sterile.

Table 1.2: Bacterial meningitis: (treatment continued) subsequent therapy after isolation of organisms (age 2 months–12 years).

Pathogen	Drugs of choice	Alternative drugs	Duration of therapy
Streptococcus pneumoniae			
• Penicillin sensitive	Crystalline penicillin or ampicillin	Ceftriaxone and cefotaxime	14 days
• Intermediate resistance to penicillin	Vancomycin + ceftriaxone or cefotaxime	Meropenem	14 days
• Highly resistant	Add rifampicin	Fluoroquinolone (moxi)	14 days
Haemophilus influenzae type b	Ceftriaxone (+ dexamethasone for first 2–4 days)	Chloramphenicol, aztreonam, ciprofloxacin	10 days
Neisseria meningitidis	Cefotaxime or ceftriaxone	Chloramphenicol, meropenem, fluoroquinolone (Moxifloxacin)	7–10 days
Staphylococcus aureus	Vancomycin	Linezolid (if methicillin resistant)	3 weeks
Pseudomonas	Ceftazidime + aminoglycoside or Cefepime + genta	Meropenem + aminoglycoside; Aztreonam + genta	3 weeks

Contd...

Contd...

Pathogen	Drugs of choice	Alternative drugs	Duration of therapy
Gram-negative (*E. coli*, other Enterobacteriaceae)	Ceftazidime or cefepime + gentamicin	Meropenem + cipro	3 weeks or at last 2 weeks after CSF sterilization
Staphylococcus epidermidis	Vancomycin	Linezolid	2–3 weeks
Enterococcus • Ampicillin susceptible • Ampicillin resistant • Ampicillin and vancomycin resistant	• Ampicillin + gentamicin • Vancomycin + gentamicin • Linezolid		

Brain Abscess

Infants and Children

- *Initial*: Vancomycin + cefotaxime or ceftriaxone + metronidazole IV
- *Alternative*: Meropenem IV + vancomycin
- Subsequently as per pus culture sensitivity:
  - *Duration of antibiotic therapy:* 4-6 weeks.

Neonatal Meningitis with Brain Abscess

- *Initial*: Meropenem + aminoglycoside IV
- *Subsequently*: As per aspirated pus culture and sensitivity.

Encephalitis

(Herpes simplex virus)
See section "Viral infections".

GASTROINTESTINAL INFECTIONS

Acute Gastroenteritis

Rotavirus and enterotoxigenic *E. coli* are responsible for nearly half, cholera for about 5-10% and *Salmonella* for about 3-7% cases of acute diarrhea in Indian children. *Giardia lamblia* is an uncommon cause. Several other bacteria; viruses and parasites also induce acute diarrhea.

Dysentery is caused largely by *Shigella* intestinal infection. Other causes for it are infection by *Entamoeba histolytica*, enteroinvasive and enterohemorrhagic *E. coli*, *Salmonella*, and *Campylobacter jejuni*.

Role of Antibiotic in Therapy

Antimicrobial agents have no role in treatment of diarrhea caused by *Rotavirus* and other viral intestinal infections. Antimicrobial therapy is chiefly indicated for cases of acute bloody diarrhea (caused mostly by *Shigella* infection), suspected cases of cholera and for infrequent cases of diarrhea due to protozoal (*E. histolytica* and *Giardia*) infection.

Dysentery due to Shigella Infection

In view of widespread increasing resistance of *Shigella* organisms to different antibiotics, the preferred agents are now considered to be as follows:
- Ciprofloxacin 30 mg/kg/day div in BD PO × 3 days; watch clinical response closely for 48 hours
- In case of failure of response to ciprofloxacin, in moderately ill cases, switch to cefixime 8–10 mg/kg/day div in BD PO
- In a sick child, better initiate treatment with IV Ceftriaxone instead of ciprofloxacin. Ceftrioxone 50–100 mg/kg/day div in BD IV × 3–5 days.

Cholera

- Antibiotics are recommended in children having moderate-to-severe dehydration
- Tetracycline 12.5 mg/kg/dose (max 500 mg/dose) four times a day PO × 3 days
- Or erythromycin 12.5 mg/kg/dose (max 250 mg) × four times a day × 3 days PO
- Or azithromycin 20 mg/kg (max 1 g) as a single dose PO
- Or doxycycline 2–4 mg/kg single dose PO
- Or ciprofloxacin 20 mg/kg (max 1g) as a single dose PO.

Salmonella Gastroenteritis (Nontypical Species)

Antibiotics are not indicated routinely in uncomplicated cases.

Indications for use: Infants (≤3 months of age) and other children who are at an increased risk of a disseminated disease, such as, children on immunosuppressive and corticosteroid therapy, patients suffering from acquired immunodeficiency syndrome (AIDS), malignancies, malaria, and malnutrition.

Treatment: As described earlier under Dysentery.

Helicobacter pylori Gastritis

At least two antibiotics + one potent proton pump inhibitor (Table 1.3).

Perirectal Abscess

Clindamycin + gentamicin or cefotaxime or ceftriaxone.

Table 1.3: First-line options for *Helicobacter pylori* gastritis.		
Drug	Dosage	Duration
i. Amoxicillin	50 mg/kg/day (max 1 g/dose BID)	14 days
+ Clarithromycin	15 mg/kg/day (max 500 mg/dose BID)	14 days
+ Omeprazole*	1 mg/kg/day (max 20 mg/dose BID)	1 month
ii. Amoxicillin	50 mg/kg/day (max 1 g/dose/BID)	14 days
+ Metronidazole	20 mg/kg/day (max 500 mg/dose BID)	14 days
+ Omeprazole*	1 mg/kg/day (max 20 mg/dose BID)	1 month
iii. Clarithromycin	15 mg/kg/day (max 500 mg/dose BID)	14 days
+ Metronidazole	20 mg/kg/day (max 500 mg/dose BID)	× 14 days
+ Omeprazole*	1 mg/kg/day (max 20 mg/dose BID)	1 month
*Omeprazole or lansoprazole or any other proton pump inhibitor		

Skeletal Infections

Arthritis (Septic)

- **Infants <3 months** (*S. aureus*, Enterobacteriaceae, Group B *Strep*)
  Oxacillin or nafcillin + cefotaxime or ceftriaxone IM/IV
  - *If MRSA*: Vancomycin + cefotaxime or ceftriaxone IM/IV.
- **Children** (3 months–14 years) (*S. aureus*, Hib, *S. pyogenes S. pneumoniae*, gram-negative bacilli, and others)
  - Vancomycin + cefotaxime or ceftriaxone or ceftizoxime.

Osteomyelitis (Acute)

- *Neonate: See* section "Neonatal Infections"
- *Children <5 years:* (*S. aureus*, *Streptococcus*, Hib) Cloxacillin or clindamycin + cefotaxime or ceftriaxone
- *Children >5 years*: (*Staph, Strep*) Cloxacillin or nafcillin or cefazolin IV
- *Duration of treatment*: 4–6 weeks or more
- *If MRSA*: Vancomycin or clindamycin instead of cloxacillin.

Osteomyelitis (Chronic)

Staphylococcal:
- *Initial*: Cloxacillin or nafcillin IV
- *For MRSA*: Vancomycin or clindamycin IV
- *Later*: Cloxacillin or first generation cephalosporin PO (cephalexin, cefadroxil, and cefazolin).

Osteomyelitis of the Foot-puncture Wound

Pseudomonas:
- Ceftazidime IV/IM or ticarcillin IV plus tobramycin or amikacin IV × 10 days
- *Alternative*: Meropenem or cefepime IV OR ticarcillin-clavulanate.

GENITOURINARY AND SEXUALLY TRANSMITTED INFECTIONS

Acute cystitis (uncomplicated lower UTI without urinary tract obstruction) (*E. coli, Klebsiella, Proteus* species, *Enterobacter*)

- Initial (before results of urine culture): Cotrimoxazole/trimethoprim @ 8–10 mg/kg/day PO × 3–5 days
- After results of culture:
  - If organisms on culture sensitive to it, continue cotrimoxazole × 7–10 days
- Or nitrofurantoin 5–7 mg/kg/div in TID/QID × 7–10 days
- Or amoxicillin 50 mg/kg/day div in TID/QID × 7–10 days
- Or cefixime 8–10 mg/kg/day div in BD × 7–10 days
- Or amoxicillin-clavulanate (30–50 mg of amoxicillin/kg/day) div in BD × 7–10 days.

Since it is difficult to distinguish between cystitis and pyelonephritis in infants and children below the age of 5 years, all cases of urinary tract infection (UTI) in this age group should be treated for 14 days.

Acute Pyelonephritis

(*E. coli, Proteus, Klebsiella* species, *Staphylococcus saprophyticus, Enterococcus*, and others)

It is advisable to choose the initial drug (on empirical basis before receipt of urine culture report) on the basis of known drug sensitivity of the likely source of infection:

Uropathogenic *E. coli*, the most common causative pathogen, in the community, or

That of locally prevalent flora in the institution or pediatric intensive care unit (PICU)

Initial (common choice): Ceftriaxone or cefotaxime IV or ampicillin + gentamicin IV

Later: As per antibiotic sensitivity of the organisms grown on culture

- Oral cefixime for gram-negative organisms almost as good as parenteral ceftriaxone (except against *Pseudomonas*)
- Ciprofloxacin—a good alternative agent for *Pseudomonas*. Levofloxacin is a good alternative quinolone

- Do not use nitrofurantoin in a child with febrile UTI (inadequate renal tissue concentration).

Second line treatment for complicated UTI:
- Piperacillin tazobactam 90 mg/kg/dose q 6 h IV or IM or Meropenem 20–40 mg/kg/dose q 8 h × 10–14 days.
- *Suspected urosepsis, child vomiting, infant <1 month*: Parenteral drugs IV/IM × 10–14 days
  - *Older children*: Initially parenteral, may give PO following improvement, total of 10–14 days.

Renal or Perinephric Abscess

Cloxacillin or nafcillin + gentamicin or ceftriaxone/cefotaxime.

Epididymitis

(Young children—*E. coli* and *S. aureus*; older children—gonorrhea and *Chlamydia*)

Cefuroxime or cefotaxime or ceftriaxone × 7–10 days.

Add cloxacillin if suspected *S. aureus* infection. If *C. trachomatis* infection is suspected in sexually active adolescents or adults, add azithromycin or erythromycin or doxycycline

Vaginal Infections

- *Bacterial vaginosis*: Metronidazole × 7 days or single large dose
- *Group A strep. infection:* Penicillin V × 10 days PO
- *Vulvovaginal candidiasis:* See section "Fungal infections".

Trichomoniasis

See section "Protozoal and other parasitic infections".

Chancroid

(*Haemophilus ducreyi*)
Ceftriaxone 250 mg IM, single dose or azithromycin 1 g PO, single dose.

Chlamydia trachomatis

- Erythromycin (or in >7 years old—doxycycline) × 7 days
- *Alternative (in adults):* Azithromycin 1 g PO, single dose

Gonorrhea

- Uncomplicated urogenital, anorectal, and pharyngeal infection
   i. Ceftriaxone 250 mg IM single dose + azithromycin 1 g PO once or
   ii. Cefixime 400 mg PO once + azithromycin 1 g PO once or
   iii. Ceftriaxone 250 mg IM single dose + doxycycline 100 mg BD PO × 7 days
       ▫ *Alternative to ceftriaxone*: Cefotaxime 500 mg IM; or ceftizoxime 500 mg IM
- *Disseminated gonococcal infection:*
   - Ceftriaxone 1 g/day IM × 7-14 days + azithromycin 1g PO single dose
- *Gonococcal conjunctivitis*: Ceftriaxone 1 g IM single dose
- *Gonococcal meningitis:* Ceftriaxone 1-2 g IV q 12 hr × 10-14 days
- *Gonococcal endocarditis:* Ceftriaxone 1-2 g IV q 12 hr × 4 weeks or more.

Note: Concurrent therapy in these patients must be done for *Chlamydia* infection.

Syphilis

- *Congenital: See* section "Neonatal infections"
- *Early:* Primary, secondary, or latent <1 year
   - Benzathine penicillin single dose IM (50,000 U/kg, max 2.4 million units)
   - *Alternative*: For nonpregnant penicillin allergic patients—tetracycline 500 mg dose QID PO or doxycycline 100 mg BID × PO × 14 days

- Syphilis >1 year duration:
    - Benzathine penicillin IM once weekly × 3 doses (50,000 U/kg, max 2.4 million units, divided over two injection sites)
    - *Alternative*: For penicillin allergic patients—doxycycline PO × 4 weeks (4 mg/kg/day, max. 200 mg/day div in BID)

Neurosyphilis

Penicillin G IV (2.5 lac U/kg/day, max 24 million U/day div Q 6 hr) × 10–14 days.

MISCELLANEOUS SYSTEMIC INFECTIONS

Bacteremia or Sepsis

- **Neonate:** *See* section "Neonatal infections"
- **Infants <3 months:**
    - *Community-acquired pathogens*: *Pneumococcus*, Hib, *N. meningitides*, *Salmonella*, *E. coli*, *S. aureus*, and other late-onset neonatal sepsis organisms, such as Group B *Streptococcus* and *Listeria*.
        a. *Initial empiric treatment*: Ceftriaxone or cefotaxime + ampicillin IV
        b. (If meningitis suspected, add vancomycin IV) to treatment as given above
        c. *Suspected S. aureus infection*: Cefotaxime + cloxacillin or nafcillin or clindamycin
        d. *Herpes simplex infection*: Acyclovir IV.
- **Sepsis in older infants and children:**
    - *Community-acquired infection*: *S. pneumoniae*, *N. meningitides*, *Salmonella*, Hib in children age <5 years
        - *Initial*: Ceftriaxone or cefotaxime
        - *Later*: As per blood culture and sensitivity findings
    - *Nosocomial sepsis*
        - Initial: Ceftriaxone or cefotaxime or piperacillin-tazobactam + aminoglycoside

◘ Add vancomycin, if coagulase-ve staphylococcal or penicillin-resistant pneumococcal infection is suspected.

Typhoid Fever

While planning treatment for typhoid fever watch for multi-drug resistant *S. typhi* infection. Many *S. typhi* organisms are now resistant to chloramphenicol, cotrimoxazole, ampicillin, and amoxicillin. As such, these drugs are not recommended today for initial use on empirical basis. These may be considered later, if the organisms are found fully susceptible on culture.

If *S. typhi* organisms are found to be resistant to nalidixic acid on culture, nalidixic acid resistant *S. typhi* (NARST), it suggests that fluoroquinolone drugs (ciprofloxacin and ofloxacin) would not be clinically effective even if the organisms exhibit in vitro sensitivity to them.

Nalidixic acid and norfloxacin do not achieve adequate blood concentration after oral administration and should not be used. Ciprofloxacin and ofloxacin* are effective in some cases but their use has not been approved by the Drug Controller General of India for patient under 18 years of age except when the child is resistant to all other recommended drugs and is suffering from life-threatening infection.

- **For cases of uncomplicated enteric fever (OPD cases):**
    - *Cefixime:* 15–20 mg/kg/day div q 12 h PO × 14 days (*first-line drug*)
    - *Azithromycin:* 10–20 mg/kg/day (max 1 g/day) OD PO × 7–14 days. To continue till one week post-fever defervescence
    - *Amoxicillin:* 75–100 mg/kg day div q 6 h PO × 14 days (*if organisms sensitive*)
    - *Trimethoprim-sulfamethoxazole (TMP-SMX):* 8 mg, TMP, 40 mg SMX/kg/day div q 12 h PO × 14 days (*if organisms sensitive*)
    - *Chloramphenicol:** 50–75 mg/kg/day div q 6 h PO × 14 days (*if organisms sensitive*)

To be used with caution.

- **For cases of severe enteric fever (requiring parenteral therapy):**
  - *First line:*
    Ceftriaxone: 75–100 mg/kg/day div q 24 h/12 h IV/IM × 14 days
  - or *Cefotaxime*: 100 mg/kg/day div q 6 h IV/IM × 14 days
    (On resolution of fever following IV use of ceftriaxone or cefotaxime, these may be replaced by oral cefixime 20 mg/kg/day—continue till one week after subsidence of fever)
  - or *Ciprofloxacin*: 15–20 mg/kg/day div q 12 h IV × 10–14 days (max 800 mg/day)
  - or *Ofloxacin:* 15–20 mg/kg/day div q 12 h IV × 10–14 days; continue for 1 week post-fever defervescence)
  - *If organisms sensitive*; may use:
    - Chloramphenicol: 50–75 mg/kg/day × 14 days, or
    - Ampicillin: 100 mg/kg/day × 14 days or
    - Trimethoprim-SMX: 8 TMP, 40 SMX mg/kg/day × 14 days.
  - *Second line:*
- Some authorities recommend that in severe cases requiring hospitalization, a third generation cephalosporin (ceftriaxone or cefixime) may be used in combination with a quinolone (ciprofloxacin or ofloxacin) or with azithromycin.
- *For non-responders, serious cases (may use):*
  - Aztreonam: 90–120 mg/kg/day div q 6–8 h IV/IM × 14 days

Adjunctive use of dexamethasone initially 3 mg/kg followed by 1 mg/kg every 6 hours for 48 hr and then gradual reduction of dose over next 3 days has been found useful in severe cases of typhoid fever, presenting with delirium, obtundation, stupor, coma or shock, alongwith other supportive treatment.

Shorter duration of therapy with some antibiotics has been found to be equally effective by some workers. It is generally recommended that antibiotic therapy should be continued for 5–7 days after the child becomes afebrile.

Peritonitis

- **Acute primary peritonitis** (without a demonstrable intra-abdominal source) (usually monomicrobial) common: pneumococci, group A streptococci, staphylococci, gram-ve enteric bacteria.
  Treatment
  Initial: Cefotaxime IV
  Later: As per culture sensitivity findings
  For resistant pneumococci: Vancomycin
  Duration of treatment: 10-14 days
- **Acute secondary peritonitis** (due to entry of enteric bacteria into the peritoneal cavity through a necrotic defect in wall of the intestines/other viscus) (usually polymicrobial infection)
  Treatment
  Initial choice of antibiotic:
  - For lower GIT perforation cases.
    Ampicillin, gentamicin + clindamycin or metronidazole
  - For peritoneal catheter-related peritonitis
    Intraperitoneal cefepime or cefazolin + ceftazidime
  Later: As per antibiotic sensitivity of peritoneal fluid isolate.

Endocarditis

- *Unknown organisms (no prosthetic valve); empirical therapy:*
  - *Initial*: Vancomycin + gentamicin (4-6 weeks)
  - *Later*: As per antibiotic sensitivity of cultured organisms
- *Strep. viridans and Streptococcus bovis:*
  - Penicillin G or ceftriaxone + gentamicin IV
  - *If penicillin allergy*: Vancomycin + gentamicin IV
- *Staphylococcus aureus and S. epidermidis:*
  Cloxacillin or nafcillin + gentamicin
  Or vancomycin + gentamicin (if MRSA).

Pericarditis (Purulent)

- Empiric (*S. aureus*, Hib, *Strep pneumoniae*, Group A streptococci and gram-negative organisms)
    - *Initial*: Vanco + cefepime
    - *Later*: As per pericardial fluid cultured organism's antibiotic sensitivity.
- *Staphylococcus aureus*
    - Cloxacillin or cefazolin IV; vancomycin (if methicillin-resistant) IV × 3–4 weeks
    - *Alternative*: Imipenem.

Pericarditis (Tuberculous)

See section "Treatment of tuberculosis".

Tetanus

- Penicillin G IV (200,000 U/kg/day div q 6 h) × 10–14 days or metronidazole IV (30 mg/kg/day div q 8 h) × 10–14 days
- *Tetanus immunoglobulin (TIG) or tetanus antitoxin (TA):* For details see under section on "Vaccines and immunoglobulins".

Septic Shock Syndrome

Critically Ill Child with Severe Sepsis and Septic Shock

Guiding principles for initial presumptive therapy:
- Provide coverage for MRSA
- If suspected GIT source (e.g. burst appendicitis) or genitourinary infection—cover for enteric organisms
- Immunocompromised child—cover for *Pseudomonas* infection
- Modify later depending upon culture reports and patient's response.

Immunocompetent Children >28 Days of Age

- Ceftriaxone or cefotaxime + vancomycin or teicoplanin

- If suspected genitourinary source → Add aminoglycoside (genta or amika)
- If suspected GIT source → Add piperacillin-tazobactam or clindamycin or metronidazole.

Immunosuppressed >28 Days of Age or Risk of Pseudomonas Species Infection

- Ceftazidime or cefepime + vancomycin or teicoplanin
- If extended-spectrum β-lactamases (ESBL) resistant organisms present → add aminoglycoside or carbapenem. Carbapenem addition preferable, if any broad spectrum antibiotic received within 2 weeks, such as third generation cephalosporin, aminoglycoside, or fluoroquinolone.

Allergic to Penicillin or Recently Received Broad-Spectrum Antibiotic

- Vancomycin or teicoplanin + meropenem
- *Alternative to meropenem*: (i) aztreonam or (ii) ciprofloxacin + clindamycin.

Patient at Increased Risk of Fungal Infections

- Immunocompromised with persistent fever on broad-spectrum antibiotics or
- With an identified fungal source
  Add the following antifungals to the antimicrobial regimen:
- Liposomal amphotericin B or
- Caspofungin or micafungin or anidulafungin.

Patients with Risk Factors for Rickettsial Infection (Travel to or Reside in an Endemic Region)

- Add doxycycline or tetracycline to the antibiotic regimen
- Besides use of appropriate antibiotic, treat or control source of infection, e.g. by drainage of pus, removal of infected viscus or catheter.

Duration of Antibiotic Therapy for Sepsis

- *If no complication:* 7–10 days
- *Longer course recommended*: If slow clinical response; undrainable foci of infection; *S. aureus* bacteremia; some fungal and viral infections; or immunologic deficiency.

If MRSA infection suspected: Empirical therapy recommended with vancomycin; If minimum inhibitory concentration (MIC) value for MRSA isolates 12 mg/mL—use daptomycin. Linezolid should not be used for empirical therapy.

CHAPTER 2

Antibiotic Therapy in Neonatal Infections

NEONATAL SEPSIS AND MENINGITIS
Causative Organisms

As per hospital-based studies, the predominant organisms responsible for neonatal sepsis and meningitis in India are *Escherichia coli*, *Klebsiella*, *Staphylococcus aureus*, *Pseudomonas*, and *Acinetobacter*.

Besides these, the organisms that most often cause nosocomial infection in neonatal units, especially in neonatal intensive care unit (NICU) (resulting in late-onset neonatal sepsis) are coagulase negative staphylococci/methicillin-resistant staphylococci, anaerobes, *enterococci*, *Candida*, and *Serratia*.

Choice of Antibiotics

The initial empirical choice of antibiotics for treatment of neonatal sepsis and meningitis is determined by:
- The timing and likely source of infection
- Spectrum of pathogens causing neonatal infection in the concerned unit/region/community
- Antimicrobial susceptibility of suspected causative pathogens, and
- Presence or absence of meningeal involvement.

Note: For dosage of recommended drugs see section "Dosage of Antimicrobial Agents in Neonates"; for information regarding mode of use, side effects, etc. see under individual drug in the section "Pediatric Drug Formulary".

Initial Empirical Therapy

- *Early-onset neonatal sepsis (within 72 hours of birth) when resistant organisms unlikely:*

Neonatal sepsis	Neonatal meningitis
Ampicillin + gentamicin or cefotaxime	Cefotaxime (+ ampicillin; for possible *Listeria* infection) + gentamicin

- *Late-onset neonatal sepsis (due to nosocomial infection in nursery/NICU) when resistant organisms likely:*

  The empirical initial choice of antibiotics in these cases is largely determined by the bacterial flora encountered in that particular NICU and their antibiotic sensitivity pattern. For example, in case of prevalent coagulase negative or methicillin-resistant *S. aureus* (MRSA) infection, combine vancomycin (instead of ampicillin) with an aminoglycoside.

Neonatal Meningitis

- Empirical treatment

First line	Inj. ampicillin +	100 mg/kg/dose	<7 days × 12 hrly IV × 3 wk >7 days × 8 hrly IV × 3 wk
	Inj. gentamicin	5–7.5 mg/kg/dose	<7 days 5 mg/kg × 24 hrly IV × 3 wk >7 days 7.5 mg/kg × 24 hrly IV × 3 wk
Second line	Inj. cefotaxime +	50 mg/kg/dose	<7 days 12 hrly × 3 wk > 7 days 8 hrly × 3 wk
	Inj. gentamicin	5–7.5 mg/kg/dose	<7 days 5 mg/kg × 24 hrly × 3 wk >7 days 7.5 mg/kg × 24 hrly IV × 3 wk

- Following isolation of the causative organisms on blood/CSF culture and establishment of their sensitivity pattern, the most appropriate antibiotic with comparatively narrow spectrum should be preferred. The use of very broad spectrum antimicrobial agents should be kept in reserve for patients with infections by highly resistant organisms.

- *Staphylococcus aureus*:

  Cloxacillin/nafcillin + aminoglycoside for possible coexisting infection with gram-negative organisms

- *MRSA and coagulase – negative staphylococci*:

  Vancomycin + aminoglycoside for possible coexisting infection with gram-negative organisms

- *Pseudomonas*:
  Ceftazidime/piperacillin-tazobactam/ticarcillin-clavulanate) + aminoglycoside
  Alternative: Meropenem + aminoglycoside

- *Enterococci*:
  - Ampicillin/vancomycin + aminoglycoside
  - *For vancomycin resistant*: Linezolid/tigecycline

- *Listeria monocytogenes*:
  Ampicillin + gentamicin

- *Anaerobic infection*:
  Clindamycin or metronidazole intravenous (IV)

- *Gram-negative enteric bacteria*:
  - *For neonatal sepsis*: Ampicillin + aminoglycoside
  - *For neonatal meningitis*: Cefotaxime + aminoglycoside
    Alternative: Ceftazidime + aminoglycoside
  - *For bacteria resistant to cephalosporins and aminoglycosides*: Meropenem or cefepime IV

- *Bacteroides fragilis meningitis*:
  Metronidazole IV

- Group-A and Group-B streptococcal infection:
  Penicillin G IV

- Herpes meningoencephalitis:
  Acyclovir IV

- *Enteroviral infections* (meningoencephalitis, hepatitis, carditis):
  Pleconaril.

Duration of Antibiotic Therapy

Neonatal sepsis: 10–14 days (or at least 5–7 days after clinical response). A blood culture after 24–48 hours of therapy should be negative. If culture is positive, consider change in antibiotics, extension in duration of therapy, and exclude the presence of a complicating factor, such as, an infected indwelling catheter, an occult abscess, subtherapeutic drug levels, or resistant organisms.

- *Neonatal meningitis*: 21 days (or at least 10–14 days after sterilization of CSF, whichever is longer, especially in cases of Gram-negative meningitis); 28 days in cases of complicated infection.
- *Staphylococcal infection*: 3 weeks or longer.

NEONATAL PNEUMONIA

- *Pneumonia during first 7–10 days*:
  - Ampicillin + aminoglycoside/cefotaxime × 10–14 days (at least 5–7 days after clinical response)
- *Nosocomial pneumonia*:
  (Usually after 7–10 days in NICU)
  - *Empirical*: Vancomycin/ampicillin + cefotaxime/aminoglycoside
- Group-B *Streptococcus*:
  - Penicillin G or ampicillin IV/IM × 10–14 days
- *S. aureus*:
  - Cloxacillin IV/IM × 21 days; for methicillin-resistant *Staphylococcus:* Vancomycin IV × 21 days
- *Pseudomonas*:
  - Aminoglycoside + ceftazidime/ticarcillin × 14 days or more
- *Chlamydia trachomatis*:
  - Erythromycin oral (PO) × 14–21 days or azithromycin PO
- *Ureaplasma urealyticum*:
  - Erythromycin × 10 days or clarithromycin × 10 days
- *RSV (respiratory syncytial virus) pneumonia*:
  - Aerosolized ribavirin.

SKIN AND SOFT TISSUE INFECTIONS

Impetigo/Pustules (*S. aureus*)

Mild cases: Mupirocin/bacitracin topical application alone
Moderate infection: Cloxacillin/cephalexin or cefadroxil PO
Extensive lesions or infant ill:
Initial: Cloxacillin IV; later parenteral antibiotic as per culture sensitivity findings;
 If MRSA: Vancomycin or linezolid × 7–10 days

Cellulitis

(*Streptococcus, S. aureus*, gram-negative enteric bacilli)
Cloxacillin + aminoglycoside IV/IM
Or Cloxacillin + cefotaxime IV/IM

Omphalitis and Necrotizing Funisitis

(Gram-negative bacilli, *S. aureus*, *Klebsiella* species, *Streptococcus pyogenes*)
Initial empiric: Cloxacillin + aminoglycoside
Alternative: Cefotaxime + clindamycin
Later: As per organism's culture and sensitivity findings
Duration of treatment: 10–14 days.

Breast Abscess

Initial: Cloxacillin IV/IM × 5–7 days
If gram-negative infection (as seen on Gram's stain/culture of pus): Cefotaxime IV.

OTITIS MEDIA

(*S. aureus*, gram-negative enteric bacteria, others)
Initial empiric: Cefotaxime, amoxicillin-clavulanate
Later: As per sensitivity of identified causative organism.

OSTEOMYELITIS, SEPTIC ARTHRITIS

(*S. aureus*, group-B *Streptococcus*, gram-negative enteric bacilli):

- *Initial*: Cloxacillin or nafcillin + cefotaxime/other third-generation cephalosporin IV
- *Later*: As per culture and sensitivity report; if MRSA: Vancomycin + cefotaxime/other third-generation cephalosporin IV
- *Duration of treatment*: 6 weeks.

URINARY TRACT INFECTION

Empiric

- *Initial*: Ampicillin + aminoglycoside (gentamicin or amikacin)
  Or Ampicillin + cefotaxime × 10–14 days
- Later as per urine culture and sensitivity findings.

If *Pseudomonas aeruginosa* infection
- Ceftazidime IV/IM + aminoglycoside.

TETANUS

Penicillin G IV (100,000–200,000 U/kg/day) div q 4–6 hours × 10–14 days + tetanus immune globulin (TIG)/tetanus antitoxin (*see* section on "Immunization")

CONGENITAL SYPHILIS

Without CNS Infection or with CNS Infection

- Aqueous crystalline penicillin G:
  Age 1 week or less: 50,000 U/kg/dose q 12 hours IV
  Older than 1 week: 50,000 U/kg/dose q 8 hours IV × for a total of 10 days
  Or
- Procaine penicillin G:
  - 50,000 U/kg OD IM × 10 days.

CONGENITAL TOXOPLASMOSIS

Without Active Chorioretinitis

- Pyrimethamine 2 mg/kg/day div in BID PO × 2 days, then 1 mg/kg/day OD PO × 2–6 months and then 1 mg/kg/day

div in once × alternate days to complete 1 year of therapy
PLUS
- Sulfadiazine 100 mg/kg/day div in BID × 1 year
  PLUS
- Folinic acid (leucovorin) 5–10 mg thrice weekly × 1 year

When active chorioretinitis involving macula or CSF protein >1,000 mg/dL

Treatment as at "without active chorioretinitis" above *PLUS* prednisone 1 mg/kg/day div in TID PO. Only for a limited period when there is an active inflammation.

CHAPTER 3
Spectra and Effectiveness of Various Antimicrobial Agents

While some antibiotics have limited ability to eradicate a certain group of microorganisms, they are ineffective against many others. It is vital that the clinicians are well informed about the true capabilities of different antibiotics to enable their logical, efficient use in the treatment of different types of infections. The spectrum of effectiveness and resistance pattern of different antibiotics against various common organisms is shown in Table 3.1.

Table 3.1: Spectrum of effectiveness of various antibiotics.

S. No.	Antibiotics	Common susceptible organisms	Common resistant organisms
I. (A)	**Penicillins (β-lactam antibiotics):**		
(i)	Penicillins (Penicillin G, Penicillin V)	Streptococci (Group A, B, C, G) *Streptococcus pneumoniae* *Listeria* *Neisseria meningitidis* (Note: Penicillin V is not effective against *Listeria* *N. meningitidis*)	*Staphylococci* *Haemophilus influenzae* *Escherichia coli*, other Enterobacteriaceae *Pseudomonas aeruginosa* *Legionella* species *Mycoplasma pneumoniae*
(ii)	Ampicillin (ampicillin, amoxicillin)	Streptococci (Group A, B, C, G) *S. pneumoniae* *Listeria* *N. meningitidis* Enterococcus *Proteus mirabilis* *H. influenzae* ± (β-lactamase negative) *E. coli* (±) *Salmonella* species (±) *Shigella* species (±)	Staphylococci Many Enterobacteriaceae *P. aeruginosa* *Bacteroides fragilis* *Klebsiella* *Chlamydia* *M. pneumoniae* *Legionella* species

Contd...

Contd...

S. No.	Antibiotics	Common susceptible organisms	Common resistant organisms
(iii)	Penicillin and (β)-lactamase inhibitor combination (amoxicillin-clavulanate, ampicillin-sulbactam)	Streptococci (Group A, B, C, G) S. pneumoniae Staphylococcus aureus (MSSA) E. coli, Klebsiella N. meningitidis H. influenzae B. fragilis Listeria (sensitive to ampicillin-sulbactam)	Pseudomonas S. aureus (MRSA) Enterobacter spp. Serratia spp.
(iv)	Antistaphylococcal penicillins (cloxacillin, dicloxacillin, methicillin, nafcillin, oxacillin)	S. aureus (methicillin sensitive) Streptococci	Gram-negative organisms S. aureus (methicillin resistant) Enterococcus Staphylococcus (coagulase-negative)
(v)	Antipseudomonal penicillins • Piperacillin, ticarcillin, mezlocillin, azlocillin	Same organisms as ampicillin + Pseudomonas E. coli Serratia Enterobacter Bacteroides Klebsiella	Same as ampicillin (except Pseudomonas and Klebsiella)

Contd...

Contd...

S. No.	Antibiotics	Common susceptible organisms	Common resistant organisms
I. (B)	Beta-lactamase inhibitor combinations Piperacillin – tazobactam Ticarcillin – clavulanate	Broad spectrum: Pseudomonas Streptococci S. aureus (MSSA) N. meningitidis H. influenzae Acinetobacter E. coli Proteus mirabilis Klebsiella Enterobacteriaceae (some) B. fragilis	Listeria Chlamydia spp. Mycoplasma pneumoniae S. aureus (MRSA)
II.	Cephalosporins (β-lactam antibiotics):		
(i)	First generation: Cephalexin Cefadroxil Cefazolin	Streptococci (Group A, B, C, G) S. pneumoniae Streptococcus viridans S. aureus (methicillin-sensitive MSSA) E. coli Klebsiella Proteus mirabilis	Many gram-negative: Pseudomonas Enterococcus S. aureus (MRSA)

Contd...

Contd...

S. No.	Antibiotics	Common susceptible organisms	Common resistant organisms
(ii)	*Second generation:*		
	(a) Cefaclor Cefuroxime axetil Cefprozil Cefotetan	Streptococci (Group A, B, C, G) *S. pneumoniae* *S. viridans* (except cefprozil) Staphylococcus (MSSA) *E. coli* *Proteus mirabilis* *Klebsiella* *H. influenzae*	*Enterococcus* *Pseudomonas* Staphylococcus (MRSA) Staphylococcus coagulase-negative Anaerobes
	(b) Cefuroxime (parenteral)	Above organisms + *N. meningitidis*	Above organisms except *N. meningitidis*
	(c) Cefoxitin	Above organisms + *B. fragilis*	Above organisms except *B. fragilis*

Contd...

Contd...

S. No.	Antibiotics	Common susceptible organisms	Common resistant organisms
(iii)	*Third generation:*		
	(a) Cefotaxime Ceftriaxone	Streptococci H. influenzae N. meningitidis Salmonella, Shigella E. coli Other Enterobacteriaceae Staphylococcus (MSSA) Klebsiella species Proteus mirabilis	Enterococci Listeria P. aeruginosa B. fragilis Staphylococcus (MRSA)
	(b) Cefpodoxime/ Cefdinir (PO)	Streptococci H. influenzae Salmonella Shigella S. pneumoniae N. gonorrhoeae Klebsiella E. coli, Proteus mirabilis Staphylococcus (MSSA)	Neisseria Pseudomonas Listeria Enterococci

Contd...

Contd...

S. No.	Antibiotics	Common susceptible organisms	Common resistant organisms
	(c) Cefixime	E. coli Proteus mirabilis H. influenzae Salmonella Shigella Streptococci A, B, C, G S. pneumoniae Klebsiella species	S. aureus Pseudomonas B. fragilis
	(d) Ceftibuten (PO)	Streptococci A, B, C, G H. influenzae E. coli Salmonella Shigella Proteus mirabilis	S. pneumoniae ± S. viridans Enterococcus S. aureus Pseudomonas

Contd...

Contd...

S. No.	Antibiotics	Common susceptible organisms	Common resistant organisms
(e)	Ceftazidime	*Pseudomonas* Streptococci A, B, C, G *S. pneumoniae* *H. influenzae* *E. coli* Other Enterobacteriaceae *Klebsiella* species	*S. aureus* *Neisseria* *B. fragilis*
(f)	Ceftizoxime	Streptococci A, B, C, G *S. pneumoniae* *S. viridans* *Staphylococcus* (MSSA) *H. influenzae* *E. coli* *Proteus mirabilis* Other Enterobacteriaceae *Staphylococcus* (MSSA) *Klebsiella* species	*Pseudomonas* *Neisseria* Anaerobes

Contd...

Contd...

S. No.	Antibiotics	Common susceptible organisms	Common resistant organisms
	(g) Cefoperazone	Pseudomonas ± Streptococci H. influenzae Staphylococcus (MSSA) Klebsiella species Salmonella E. coli Other Enterobacteriaceae	S. aureus (MRSA) Listeria B. fragilis
(iv)	Fourth generation:		
	Cefepime Cefpirome	Streptococci H. influenzae N. meningitidis E. coli Other Enterobacteriaceae Staphylococcus (MSSA) Pseudomonas Klebsiella species Salmonella Shigella	S. aureus (MRSA) Listeria B. fragilis Clostridium difficile Enterococcus faecalis

Contd...

Contd...

S. No.	Antibiotics	Common susceptible organisms	Common resistant organisms
III.	Fluoroquinolones:		
	(a) Ciprofloxacin, Ofloxacin, Norfloxacin	(i) Gram-negative organisms E. coli, Proteus mirabilis H. influenzae Salmonella Shigella Klebsiella Neisseria Chlamydia M. pneumoniae (ii) Pseudomonas Listeria (moderately sensitive to ciprofloxacin)	Streptococci (Group A, B, C, G) S. pneumoniae Enterococcus Anaerobes Staphylococcus (MRSA) Pseudomonas (except ciprofloxacin)
	(b) Pefloxacin	Gram-negative organisms (as with quinolones at (a) above	As with quinolones at (a) above

Contd...

Contd...

S. No.	Antibiotics	Common susceptible organisms	Common resistant organisms
	(c) Gatifloxacin Moxifloxacin Trovafloxacin Levofloxacin Sparfloxacin	Gram-negative organisms as with quinolones at (a) above Streptococci (Group A, B, C, G) S. pneumoniae S. viridans Staphylococcus (MSSA) M. pneumoniae Chlamydia species Anaerobes (some)	Pseudomonas Anaerobes (some)
IV.	Aminoglycosides: Gentamicin Tobramycin Amikacin Netilmicin	E. coli Proteus mirabilis H. influenzae Klebsiella Pseudomonas Serratia, Enterobacter	Gram-positive organisms Anaerobes Some Pseudomonas N. meningitidis M. pneumoniae

Contd...

Contd...

S. No.	Antibiotics	Common susceptible organisms	Common resistant organisms
V.	**Macrolides:**		
	(a) Erythromycin Roxithromycin Clarithromycin	Streptococci M. pneumoniae Corynebacterium diphtheriae Listeria Bordetella pertussis Chlamydia Legionella Staphylococcus (MSSA)* H. influenzae*	Gram-negative P. aeruginosa B. fragilis
	(b) Azithromycin	Above organisms + Salmonella typhi	As above except S. typhi
VI.	**Tetracyclines:**		
	Tetracycline Doxycycline Minocycline	Chlamydia Rickettsia species Mycoplasma Some anaerobes S. pneumoniae V. cholerae Campylobacter	Staphylococcus Many Enterobacteriaceae Enterococcus Pseudomonas

Contd...

Contd...

S. No.	Antibiotics	Common susceptible organisms	Common resistant organisms
VII.	Chloramphenicol:	Streptococci (Group A, B, C, G) S. pneumoniae H. influenzae Salmonella ± Shigella ± N. meningitidis E. coli Chlamydia species M. pneumoniae Anaerobes (some)	Staphylococcus Many Enterobacteriaceae Pseudomonas
VIII.	Trimethoprim-sulfamethoxazole:	S. aureus (MSSA) S. pneumoniae E. coli ± Salmonella ± Shigella ± H. influenzae ±	Streptococcus (A, B, C, G) Pseudomonas Enterococcus Anaerobes

Contd...

Contd...

S. No.	Antibiotics	Common susceptible organisms	Common resistant organisms
IX.	*Clindamycin (lincosamide):*		
		Gram-positive streptococci *S. aureus* (MSSA) Some anaerobes	Gram-negative *Enterococcus*
X.	*Glycopeptides: Vancomycin, teicoplanin, Telavancin (lipoglycopeptide):*		
		Streptococci A, B, C, G *S. pneumoniae* *Staphylococcus* (MSSA and MRSA) *Enterococcus faecalis* *C. difficile* *Listeria*	Gram-negative *Pseudomonas*
XI.	*Carbapenems (β-lactam antibiotics):*		
	Imipenem* Meropenem Ertapenem	Broad spectrum Gram-positive cocci Gram-negative organisms *Pseudomonas* (except Ertapenem) Anaerobes, *Listeria*	*Staphylococcus* (MRSA) *Enterococci* (many)

Contd...

Contd...

S. No.	Antibiotics	Common susceptible organisms	Common resistant organisms
XII.	Aztreonam (monobactam):	Gram-negative aerobes *Pseudomonas* Enterobacteriaceae	Gram-positive cocci Anaerobes
XIII.	Metronidazole:	Anaerobes	Gram-positive Gram-negative
XIV.	Rifampin:	*Mycobacterium tuberculosis* *Mycobacterium leprae* *N. meningitidis* *H. influenzae* *Staphylococcus* (MSSA and MRSA)	*Salmonella* *Shigella* *Pseudomonas*
XV.	Linezolid (oxazolidinone); daptomycin (lipopeptide):	Streptococci (Group A, B, C, G) *S. pneumoniae* *S. aureus* (MSSA) *S. aureus* (MRSA)	Gram-negative organisms (including *E. coli, Salmonella, Shigella, Proteus, P. aeruginosa, N. meningitidis,* others)

Contd...

Contd...

S. No.	Antibiotics	Common susceptible organisms	Common resistant organisms
	Linezolid, Daptomycin (Contd)	Staphylococcus epidermidis Enterococcus faecalis Listeria monocytogenes	
XVI.	Tigecycline (glycylcycline):	Gram-positive streptococci, S. aureus (MSSA) S. aureus (MRSA) Listeria monocytogenes H. influenzae E. coli E. coli/Klebsiella species ESBL + E. coli/Klebsiella species KPC + Enterobacter species Salmonella species Shigella species B. fragilis Chlamydia M. pneumoniae	Enterococci (Vancomycin resistant) Pseudomonas aeruginosa

Contd...

Contd...

S. No.	Antibiotics	Common susceptible organisms	Common resistant organisms
XVII.	Colistin (colistimethate):	E. coli Klebsiella species E. coli/Klebsiella ESBL + E. coli/Klebsiella KPC + Enterobacter species Pseudomonas Acinetobacter species	Gram-positive cocci Listeria N. meningitidis Proteus vulgaris
XVIII.	Fosfomycin:	S. pneumoniae S. aureus (MSSA and MRSA) E. coli Klebsiella P. vulgaris Serratia marcescens	Listeria monocytogenes Pseudomonas Acinetobacter species

Contd...

Contd...

S. No.	Antibiotics	Common susceptible organisms	Common resistant organisms
XIX.	Nitrofurantoin:	Streptococci (A, B, C, G) S. pneumoniae Enterococcus faecalis S. aureus (MSSA and MRSA) E. coli Salmonella Shigella	Pseudomonas P. vulgaris S. marcescens Chlamydophila species
XX.	Fusidic acid:	Enterococcus faecalis S. aureus (MSSA and MRSA) S. epidermidis N. gonorrhoeae; N. meningitidis	E. coli Klebsiella Salmonella Shigella

Contd...

Contd...

S. No.	Antibiotics	Common susceptible organisms	Common resistant organisms
XXI.	Telithromycin (ketolide)	Streptococci (A, B, C, G) S. aureus (MSSA) Listeria monocytogenes M. pneumoniae Rickettsia species	S. aureus (MRSA) Gram-negative

(ESBL: extended-spectrum beta-lactamase; MRSA: methicillin-resistant *Staphylococcus aureus*; MSSA: methicillin-sensitive *Staphylococcus aureus*)

Note:

* Clarithromycin and azithromycin have greater antibacterial activity against *Staphylococcus* (MSSA) and *Haemophilus influenzae* as compared to erythromycin.

Meropenem and Imepenem are third-line agents preferably reserved for serious infections due to multiple resistant strains, e.g. those with ESBL (with extended spectrum beta-lactamases).

4 Preferred Antimicrobial Agents against Selected Bacteria

Table 4.1 lists drugs of choice and alternatives for empirical use against selected commonly encountered bacteria. It is based on generally observed sensitivity pattern of different bacteria to various antibiotics. Clinicians must, however, take into due consideration the locally prevalent antibiotic sensitivity/resistance pattern of organisms in their region, community and institution to arrive at the appropriate choice of antimicrobial agents in their clinical practice. The choice of appropriate antibiotic in an individual case would also be influenced by the site and severity of infection, presence of any coexisting morbid conditions and patient's immunologic status. As far as possible, first-line simple antibiotic, which would suffice in the particular case, should be chosen for treatment instead of the strong second-line one.

Table 4.1: Drugs of choice and alternatives for empirical use against selected commonly encountered organisms.

Organism and the common clinical illness	Drug of choice	Alternative	#Other effective agents
Bacteroides fragilis Peritonitis, sepsis, abscesses, appendicitis	Metronidazole Clindamycin	Piperacillin-tazobactam Ticarcillin/clavulanate	Meropenem, imipenem
Bordetella pertussis Pertussis	(for age >1 month Erythromycin Clarithromycin	For <1 month azithromycin	For children aged >2 months TMP-SMX
Brucella spp. Brucellosis	Doxy + genta	Doxy + RIF or TMP-SMX + genta	Doxy + RIF + genta
Campylobacter jejuni Diarrhea	Erythromycin, azithromycin	Ciprofloxacin	TMP-SMX
Chlamydia trachomatis Urethritis, vaginitis (in adolescents)	Erythro, azithro	Ofloxacin, levofloxacin	

Contd...

Contd...

Organism and the common clinical illness	Drug of choice	Alternative	*Other effective agents
Clostridium difficile Antibiotic associated colitis	Mild illness: Metronidazole (PO)	Moderate, severe illness vancomycin (PO)	Bacitracin (PO)
Clostridium tetani Tetanus	Penicillin G, metronidazole	Erythromycin, tetracycline, doxy	
Corynebacterium diphtheriae Diphtheria	Erythromycin (+ antitoxin)	Penicillin G/Procaine Penicillin	
Eikenella corrodens Human bite wounds, abscesses, meningitis	AM-CL, ampicillin	TMP-SMX, FQ, Penicillin G	(Resistant to: cephalexin, clindamycin, erythromycin, metronidazole)
Escherichia coli (E. coli) UTI; not hospital acquired	2nd/3rd gen. cephalosporin	Amp/Amox/TMP-SMX	
Sepsis, pneumonia, hospital-acquired UTI	Ceftriaxone/cefotaxime + aminoglycoside		

Contd...

Contd...

Organism and the common clinical illness	Drug of choice	Alternative	*Other effective agents
E. coli – Meningitis	Ceftazidime/cefepime + aminoglycoside	Meropenem + ciprofloxacin	
E. coli – Diarrhea	See under 'Gastrointestinal Infections' in Chapter 1 (Guidelines for Antimicrobial Therapy)		
Enterococcus spp. Endocarditis, UTI	Ampicillin + aminoglycoside	Vancomycin + aminoglycoside	For vancomycin resistant: Linezolid, daptomycin, tigecycline
Haemophilus ducreyi Chancroid	Azithro/ceftriaxone	Erythro, ciprofloxacin	
Haemophilus influenzae URI, non-life-threatening	AM-CL, Ceph 2/3	Ampicillin, Amoxycillin	
Meningitis, epiglottitis, pneumonia, arthritis	Ceftriaxone, cefotaxime	Amoxy-clavulanate	
Helicobacter pylori	See under treatment of H. pylori infection		

Contd...

Contd...

Organism and the common clinical illness	Drug of choice	Alternative	#Other effective agents
Klebsiella spp. UTI	Fosfomycin	Nitrofurantoin	
Sepsis, pneumonia, meningitis	Imipenem, meropenem	Cefepime Fluoroquinolone	(Use most narrow spectrum effective agent as per culture) Colistin
Listeria monocytogenes Sepsis, meningitis	Ampicillin + gentamicin	TMP-SMX, erythromycin	Aminoglycoside + vancomycin
Moraxella catarrhalis Sinusitis, otitis, bronchitis	AM-CL, 2nd/3rd ceph, TMP-SMX	Azithro, clarithro	Erythro and quinolones
Mycoplasma pneumoniae Pneumonia	Erythro, azithro, clarithro	Doxycycline	
Neisseria gonorrhoeae Gonorrhea	Ceftriaxone/ cefotaxime + doxycycline or azithromycin	Cefixime + azithro/ doxycycline	

Contd...

Organism and the common clinical illness	Drug of choice	Alternative	#Other effective agents
Neisseria meningitidis Meningitis, sepsis	Penicillin G, ampicillin	Ceftriaxone, cefotaxime,	If β-lactam allergy, ciprofloxacin, chloramphenicol
Pasteurella multocida Sepsis, abscesses, animal bite wound	Penicillin G, AMP, amox, cefuroxime	Doxy, levo, moxi, TMP-SMX	Ceftriaxone, cefpodoxime
Proteus mirabilis UTI, sepsis, meningitis	Ampicillin, amoxy	Carbapenems, cephalosporins	Fluoroquinolones
Pseudomonas aeruginosa (i) Urinary infection	An antipseudomonal penicillin,* ceftazidime, cefepime imipenem, meropenem, tobramycin, ciprofloxacin, aztreonam	Piperacillin-tazobactam + aminoglycoside	
(ii) Serious infections: sepsis, meningitis	**Antipseudomonal penicillin-β-lactam combination + tobramycin or ciprofloxacin ** Ticarcillin-clavulanate/ Piperacillin-tazobactam	Meropenem, Aztreonam	

Contd...

Contd...

Organism the Common clinical illness	Drug of choice	Alternative	#Other effective agents
Salmonella typhi[a] Typhoid fever, sepsis	(Severe typhoid) Ceftriaxone, cefotaxime, FQ	Cefixime, azithro, TMP-SMX (for outpatient treatment)	Chloramphenicol, amox
Shigella sp.[#b] Dysentery	Cefixime Ceftriaxone, ciprofloxacin	Azithromycin	
Staphylococcus aureus (Methicillin-sensitive)	Cloxacillin/nafcillin	Clinda, vanco	
(Methicillin-resistant)	Vancomycin + gentamicin (for severe infection)	(For mild infection: Clinda, trimethoprim-sulfamethoxazole) (for very severe infection: linezolid, daptomycin)	
Staphylococcus epidermidis	Vancomycin	FQ	
Staphylococcus saprophyticus	Ceph oral; AM-CL	FQ, TMP-SMX	

Contd...

Contd...

Organism the common clinical illness	Drug of choice	Alternative	#Other effective agents
Strep. (Group A, B, C, G, F) (*Streptococcus pyogenes*) Penicillin-sensitive			
(i) Pharyngitis, impetigo, adenitis	Penicillin V or amoxicillin, or benzathine penicillin	Macrolide, ceph 1, clindamycin	
(ii) Pneumonia, sepsis, meningitis	Penicillin G, ampicillin	A first-generation ceph, vancomycin	
(For serious group B infection)	Penicillin G ± gentamicin	Ampicillin + gentamicin	
(For serious group A infection)	Penicillin G ± clindamycin		
Streptococcus pneumoniae (i) Penicillin-sensitive	Amoxicillin Penicillin G	Ceftriaxone/cefotaxime A macrolide, clinda, cefpodoxime, cefdinir, TMP-SMX	
(ii) Penicillin-resistant	Vancomycin, rifampicin in meningitis cases, cefotaxime/ ceftriaxone	For non-meningeal infection: Cefotaxime, ceftriaxone, high dose AMP	Linezolid
Vibrio cholerae	Doxy or tetracycline	Erythromycin, azithromycin, ciprofloxacin	Quinolones effective for *V. cholerae* 01 and 0139 strains

Contd...

Contd...

Organism the Common clinical illness	Drug of choice	Alternative	#Other effective agents
Yersinia enterocolitica mild cases	Ciprofloxacin; or TMP-SMX	Fluoroquinolones	
for systemic infection and very young:	Ceftriaxone (other parenteral 3rd gen ceph) + aminoglycoside		

*Antipseudomonal penicillins: Piperacillin, ticarcillin, mezlocillin, azlocillin
** Antipseudomonal penicillins-β-lactam combination: Ticarcillin clavulanate, Piperacillin-tazobactam.
#The list of other effective agents is not complete, only some of them have been listed.
(Amox: amoxicillin; clinda: clindamycin; AM-CL: amoxicillin clavulanate; AM-SB: ampicillin-sulbactam; AMP: ampicillin; azithro: azithromycin; CARB: carbapenem; clarithro: clarithromycin; ceph 1, 2, 3: first, second, third generation cephalosporin; CIP: ciprofloxacin; doxy: doxycycline; erythro: erythromycin; FQ: fluoroquinolones; gati: getifloxacin; IMP: imipenem; levo: levofloxacin; MER: meropenem; moxi: moxifloxacin; genta: gentamicin; Pip-Tz: piperacillin-tazobactam; RIF: rifampicin; teico: teicoplanin; TMP-SMX: trimethoprim-sulfamethoxazole; UTI: urinary tract infection; vanco: vancomycin)
#a & #bFor details see under diseases in Chapter 1.

RESERVE ANTIMICROBIALS

These drugs are held in reserve to maintain their effectiveness in treating certain difficult situations by reducing the spread of microbial resistance.

Carbapenems (Imipenem-cilastatin, Meropenem, Ertapenem)

Special indications:
- Severe sepsis (more than one organ failure of recent onset and/or elevated serum lactate level)
- Clinical failure of other antibiotics over 48 hours (worsening inflammatory markers, unresolving fever, new/worsening hemodynamic instability)
- Underlying severe immune suppression, e.g. neutropenia, immunosuppressive therapy, diabetic ketoacidosis
- Infections (e.g. bacteremia, intra-abdominal infections, nosocomial pneumonia, etc.) caused by gram-negative bacteria (*E. coli*, *Klebsiella*, *Enterobacter* spp., *Pseudomonas aeruginosa*) resistant to other classes of antibiotics and susceptible only to carbapenems on culture and sensitivity studies.

Linezolid (Intravenous and Oral)

For restricted use only:
- Glycopeptide-insensitive *Staphylococcus aureus*
- Vancomycin-resistant Enterococcus
- For IV/oral switch from IV vancomycin [used for methicillin-resistant *Staphylococcus* (MRS) or methicillin-resistant *Staphylococcus epidermidis* (MRSE)] to oral linezolid on discharge when rifampicin-trimethoprim combination is inappropriate.
- As home/outpatient parenteral antibiotic therapy for skin and soft tissue infections as an alternative to IV teicoplanin.

Colistin

Indications:
- Pan-resistant organisms as per culture report with evidence of invasive disease—fever/leukocytosis/elevated procalcitonin (PCT) or culture from a sterile site.
- Clinical failure of all other classes of antibiotics over 75 hours.

Rifampicin

Indications:
- For treatment of tuberculosis as a part of 4-drug regimen
- Treatment of mycobacteria
- Chemoprophylaxis of meningococcal meningitis.

Note: Rifampicin not to be used alone as an antibacterial.

Aminoglycosides

Criteria for use:
- Only as a part of initial empiric regimen of a combination therapy to step down to single drug after culture report
- Other safer drug option not available on culture report
- Not to be used if focus of infection in lung or anaerobic abscess.

Vancomycin

Drug of choice for inpatient treatment of following infections:
- Serious (e.g. bacteremia, osteomyelitis) coagulase negative Staphylococcus and methicillin-resistant *Staphylococcus aureus* (MRSA) infections and penicillin-resistant enterococcal infections
- Empiric therapy in febrile neutropenia patients not responding to first-line therapy
- Continuous ambulatory peritoneal dialysis (CAPD) associated peritonitis
- Prosthetic value endocarditis.

Teicoplanin

It is a suitable alternative to vancomycin for all indications for vancomycin, except meningitis.

- Patients on outpatient parenteral therapy with glycopeptide loading doses
- Inability to tolerate vancomycin
- Oncology/hematology patients
- Rare cases of vancomycin resistant and teicoplanin sensitive.

TREATMENT OF MULTIDRUG-RESISTANT BACTERIAL PATHOGENS

- MRSA
- Vancomycin-resistant *Enterococcus*
- Extended-spectrum β-lactamases (ESBL) producing Enterobacteriaceae
- Carbapenem-resistant Enterobacteriaceae.

Treatment of Methicillin-resistant *Staphylococcus aureus*

- Resistant to all penicillins, cephalosporins, and macrolides
- May be sensitive in vitro but do not use: Fluoroquinolones, aminoglycosides, CM, doxycycline
- Avoid rifampicin (except for tuberculosis, other mycobacterial diseases).
- Drugs of choice:
  - Vancomycin, teicoplanin (glycopeptides)
  - Linezolid: for skin and soft tissue infections
  - Mupirocin local intranasal application—for eradicating nasal carriage
  - Daptomycin: For complicated skin infection; for *S. aureus* bacteremia. NOT FOR treatment of pneumonia as it gets inactivated by pulmonary surfactant and has poor lung penetration.

Treatment of Vancomycin-resistant *Enterococcus*

Linezolid: Only drug specifically approved for vancomycin-resistant Enterococcus-bloodstream infection
　　Other approved drugs for specific situations:
- Nitrofurantoin: for uncomplicated urinary tract infection
- Fosfomycin: Urinary tract infection susceptible isolates
- Streptomycin + Ampicillin: for enterococcal endocarditis by susceptible organisms
- Ampicillin (high dose)—for susceptible strain isolates.

Treatment of ESBL-producing *Enterobacteriaceae*

Drugs of choice for serious infections caused by these agents:
- Carbapenems (Ertapenem, meropenem, imipenem)
- For mild infections when ESBL susceptible in vitro—piperacillin-tazobactam, cefoperazone-sulbactam—use group 1 carbapenems.

Note: These organisms resistant to most broad-spectrum antibiotics. Do not use even if in vitro sensitive to all penicillins, cephalosporins (including cefepime, cefpirome), aztreonam.

Treatment of Carbapenem-resistant Enterobacteriaceae (Extremely Drug Resistant)

- **Tigecycline:** Active in vitro
  Licensed for use in complicated skin and first-time infection and complicated intra-abdominal infection
- **Colistin**—successful in some cases
  Some strains may be susceptible to CM, ciprofloxacin, cotrimoxazole.

CHAPTER 5

Antimicrobial Chemoprophylaxis in Patients/Contacts

ANTIBACTERIAL CHEMOPROPHYLAXIS

Disease/pathogen	Recommended drug and its dose
Diphtheria For protection of contacts	Erythromycin 40–50 mg/kg/day div q QID (max 2 g/day) × 7 days or benzathine penicillin <6 years: 0.6 million IU single dose >6 years: 1.2 million IU single dose
Pertussis (*Bordetella pertussis*) For protection of household and close contacts	Erythromycin 40–50 mg/kg/day div q QID (max 2 g/day) × 14 days + immunoprophylaxis (see in Chapter 29)
Malaria (Plasmodia) For protection of an individual	See in Chapter 7
Meningitis (*Neisseria meningitidis*) For protection of contacts	Rifampicin *For children >1 month*: 10 mg/kg/dose q 12 h (max dose 600 mg) × 4 doses *For infants 0–1 month* 5 mg/kg/dose q 12 h × 4 doses or ceftriaxone <15 year: 125 mg IM single dose >15 year: 250 mg IM single dose or ciprofloxacin >18 year: 500 mg PO single dose

Contd...

Contd...

Disease/pathogen	Recommended drug and its dose
Meningitis (Haemophilus influenzae type b) For protection of contacts	Rifampicin For children >1 month 20 mg/kg/day (max 600 mg) div q OD PO × 4 days For infants up to 1 month 10 mg/kg/day div q OD PO × 4 days
Rheumatic fever (Streptococcus group A) For protection of patient #(Secondary prophylaxis to prevent recurrence)	Benzathine penicillin < 27 kg : 600,000 every 3–4 weeks IM ≥27 kg 1–2 million units every 3–4 weeks IM; Or penicillin V <5 yr: 125 mg dose q BID PO ≥ 5 yr: 250 mg dose q BID PO Or sulfadiazine/sulfisoxazole < 27 kg: 500 mg OD PO ≥27 kg: 1 g OD PO Or erythromycin 250 mg q BID (for patients allergic to penicillin)
Recurrent urinary tract infection For protection of patient	Cotrimoxazole 2 mg of trimethoprim (TMP)/10 mg of sulfamethoxazole/kg/day div q OD HS PO Or nitrofurantoin 1–2 mg/kg/day div q OD; Or nalidixic acid 30 mg/kg/day div q 12 h PO
Tuberculosis (Mycobacterium tuberculosis) For protection of patient/ contacts	See in Chapter 6
Sickle cell disease, functional or anatomic asplenia For prevention of pneumococcal sepsis in patient	Penicillin V *Up to age 3 years*: 125 mg/dose BID; *then*: 250 mg/dose BID; until at least 5 years of age Or Erythromycin 10 mg/kg/dose BID; (in penicillin allergy cases)

Contd...

Disease/pathogen	Recommended drug and its dose
Bacterial endocarditis[#] *For protection of patient* (i) Prior to dental and upper respiratory tract surgical procedures	**A. PO** Amoxicillin: 50 mg/kg, max. 2 g (adult dose) 1 hr before procedure ***If penicillin allergy*** Clindamycin: 15 mg/kg, max 500 mg (adult dose) 1 hr before procedure Or cephalexin: 50 mg/kg, max 2 g (adult dose) 1 hr before procedure Or azithromycin/clarithromycin 15 mg/kg, max 500 mg (adult dose) 1 hr before procedure Or **B. Parenteral** Ampicillin: 50 mg/kg IM or IV, max 2 g (adult dose); 30 min before procedure ***If penicillin allergy*** Clindamycin: 20 mg/kg IM/IV, max. 600 mg (adult dose); 30 min before procedure Or cefazolin: 50 mg/kg IM or IV max 1 g (adult dose); 30 min before procedure
(ii) *Prior to gastrointestinal tract and genitourinary tract procedures*	Not recommended now

[#]*For duration of secondary prophylaxis in patients of rheumatic fever, (Table 5.1).*
Note: Do not use cephalosporins if immediate type of hypersensitivity reaction to penicillin (urticaria, angioedema or anaphylaxis) has been observed.

ANTIVIRAL CHEMOPROPHYLAXIS

Influenza

Chemoprophylaxis—7 days
A. Child age <3 months: Oseltamivir for chemoprophylaxis not recommended

Chapter 5: Antimicrobial Chemoprophylaxis in ...

Table 5.1: Duration of secondary prophylaxis.	
Rheumatic fever without carditis	5 years or until age 21 years whichever is longer
RF with carditis but no residual heart disease	10 years or until age 21 years whichever is longer
RF carditis and residual heart disease	10 years since last episode or until age 40 years, whichever is longer, possibly lifelong
Severe carditis	Lifelong
After valve surgery	Lifelong

Age ≥3 months below 1 year: 3 mg/kg/dose OD
Age 1 year or >1 year: Oseltamivir according to body weight
15 kg or less = 30 mg OD
>15–23 kg = 45 mg OD
>23–40 kg = 60 mg OD
>40 kg = 75 mg OD

B. Zanamivir for chemoprophylaxis–7 days
   For children age 7 years and older:
   10 mg (two 5 mg inhalations) OD.

6 Drug Therapy and Prevention in Childhood Tuberculosis

INTRODUCTION

The aim of drug therapy in a child with tuberculosis (TB) is to eradicate the infection in a short time, prevent occurrence of relapses, and avoid emergence of drug resistance. Towards this end, a suitable combination of drugs is employed for appropriate lengths of time to eliminate various subpopulations of TB bacilli (such as, the extracellular, intracellular, rapidly and slow growing as well as the dormant ones) residing in different areas of the tuberculous lesion.

Initially under the Revised National Tuberculosis Control Program (RNTCP) of Government of India intermittent, thrice weekly directly observed treatment short-course (DOTS) strategy was adopted for the treatment of TB patients. Later, poor regular reporting and irregular intake of drugs by patients were considered to be contributing to increasing incidence of multiple-drug-resistant (MDR) cases of TB in the community. Subsequently, it has now been decided to employ daily regimen of anti-TB drug therapy.

For the purpose of treatment, TB cases are classified into the following categories.
- *Category I*: New cases
- *Category II*: Previously treated cases:
  - Failure to respond
  - Treatment after default
  - Relapse cases
  - Retreatment and others.

Failure to respond: A case of pediatric TB, who fails to have bacteriological conversion to negative status or fails to respond clinically or deteriorates after 12 weeks of compliant intensive phase.

Treatment after default: A patient who has taken treatment for at least 4 weeks and comes after interruption of treatment for 2 months and has active disease.

Relapse: Patient declared cured/completed therapy in past and has evidence of recurrence.

DRUG REGIMEN

The choice of anti-TB drugs and duration of therapy in different categories of patients are shown in Table 6.1 and their dosage in Table 6.2.

For ease of administration, separate pediatric and adult Fixed Drug Combination (FDC) tablets have been developed for use in intensive and continuation phase of

Table 6.1: Antituberculosis (TB) drugs and duration of therapy in different categories of patients.

Treatment category	Type of patients	TB treatment regimens		
		Intensive phase	Continuation phase	Total duration

Category I: New cases	A. Pulmonary TB:
	i. Progressive, pneumonia, collapse
	  – Endobronchial,
	  – Fibrocavitary
		2 HRZE	4 HRE	6 months

	ii. Miliary disseminated TB	3 HRZE	6 HR	9 months

	B. Extrapulmonary TB:
	i. Intestinal TB
	  – Peritonitis,
	  – Pericarditis
	  – Pleural effusion,
	  – Genitourinary TB
		2 HRZE	4 HR	6 months

Contd...

Contd...

Treatment category	Type of patients	TB treatment Regimens		
		Intensive phase	Continuation phase	Total duration
	ii. TB meningitis – Spinal TB, – Disseminated TB, – Osteoarticular TB	3 HRZE	6 HR (may extend another 3 months on case-to-case basis)	9–12 months
Category II: Previously treated cases	• Failure to respond • Relapse cases • Treatment after default • Retreatment • Others	2 HRZE S# +1 HRZE	5 HRE	8–10 months (may extend another 2 months on case-to-case basis)

Note: 2 HRZE means—2 months treatment with isoniazid (INH), rifampicin, pyrazinamide and ethambutol; S# stands for streptomycin

therapy. The schedule for their administration under RNTCP is placed in Table 6.3.

Pediatric FDC tablets composition:
- *For intensive phase*: RHZ (rifampicin, INH, pyrazinamide): 50 + 75 + 150
- *For continuation phase*: RH 50 + 75.

Adult FDC tablet composition:
- *For intensive phase*: HRZE (INH, rifampicin, pyrazinamide, ethambutol) 75/150/400/275
- For continuation phase: HRE 75/150/275.

Note: Ethambutol tablets and streptomycin injection are administered separately as per requirement in individual cases.

Role of Steroids

Adjunctive steroid therapy is recommended in case of tuberculous meningitis, pericarditis, massive pleural effusion

Table 6.2: Dosage of anti-tuberculosis (TB) drugs.

Drug	Daily dosage (mg/kg)	Maximum dose per day daily regimen	Intermittent thrice weekly dosage under RNTCP	Maximum per day dose in intermittent thrice weekly regimen
Isoniazid (H)	10 mg/kg (10–12 mg/kg)	300 mg/day	15 mg/kg	300 mg/day
Rifampicin (R)	10 mg/kg (10–12 mg/kg)	600 mg/day	15 mg/kg	600 mg/day
Ethambutol (E)	20 mg/kg (15–25 mg/kg)	1,600 mg/day	30 mg/kg	1,600 mg/day
Pyrazinamide (Z)	30 mg/kg (30–35 mg/kg)	2,000 mg/day	35 mg/kg	2,000 mg/day
Streptomycin (S)	15 mg/kg	1 g/day	30 mg/kg	1 g/day

(RNTCP: Revised National Tuberculosis Control Program)
Note: For more details regarding dosage, precautions, and side effect of above drugs, see under Section 4: Pediatric Drug Formulary.

Table 6.3: Drug schedule using Fixed Drug Combination (FDC) tablets under Revised National Tuberculosis Control Program (RNTCP).

	Intensive phase		Continuation phase		
Weight band (kg)	RHZ tablets (pediatric)	Ethambutol 100 mg tablets	RH tablets (pediatric)	Ethambutol 100 mg tablets	Injection Streptomycin (mg)
4–7	1	1	1	1	100 mg
8–11	2	2	2	2	150 mg
12–15	3	3	3	3	200 mg
16–24	4	4	4	4	300 mg
25–29	3 + 1 Adult	3	3 + 1 Adult	3	400 mg
30–39	2 + 2 Adult	2	2 + 2 Adult	2	500 mg

with respiratory distress, miliary TB with hypoxemia, endobronchial TB, mediastinal compression syndrome, and tuberculoma with neurologic manifestations. Prednisone 2 mg/kg in one to two divided doses orally daily for 2–4 weeks followed by gradual tapering over 2 weeks.

PREVENTIVE THERAPY

Child in Contact with an Adult with Pulmonary Tuberculosis

Firstly, such child must be examined and investigated for any evidence of having developed TB infection. If so, he should be given requisite treatment and properly followed up. If there is no evidence of infection, he should be provided isoniazid (INH) prophylaxis at a dose of 10 mg/kg/day for 6 months.

Other Indications for Chemoprophylaxis

- All HIV infected children who are tuberculin (Mantoux) test positive (over 5 mm induration) or had a known exposure to an infectious TB case.
- All tuberculin test positive children who are receiving immune suppressive therapy.
- A child born to mother who had TB in pregnancy after excluding congenital TB.

MANAGEMENT OF INFANT BORN TO MOTHER WITH TUBERCULOSIS

Firstly, infant should be screened for evidence of TB by physical examination, tuberculin test, and X-ray chest. If there is no evidence of disease, INH prophylaxis should be commenced at dose of 10 mg/kg/day.

After 3 months, the child should be examined for evidence of TB and a repeat tuberculin test is done. If tuberculin test is negative and there is no evidence of disease, the infant should be immunized with bacillus Calmette-Guérin (BCG) vaccine and INH can be stopped.

If tuberculin test is positive but the infant is asymptomatic, INH prophylaxis should be continued for another 3 months (total 6 months).

An infant with congenital TB should be treated as outlined for New Cases in Table 6.1.

CHAPTER 7

Malaria: Treatment and Chemoprophylaxis

DRUG THERAPY IN MALARIA

It should be tailored according to the species and resistance pattern of the *Plasmodium* organisms responsible for causing malaria in the concerned region.

Treatment of Uncomplicated *Plasmodium vivax* Malaria

- *Chloroquine PO*: Initial 10 mg base/kg (maximum dose 600 mg); followed by 5 mg (maximum 300 mg base) at 6, 24, and 48 hours. Total dose 25 mg/kg.
- Chloroquine to be followed by primaquine in dose of 0.25 mg/kg/day once daily for 14 days for prevention of relapse (radical cure).

Precautions

It is recommended that chloroquine should not be administered on empty stomach and while the child is having high fever. Temperature should be brought down before its administration. If vomiting occurs within 45 minutes of a dose of chloroquine, repeat this dose after control of vomiting by use of an antiemetic such as, ondansetron/domperidone.

It is desirable that prior to administration of primaquine, the child should be screened for glucose-6-phosphate dehydrogenase (G6PD) deficiency in view of risk of development of hemolytic anemia in G6PD deficient cases, and he should be closely watched during its use. In patients with borderline G6PD deficiency, primaquine should be administered in modified dose of 0.6–0.8 mg/kg once weekly for 6 weeks. It should not be administered to those with severe G6PD deficiency. Primaquine is contraindicated in infants (under 1 year), pregnant, and breastfeeding women.

Treatment of Uncomplicated *P. falciparum* Malaria

Artemisinin Combination Therapy

Artemisinin combination therapy (ACT) is recommended for all confirmed cases of *Plasmodium falciparum* infection found by microscopy or rapid diagnostic test (RDT). It consists of an artemisinin derivative combined with a long-acting antimalarial. The ACT recommended in the National Malaria Control Program all over India (except north-east states) is ACT-SP (i.e. artesunate + sulfadoxine-pyrimethamine).

For north-eastern states, the recommended combination is ACT-AL (artemether + lumefantrine). Primaquine is simultaneously employed in both cases.

The dosage schedule for ACT–SP combination for management of *P. falciparum* cases is as follows.

Artesmate 4 mg/kg PO OD × 3 days

+ Sulfadoxine pyrimethamine single dose on day 1 PO (Sulfadoxine 25 mg/kg and pyrimethamine 1.25 mg/kg).

(***Note***: Monotherapy of oral artemisinin derivatives is banned in India)

Reference: National Institute of Malaria Research & National Vector Borne Disease Control Programme, Delhi. (2014). Guidelines for Diagnosis & Treatment of Malaria in India 2014. [online] Available from http://www.mrcindia.org/Diagnosis%20of%20Malaria%20pdf/Guidelines%202014.pdf. [Accessed September, 2018].

Antimalarial Therapy in Severe and Complicated *P. falciparum* or *P. vivax* Malaria

Severe malaria is a medical emergency in children. In case of strong clinical suspicion, start antimalarial therapy promptly even if initial blood smear examination is negative for malarial parasites. Repeated blood smear examination and/or rapid antigen detection tests should be done in an effort to confirm the diagnosis. Effective therapy is comprised of—(1) antimalarial chemotherapy, (2) supportive management, and (3) management of complications.

Note: *According to WHO, the term "Severe Malaria" refers to those symptomatic malaria infections, which can lead to death if not treated appropriately. It may manifest as cerebral malaria (acute encephalopathy with unarousable coma), generalized convulsions, severe normocytic normochromic anemia, acute renal failure, pulmonary edema, hypoglycemia, hypotension/shock (algid malaria), bleeding/disseminated intravascular coagulation (DIC), acidemia/acidosis, hemoglobinuria, jaundice, hyperparasitemia (parasite count over 250,000/μL or more than 5% RBC infected).*

Antimalarial Drug Therapy in Severe and Complicated Malaria

Parenteral artemisinin derivatives or quinine are recommended as specific antimalarial therapy.

Initial:
- ***Artesunate IV/IM***:
  Artesunate 2.4 mg/kg intravenous (IV) or intramuscular (IM) (maximum 120 mg) at admission to be followed by one dose 1.2 mg/kg/dose (maximum 60 mg) at 12 hours and 24 hours and then 1.2 mg/kg once daily. Artesunate powder 60 mg per ampoule is dissolved in 0.6 mL of 5% sodium bicarbonate, and diluted to 3–5 mL with 5% dextrose. The calculated recommended dose is then immediately given by IV push/IM in anterior thigh. Parenteral artesunate is continued for 6 days or changed earlier when patient can take medicines orally. He is then shifted to ACT-SP oral combination therapy of artesunate plus sulfadoxine–pyrimethamine described earlier.

- *Or Quinine IV*:
  Quinine salt 20 mg/kg diluted in 10 mL/kg of 5% dextrose or dextrose normal saline is administered as IV infusion over a period of 4 hours. The infusion rate should not exceed 5 mg/kg body weight per hour. It is to be followed by maintenance dose of quinine salt 10 mg/kg by infusion (over 2 hours) every 8 hours (calculated from the beginning of previous infusion). If parenteral quinine therapy needs to be continued beyond 48 hours, dose should be reduced to 7 mg/kg every 8 hours. Shift to oral quinine sulfate as soon as possible to complete a course of 7 days (parenteral + oral).

- *Or quinine IM*:
  If quinine cannot be administered through properly controlled IV infusion, same dose of quinine salt can be administered by IM injection. Each dose (as recommended above) should be split in two halves. One half component should be injected in anterior thigh on one side and the other half in the anterior thigh on the other side (not in buttock)

- *Or Artemether IM*:
  Artemether IM 3.2 mg/kg on admission, then 1.6 mg/kg per day OD. Once the patient is able to swallow, complete treatment by giving a course of artesunate plus sulfadoxine-pyramethamine.

For follow-up treatment:
Once the patient can tolerate oral therapy after either artesunate or artemether parenteral therapy (for at least 24 hours), further follow-up treatment should be with ACT-SP combination as described earlier.

It is worthy of note that patients, who initially received parenteral quinine, should also be treated subsequently with full course of oral ACT.

Note: Uncommon cases of severe malaria due to *P. vivax* infection should be treated like severe *P. falciparum* malaria. In these cases, primaquine should be given for 14 days for preventing relapse after the patient recovers from acute illness.

CHEMOPROPHYLAXIS AGAINST MALARIA

Chemoprophylaxis is recommended for travelers from nonendemic areas to endemic malarious area. Before prescribing for prophylaxis, latest information about drug resistance pattern in that area must be taken into account.

- *For chloroquine susceptible area*:
  Chloroquine phosphate 5 mg base/kg maximum 300 mg; once weekly. Start 1–2 weeks prior to departure, continue for 4 week after last exposure.
- *For chloroquine resistance area:*
  Mefloquine, doxycycline, or malarone tablets
  (i) *Mefloquine 250 mg (228 mg base) per tablet (for long-term prophylaxis— >6 weeks)*:
    ▫ *<10 kg*: 4.6 mg base (5 mg salt)/kg/once weekly
    ▫ *10–19 kg*: ¼ tablet/once weekly
    ▫ *20–30 kg*: ½ tablet/once weekly
    ▫ *31–45 kg*: ¾ tablet/once weekly
    ▫ *>45 kg*: 1 tablet once weekly.

  Start 1–2 week prior to departure and continue for 4 weeks after return.

  (ii) *Doxycycline (for short-term chemoprophylaxis—<6 weeks)*:
    ▫ For children above 8 years, 1.5 mg/kg daily (maximum 100 mg)
    ▫ Start 1–2 days before departure and continue for 4 week after last exposure.
    ▫ Contraindications: History of convulsion, neuropsychiatric problems, and cardiac condition.

  (iii) *Atovaquone/proguanil (Malarone)*:
    ▫ *Pediatric tablet*: 62.5 mg atovaquone/25 mg proguanil
    ▫ *Adult tablet*: 250 mg atovaquone/100 mg proguanil
    ▫ *5–8 kg*: ½ tablet once daily (pediatric tablet)
    ▫ *9–10 kg*: ¾ tablet once daily (pediatric tablet)
    ▫ *11–20 kg*: 1 pediatric tablet once daily
    ▫ *21–30 kg*: 2 pediatric tablets once daily

- *31–40 kg*: 3 pediatric tablets once daily
- *>40 kg*: 1 adult tablet once daily.

Malarone tablet to be started 1–2 days before departure and continued for 7 days after exposure. It is not recommended for children <5 kg, and women breastfeeding infants and for those having severe renal impairment.

8 Treatment of Helminthic, Protozoal, and Other Parasitic Infections

Note: For dosage, mode of use, and other information regarding recommended drugs, see under the individual drugs in Section 4: "Pediatric Drug Formulary".

GUIDELINES FOR CHOICE OF DRUGS

Helminthic Infections

Ascariasis:
Mebendazole or albendazole or ivermectin or nitazoxanide.
 Piperazine citrate (for ascariasis complicated by intestinal or biliary obstruction).

Cutaneous larva migrans (Ancylostoma braziliense):
Ivermectin PO, albendazole PO, or thiabendazole solution topical application QID × 2–5 days.

Cysticercosis:
Albendazole or praziquantel.

Enterobius vermicularis:
See "Pinworm infection"

Echinococcosis:
See "Tapeworm infection"

Filariasis:
- *Wuchereria bancrofti, Brugia malayi, Brugia timori*:
  - Ivermectin + albendazole; Diethylcarbamazine drug of choice for lymphatic filariasis.
- *Tropical pulmonary eosinophilia*:
  - Diethylcarbamazine 2 mg/kg/ dose TID PO × 12–21 days.

Hookworm:
Albendazole, mebendazole, or pyrantel pamoate.

Hydatid disease:
See "Tapeworm infection"

Hymenolepis nana:
See "Tapeworm infection"

Pinworm (Enterobius vermicularis):
Mebendazole or albendazole or pyrantel pamoate.

Roundworm:
See "Ascariasis"

Schistosomiasis:
Praziquantel.

Strongyloidiasis:
Ivermectin or albendazole.

Tapeworm infections:
Taenia saginata (beef tapeworm, adult stage intestinal infection):
Praziquantel or niclosamide.

Taenia solium (pork tapeworm, adult intestinal infection):
Praziquantel or niclosamide.

Diphyllobothrium latum (adult intestinal infection):
Praziquantel or niclosamide

Hymenolepis nana (dwarf tapeworm, adult intestinal infection):
Praziquantel – Alternative; niclosamide or nitazoxanide.

Cysticercosis (intermediate stage infection of Taenia solium):
Drugs of choice: Albendazole or praziquantel;
Alternative: Surgery.

Echinococcosis (hydatid disease, intermediate stage infection of Echinococcus granulosus):
Albendazole (when cysts not amenable to PAIR or surgery) (PAIR—Percutaneous aspiration injection reaspiration).

Toxocariasis:
See visceral larva migrans

Trichinellosis (Trichinella spiralis):
Albendazole or mebendazole [plus steroids when myocarditis or central nervous system (CNS) involvement].

Trichuriasis (whipworm):
Mebendazole or albendazole or ivermectin.

Visceral larva migrans:
(*Larval infection of toxocara*)
Alternatives: Albendazole or mebendazole (corticosteroids for eye involvement).
Additional prednisone 1 mg/kg/day × 2–4 weeks helpful.

Protozoal Infections

Amoebiasis:
Asymptomatic intestinal luminal amoebiasis:
- Diloxanide furoate, paromomycin, or iodoquinol

Mild-to-moderate invasive intestinal disease (colitis):
- Metronidazole, or tinidazole.
- *Note*: As these drugs are not very effective against cysts in the intestinal lumen, follow up their treatment with one of the drugs placed under (*asymptomatic intestinal amoebiasis*) above.

  For dosage, see under individual drugs.

Fulminant intestinal disease, amoebic liver abscess, and metastatic amoebiasis:
- Metronidazole × 7–10 days followed by tinidazole × 5 days PO followed by iodoquinol or paromomycin.

Balantidiasis (Balantidium coli infection):
Metronidazole, tetracycline, or iodoquinol.

Cryptosporidiosis:
Immunocompetent patients: No specific treatment; self-limited
Immunocompromised: Nitazoxanide.

Giardiasis:
Metronidazole, tinidazole, or nitazoxanide
Alternatives: Furazolidone, paromomycin, or quinacrine.

Leishmaniasis:
First-line drug in untreated cases (*except* in Bihar, where there is high incidence of drug resistance): Sodium stibogluconate

For cases with primary treatment failure and relapse cases: Miltefosine or Amphotericin B, Liposomal amphotericin, Pentamidine.

Paromomycin topical twice daily × 10–20 days for localized cutaneous leishmaniasis (LCL).

Note: Miltefosine (oral) may be employed as first-line drug; effective and safe.

- *Malaria*:
  See Chapter 7 "Treatment and Chemoprophylaxis of Malaria".
- *Pneumocystis carinii now called Pneumocystis jirovecii (pneumonia)*:
  Cotrimoxazole
  Alternatives: Pentamidine or primaquine + clindamycin
- *Toxoplasmosis*:
  Pyrimethamine + sulfadiazine
  (Spiramycin for pregnant mother)
- *Trichomoniasis (Trichomonas vaginalis)*:
  Metronidazole or tinidazole.

Arthropod Infestations

Lice (Pediculosis):

1% permethrin cream topically once, may repeat once in 7–10 days; or lindane lotion topically once, repeat in one week (not recommended for pubic hair). For eyelash infestation, petrolatum application locally q 3–5 times/day × 8–10 days.

For persistent cases: Ivermectin 200 µg/kg PO × three doses on days 1, 2, and 10.

Scabies:

Permethrin 5% topical to entire body (including scalp in infants) × 8–12 hours before bathing, OR

Lindane (gamma benzene hexachloride—BHC) lotion 1%; apply locally over whole body below neck at bed time, bathe next morning, OR

Ivermectin 0.2 mg/kg/dose PO × once; repeat after 7 days.

Alternative: 10% crotamiton lotion—topical application overnight on days 1, 2, 3, and 8.

Drugs for Selected Viral Infections

Presently, there are few drugs with limited efficacy for treatment of some viral infections in children. These are listed in Table 9.1.

Table 9.1: Recommended drugs for treatment of viral infections.	
Type of viral infection	Recommended drugs for treatment
Cytomegalovirus (CMV)	• Ganciclovir • Valganciclovir • Foscarnet • Cidofovir
Chronic hepatitis B	• Interferon-α2b (IFN-α2b) • Lamivudine (for children > 2 years) • Adefovir dipivoxil (for children > 12 years) • Entecavir (for children > 16 years) • Tenofovir (for children > 16 years) • Peginterferon-$α_2$
Chronic hepatitis C	• Peginterferon (for children > 3 years) • IFN-α2b • Ribavirin (for children > 3 years) • Sofosbuvir (for adults) • Simeprevir (for adults)
Herpes simplex	• Acyclovir (antiviral agent of choice) • Famciclovir • Valacyclovir • Foscarnet ⎫ • Cidofovir ⎭ (for acyclovir-resistant mutants)

Contd...

Contd...

Type of viral infection	Recommended drugs for treatment
Influenza A and B	- Oseltamivir (for children > 2 weeks) - Zanamivir (for children > 7 years) - Amantidine, Rimantidine (not currently recommended due to recent widespread resistance among different strains of these viruses)
Respiratory syncytial virus (RSV)	- Ribavirin (by aerosol) (Not used much now)
Varicella-zoster virus	- Acyclovir—any age - Valacyclovir—for children 2 to < 18 years - Famciclovir ⎤ for acyclovir- - Foscarnet ⎦ resistant cases

- For dosage, mode of use, and other information regarding recommended drugs, see under the individual drugs in Section: "Pediatric Drug Formulary".

Guidelines for HIV Treatment

The currently available pediatric antiretroviral therapy (ART) for human immunodeficiency virus (HIV) infection does not eradicate the virus. It instead suppresses the virus for extended periods of time. It changes the course of the disease to a less severe chronic process with reduction in mortality and morbidity of infected infants and children.

The aims of treatment with antiretroviral drugs in HIV-infected children are to achieve and sustain full HIV ribonucleic acid (RNA) viral load (VL) suppression and restoration of normal immune function, while avoiding drug toxicity and evolution of viral drug resistance. Good immune function (CD4 + cell count) reduces the risk of opportunistic infections and incidence of various HIV infection complications. Measures are simultaneously taken to prevent development and effective treatment of any opportunistic infection developing during course of the disease.

NACO GUIDELINES FOR HIV TREATMENT

The National AIDS Control Organisation (NACO) with support from WHO, UNICEF, and Clinton Health Access Initiative, have formulated Antiretroviral Therapy Guidelines–2013. These guidelines are intended to guide pediatricians prescribing ART, as well as the team at the ART centers on the practical issues regarding treatment of HIV infection among infants and children.

Factors affecting commencement of therapy and choice of drugs include age of the child, clinical stage of the disease, immune status (CD4+ count and percentage),

Chapter 10: Guidelines for HIV Treatment

Table 10.1: Guidelines for management of HIV/AIDS in children.

Age	Clinical stage	Immunological status	Action recommended
Age below 24 months	Any	Any	Treat all
Age above 24 months	WHO stage 1	—	Watch
Age 2–5 years	WHO stage 2	CD4 below 25% as absolute CD4 count below 750 mm^3	Treat
Age above 5 years	WHO stage 2	Absolute CD4 count below 350 mm^3	Treat
Any age	WHO stage 3	Any	Treat
Any age	WHO stage 4	Any	Treat

(WHO: World Health Organization)
Note: WHO has defined staging of HIV/AIDS in children with confirmed infection into 4 clinical stages 1, 2, 3, and 4 on the basis of the child's clinical status, organ involvement, and associated infections.

magnitude of the viral load, presence of any opportunistic infections, and the type of treatment and its results, if taken earlier. Broad guidelines for approach to management of HIV/AIDS in children are placed in Table 10.1.

ANTIRETROVIRAL DRUGS

As per their mode of action, the drugs presently employed in India for treatment of HIV infection in children fall into three major classes:

1. *Nucleoside (or nucleotide) reverse transcriptase inhibitors (NRTIs)*: These drugs inhibit HIV reverse transcriptase enzyme activity, which is responsible for viral deoxyribonucleic acid (DNA) copies being transcribed from the virion RNA—an important step in the replication of HIV. There are two subgroups of NRTIs.
   i. *Thymidine analogues*: These are active against dividing cells. For example, zidovudine, stavudine, abacavir.

ii. *Nonthymidine analogues*: For example, lamivudine, didanosine. These act against resting cells which serve as a reservoir for HIV.
2. *Non-nucleoside reverse transcriptase inhibitors (NNRTIs)*: They attach to the transcriptase and reduce the activity of this enzyme thereby inhibiting replication of HIV. For example, these are nevirapine, efavirenz, etravirine and rilpivirine.
3. *Protease inhibitors (PIs)*: These agents act at a different stage in viral replication. They inhibit HIV protease enzyme, which is critical for HIV assembly. By blocking this enzyme activity, these drugs prevent package of infectious virions before they leave the infected cell. For example, lopinavir, ritonavir, nelfinavir and atazanavir.

Recently two new classes of antiretroviral drugs have become available abroad:
1. *Fusion inhibitor—Enfuvirtide*:
   This drug binds to viral Gp41, causes conformational changes that prevent fusion of the virus with CD4 cell and entry into the cell.
2. *Integrase strand transfer inhibitors (INSTIs)*: These block the enzyme that catalyzes the incorporation of the viral genome into the host's DNA, e.g. raltegravir, dolutegravir, elvitegravir.

COMBINATION THERAPY

Principle of Antiretroviral Drug Therapy

Antiretroviral therapy is designed to achieve maximal viral suppression by targeting drugs at different points in the virus life cycle, at various stages of its activation, and at all tissue sites of virus assembly.

In general, triple drug combination therapy comprising 2 NRTIs with 1 NNRTI or PI drug is employed as first-line measure. For example, it comprises a combination of zidovudine (a thymidine analogue NRTI); lamivudine (a non-thymidine NRTI) with nevirapine (NNRTI). In another combination, nevirapine (NNRTI) may be replaced by ritonavir (PI).

Chapter 10: Guidelines for HIV Treatment

The NACO guidelines provide comprehensive advice about employment of various antiretroviral drugs in different age groups under different clinical situations such as for—(1) first-line treatment, (2) second-line treatment in the event of failure of first-line treatment, (3) in case of development of adverse reaction to one of the drugs (or) presence of some concurrent infections. Information is also provided about antiretroviral drug pediatric fixed dose combination preparations, which have been developed for administration on weight-band dosing system. Besides management of HIV infection, vital information has been provided about various bacterial, viral, fungal, and parasitic infections often encountered along with it.

Considering the complexity of issues, ART for HIV infection should preferably be conducted in specialized ART centers with availability of trained physicians, requisite laboratory facilities, and proper long-term follow-up. Lifelong close adherence to prescribed therapy is essential in HIV patients.

Note: NACO Pediatric Antiretroviral Therapy (ART) Guidelines–2013, are available on line for guidance.

11. Preferred Therapy for Selected Fungal Pathogens

Note: For dosage, mode of use and other information regarding recommended drugs, see under the individual drugs in the Section: "Pediatric Drug Formulary".

ASPERGILLOSIS

- *Allergic bronchopulmonary aspergillosis* (ABPA): Itraconazole or voriconazole + systemic corticosteroids.
- *Invasive pulmonary aspergillosis (IPA) or extrapulmonary:*
  - Voriconazole or posaconazole
  - Amphotericin B lipid complex
  - Itraconazole
  - Caspofungin/micafungin.

CANDIDIASIS

- *Oral candidiasis*: Local application of either nystatin, miconazole suspension, gentian violet lotion or clotrimazole troches/lotion. For recalcitrant or recurrent infection, fluconazole single-dose PO. In breastfed infant—fluconazole single dose PO taken by mother may be effective both for mother and infant.
- *Diaper dermatitis*: Nystatin cream, powder, ointment or clotrimazole 1% cream or miconazole 2% ointment topical application (+hydrocortisone 1% cream topical × 1–2 days if significant inflammation).
- *Vulvovaginal candidiasis:*
  - Vaginal creams or troches of nystatin, clotrimazole or miconazole.
  - Single oral dose of fluconazole.

- *Oropharyngeal candidiasis:*
  Clotrimazole troches or nystatin suspension qid topical use or fluconazole PO daily (12 mg/kg/day).
- *Neonatal candidiasis (severe, invasive):*
  Amphotericin B deoxycholate 1 mg/kg/day (for infants) or fluconazole (preferred for invasive, especially urinary tract infection) 12 mg/kg/day.
- *Systemic candidiasis:*
  - Lipid-based amphotericin B 3–5 mg/kg/day IV.
  - Azoles.
    Fluconazole 12 mg/kg/day IV/PO
    or voriconazole 8 mg/kg/dose BD IV, oral maintenance 9 mg/kg/dose.
    or posaconazole 12–24 mg/kg/day div q TID.
  - Echinocandins (Broad spectrum):
    - Caspofungin 50 mg/m^2/day IV (adults 50 mg/day IV).
    - Micafungin 2–10 mg/kg/day IV (adults 100 mg/day IV).
    - Anidulafungin 1.5 mg/kg/day IV (adults 100 mg/day IV).

COCCIDIOIDOMYCOSIS

- *Primary pulmonary infection:*
  Fluconazole 6–12 mg/kg/day × 3–6 months, or
  Itraconazole 5–10 mg/kg/day × 3–6 months.
- *Diffuse pneumonia:*
  Amphotericin B initially followed by high-dose fluconazole for extended period.
- *Disseminated infection (Extrapulmonary):*
  - Noncentral nervous system, nonextensive, not rapidly progressive:
    Fluconazole or itraconazole PO.
  - Skeletal infections:
    Itraconazole.
  - Lesions rapidly progressive; in critical location
    Itraconazole or amphotericin B deoxycholate.
  - For salvage therapy:
    Voriconazole.

- Meningitis
  Fluconazole PO or itraconazole PO.
  If failure with above: Amphotericin B deoxycholate intrathecal;
  Salvage therapy with voriconazole.

CRYPTOCOCCOSIS

- *Immunocompetent patient, asymptomatic, limited to lungs:*
  Fluconazole PO 6–12 mg/kg/day × 3–12 months, or itraconazole PO 5–10 mg/kg/day div q 12 h × 3–12 months.
- *Disseminated, pulmonary or central nervous system infection in HIV-infected patients:*
  Induction therapy: Amphotericin B (0.7–1 mg/kg/day) + flucytosine (100–150 mg/kg/day) × 6–10 weeks, followed by consolidation phase—fluconazole minimum (8–10 weeks) and then continue for life (maintenance therapy).

HISTOPLASMOSIS

- *Asymptomatic/mildly symptomatic acute pulmonary histoplasmosis*
  No treatment; if no improvement in 1 month: Itraconazole or fluconazole PO.
- *Pulmonary; hypoxemic*:
  - Amphotericin B 0.7–1 mg/kg/day, or
    amphotericin B lipid complex 3–5 mg/kg/day until improvement; then continue therapy with itraconazole 5–10 mg/kg/day PO div q bid (maximum 400 mg/day × minimum 12 weeks)
  - If obstructive disease due to granulomatous mediastinal disease, treat sequentially with amphotericin and itraconazole for 6–12 months).
- *Mild mediastinal disease*: Only itraconazole PO.

12 Fluids, Electrolytes and Acid-base Management in Acute Gastroenteritis

SOME ESSENTIAL FACTS

Daily Maintenance Requirements

i. Fluid:
 0–10 kg: 100 mL/kg
 11–20 kg: 1000 mL + 50 mL/kg for each kg > 10 kg
 >20 kg: 1500 mL + 20 mL/kg for each kg >20 kg

ii. Sodium: 2–3 mEq/kg/day
iii. Potassium: 1–2 mEq/kg/day

ASSESSMENT OF DEHYDRATION IN A PATIENT WITH DIARRHEA

Based on the patient's clinical features, a patient having diarrhea is categorized as having: (i) No dehydration; (ii) Some dehydration; and (iii) Severe dehydration (Tables 12.1 and 12.2). This categorization developed by the World Health Organization (WHO) as a part of Integrated Management of Childhood Illness (IMCI) strategy has been adapted to its Indian version, named Integrated Management of Neonatal and Childhood Illness (IMNCI).

Treatment Plan A: For Cases with No Dehydration

Administration of oral rehydration solution (ORS) should be commenced early to prevent development of dehydration.

Table 12.1: Assessment of dehydration status.

Clinical signs	Group I	Group II	Group III
General condition	Well, alert	Restless, irritable	Lethargic or unconsciousness
Eyes	Normal	Sunken	Sunken
Thirst	Not thirsty, drinks normally	Thirsty, drinks eagerly	Drinks poorly, not able to drink
Skin pinch	Goes back quickly	Goes back slowly	Goes back very slowly
Criteria	All features as above	Patient has 2 or more of above signs	Patient has 2 or more above signs
Hydration status: Conclusion	No dehydration	Some dehydration	Severe dehydration
Recommended treatment plan	Plan A	Plan B	Plan C

Table 12.2: Estimated fluid deficit as per dehydration status.

Grade of dehydration	Fluid deficit as % of body weight	Fluid deficit in mL/kg body weight
No signs of dehydration	<5%	<50 mL/kg
Some dehydration	5–10%	50–100 mL/kg
Severe dehydration	>10%	>100 mL/kg

The mother is advised to administer low osmolarity ORS (now recommended by WHO and Indian Academy of Pediatrics) to (i) replace ongoing losses of fluid and electrolytes in stools and vomit as per child's age (Table 12.3) or at the rate of 10 mL/kg/stool and 2–3 mL/kg for each vomit.

The low osmolar ORS formulations (according to WHO guidelines) are now widely available in powder form in sachets of different sizes. These need to be reconstituted in clean drinking water, as per given directions, in quantities

Table 12.3: Replacement fluid for loss in stools as per the child's age.

Age	ORS replacement per stool	Amount of total ORS in a day
< 24 months	50–100 mL/stool	500 mL/day
2–10 years	100–200 mL/stool	1,000 mL/day
10 years or more	As much as wanted	2,000 mL/day

varying between 200 mL and 1 liter. Following reconstitution, it provides sodium 75 mEq/L, potassium 20 mEq/L and glucose 75 mmol/L with total osmolarity 245 mOsm/L.

Alternatives to WHO ORS

In situations when WHO ORS packets are not available or the child does not accept it for reasons of taste, home made ORS can be prepared by adding a two-finger-and-thumb pinch of common salt (0.8 g) and a 4-finger scoop (or one heaped teaspoon) of sugar (8 g) in a liter of clean drinking water. A few drops of fresh lemon juice can be added to improve its taste. Salted rice kanjee, salted lassi, and vegetable or chicken soup with salt are culturally acceptable substitutes available in most homes. In the absence of these, weak unsweetened tea, green coconut water and unsweetened fresh fruit juice may be employed. Commercial carbonated beverages, commercial fruit juice and sweetened tea are unsuitable alternatives and should not be used.

Treatment of Cases with Some Dehydration: IMNCI Treatment Plan B

For correction of fluid deficit, 75 mL/kg of ORS should be given over a period of 4 hours. In case dehydration persists, more ORS is given for full correction of deficit. Besides it, ORS is to be given for replacement of fluid losses in stools and vomit as explained under plan A.

Breastfeeds, intake of milk and other light foods as per child's age should be resumed.

Children with Severe Dehydration: IMNCI Treatment Plan C

Children with severe dehydration and shock, require urgent intravenous fluid therapy. In a child above 12 months of age, Ringer lactate should be administered at the rate of 30 mL/kg within 30 minutes and at the rate of 70 mL/kg over the next 2½ hours. In infants below 12 months, initial bolus at the rate of 30 mL/kg is given over 1 hour and 70 mL/kg over the next 5 hours. If the radial pulse is noticed to be weak or not palpable or the patient has not passed urine after the initial bolus, fluid at the rate of 30 mL/kg is repeated, and close watch kept on child's circulatory status and urinary output. Further management is done according to the child's status of hydration, electrolytes, acid-base level and clinical progress. Fluid losses through vomiting and stools are estimated every 4–6 hours and replaced by administering 5% dextrose N/2 solution at the rate of 10 mL/kg per stool and 2 mL/kg per vomit till such time the child resumes oral intake of ORS.

Metabolic Acidosis

Moderate acidosis, if present, is corrected by administration of 3 mL of 7.5% sodium bicarbonate per kg. One-half is given during first hour diluted with equal amount of distilled water or double the amount of 5% dextrose solution slowly as IV bolus, and the rest during next 7 hours. To prevent development of hypocalcemic tetany following correction of acidosis, give calcium gluconate 50 mg/kg (10% calcium gluconate 0.5 mL/kg) IV slowly separately. If mixed with fluid containing sodium bicarbonate, it will get precipitated as calcium carbonate.

Hypokalemia

For its prevention, add 1 mL 15% KCl per 100 mL of N/2 or N/5 saline in 5% dextrose solution after establishment of urinary output. For correction of hypokalemia, add 15% KCl to IV fluid not exceeding at the rate of 2 mL/100 mL (40 mEq/L) with regular monitoring of serum potassium level.

Hypernatremia

Children, especially young infants with diarrhea are liable to develop hypernatremic dehydration when they receive hypertonic drinks, such as canned fruit juices, carbonated beverages and highly salted cum sugar solution as oral rehydration therapy. Those with serum sodium more than 150 mEq/L and osmolality more than 295 mOsm/kg feel extremely thirsty and are liable to develop convulsions. Although the concentration of sodium is abnormally high in serum and extracellular fluid in cases with hypernatremic dehydration, there is total body deficit of sodium.

These children can be successfully treated with oral rehydration regimen employing low osmolar ORS or by administration of glucose electrolyte solution containing 90 mmol/L of sodium alternating with plain water. However, if the child is unable to drink orally, Ringer lactate can be initially used to treat shock and subsequently oral rehydration therapy done by use of ORS alternating with plain water.

Hypotonic Dehydration

Patients of diarrhea, who ingest only large amounts of water or watery drinks that contain very little salt, are liable to develop hyponatremia with serum sodium level below 130 mEq/L. Initially intravascular volume depletion should be corrected by administering isotonic fluid—NS or Ringer lactate.

Subsequently, 24-hour fluid needs comprising maintenance and residual deficit should be administered over 24 hours using 5% dextrose NS + 20 mEq/L KCl.

Hyponatremia should not be too rapidly corrected as overcorrection in the serum sodium concentration above 135 mEq/L is associated with an increased risk of central pontine myelinolysis.

Hyponatremic patients with neurologic symptoms (seizures) should be given an acute infusion of hypertonic (3%) saline to increase the serum sodium concentration rapidly and they should be closely monitored.

13. Treatment of Acute Hyperkalemia and Hypokalemia

ACUTE HYPERKALEMIA

Serum Potassium Level more than 5.5 mEq/L

- *Mild to moderate hyperkalemia (serum K^+ < 6.5 mEq/L):*
  - Stop all sources of intake of potassium [oral or intravenous (IV)]
  - Discontinue potassium-sparing diuretics, if child is receiving them
  - Monitor serum potassium level closely
  - Monitor electrocardiogram (ECG).
- *Severe hyperkalemia (serum K^+ level ≥ 6.5 mEq/L):*
  - Urgent ECG monitoring for assessment of cardiac effects of hyperkalemia*
  - Execute emergency management as advised in Table 13.1.

Table 13.1: Emergency management.			
Therapy	Mode of action	Onset	Duration
10% calcium gluconate 0.5–1 mL/kg (50–100 mg/kg) intravenous (IV) over 5 minutes (give over 30 minutes if patient on digitalis) May repeat	Reverses the deleterious effect of hyperkalemia on cell membrane of cardiac cells; prevents serious arrhythmias No effect on serum K^+ level	Immediate	Brief

Contd...

Contd...

Therapy	Mode of action	Onset	Duration
Sodium bicarbonate solution 7.5% 1–2 mL/kg IV over 5–10 minutes	Moves potassium into cells, lowers serum potassium level	20–30 minutes	2–4 hours
Insulin 0.1 unit/kg with 25% glucose 2 mL/kg (i.e. 1 unit/ 5 g of glucose) IV over 30 minutes	Lowers serum potassium by moving potassium into cells	Within 30 minutes	2–4 hours

*Progressive changes in ECG following increasing level of serum potassium:
- *Initially peaking of T wave*
- *As K$^+$ level increases, widening of PR interval, flattening/disappearance of P wave, widening of QRS, sine wave, first-degree heart block, ventricular dysrhythmia, and cardiac asystole.*

Dialysis (hemodialysis more effective than peritoneal dialysis) should be done:
- If all measures of emergency management described in Table 13.1 fail;
- If severe renal failure;
- If high rate of endogenous potassium release, e.g. in tumor lysis syndrome, rhabdomyolysis.

Following control of acute hyperkalemia, begin measures that remove K$^+$ from body:
- Sodium polystyrene sulfonate (Kayexalate)
  PO: 1 g/kg/dose every 6 hours or PR: 1 g/kg/dose every 2–6 hours. Retain enema in colon for at least 30–60 minutes.
- In those who are not anuric, give loop diuretic (e.g. furosemide) in high doses.

HYPOKALEMIA

Hypokalemia may develop due to gastrointestinal (GI) losses (diarrhea, vomiting, and gastric aspiration), renal losses (excessive use of diuretics, proximal or distal renal tubular acidosis, and hyperaldosteronism), or low intake which are all associated with total body potassium depletion. In cases with intracellular potassium shift (as in metabolic alkalosis, insulin therapy especially in patients with diabetic ketoacidosis, and familial hypokalemic periodic paralysis), there is no change in total body potassium.

The management of hypokalemia is greatly influenced by serum potassium level, the underlying causative factors, renal function, and the patients' ability to tolerate oral potassium.

Asymptomatic hypokalemia with serum potassium 3.0–3.5 mEq/L may be treated with oral administration of potassium at the rate of 1–4 mEq/kg/24 hrs divided over BID-QID doses. 1 mL of 15% solution of potassium chloride (KCl) provides 2 mEq of potassium. For parenteral administration, the concentration of potassium in the infusate should not exceed 40 mEq/L (i.e. 20 mL of 15% KCl/L). Potassium must be administered only when renal function is established (urine passed or its passage confirmed by urinary catheterization if necessary). In critical situations (severe hypokalemia with ECG abnormalities), potassium infusion of 0.5 mEq/kg/h may be given for 1–2 hours. The adult maximum dose is 40 mEq. The maximum concentration in peripheral IV line should not exceed 40 mEq/L. Recheck serum potassium every hour, avoid overdosage. Treat the underlying cause.

Electrocardiogram changes in hypokalemia include a flattened T wave, depressed ST-segment, lengthening of Q-Tc, and appearance of a U wave.

14 Management of Asthma

GOALS

The long-term goals of asthma management are to achieve good symptom control, maintain the child's normal activity, and minimize future risks of exacerbations, fixed airflow limitations, and adverse side effects of treatment. Achievement of these objectives involves control of factors contributing to the causation and severity of asthma and use of appropriate pharmacotherapy.

GUIDELINES FOR PHARMACOTHERAPY

For the purpose of appropriate pharmacotherapy, the severity of disease in asthmatic children is classified into four categories on the basis of the frequency and severity of symptoms and degree of functional impairment. The various categories and criteria for their classification are placed in Table 14.1.

DRUGS EMPLOYED FOR MANAGEMENT OF ASTHMA

- *Quick-reliever medications*:
  - *Short-acting β-agonists (SABAs)*: Salbutamol, levosalbutamol, terbutaline, and pirbuterol.
- *Long-term anti-inflammatory controller drugs*:
  - *Inhaled corticosteroids (ICSs)*: Budesonide, fluticasone, beclomethasone, mometasone, ciclesonide, and triamcinolone.

Table 14.1: Various categories of asthma; criteria for classification.

Category	Daytime symptoms	Nighttime	Peak expiratory flow rate
Intermittent asthma	<1 time a week, general activity unaffected	≤2 times a month	≥80% predicted; variability < 20%
Mild persistent asthma	>1 time a week but < 2 times a day	>2 times a month	≥80% predicted; variability 20–30%
Moderate persistent asthma	Daily attacks and use of bronchodilator, general activity affected	>1 time a week	>60% and < 80% predicted; variability > 30%
Severe persistent asthma	Continuous; limited physical activity	Frequent	<60% predicted; variability > 30%

- *Systemic oral corticosteroids (OCSs)*: Prednisone, prednisolone, and methylprednisolone.
- *Leukotriene receptor antagonists (LTRAs)*: Montelukast, zafirlukast.
- *Long-acting β-agonists (LABAs)*: Salmeterol, formoterol.
- *Nonsteroidal anti-inflammatory agents*: Cromolyn, nedocromil.
- Theophylline.
- *Anti-immunoglobulin E*: Omalizumab.

PRINCIPLES OF DRUG THERAPY

Children with intermittent asthma are managed with quick bronchospasm "reliever", SABAs as and when required for quick symptomatic relief. They are not administered any "controller" drugs on long-term basis.

On the other hand, persistent asthma cases are regularly administered long-term anti-inflammatory "controller" drugs. Besides exercising control of symptoms and reducing incidence of further exacerbations, they control airway inflammation and decline in lung function.

The types and amounts of daily controller medications to be used in an asthmatic child, depend upon the severity of his disease and treatment received earlier. In addition, SABAs are employed for quick relief of symptoms, as and when required.

STEPWISE TREATMENT OF ASTHMA

It is recommended that drug therapy should be done stepwise according to the severity of disease, as laid out in Table 14.2.

In a particular child, the stepwise treatment should be started at the step appropriate to the severity of his disease. Subsequently, if the child has well-controlled asthma for at least 3 months, the treatment may be lowered to a step below it while taking care to maintain good control. On the other hand, if a child has not well-controlled asthma, the therapy

Table 14.2: Stepwise treatment of asthma.

Disease category	Step	Drugs recommended
Intermittent asthma	1	Inhaled short-acting β-agonists (SABAs) as required No controller drug
Mild persistent asthma	2	Inhaled corticosteroid (ICS) low dose Or montelukast/zafirlukast Or theophylline (in children > 5 years) (SABA as required)
Moderate persistent asthma	3	Low-dose ICS + long-acting β-agonists (LABAs) Or low-dose ICS + montelukast/theophylline Or medium-dose ICS (SABA as required)
Severe persistent asthma	4	Medium-dose ICS + LABA/montelukast/theophylline
	5	High-dose ICS + LABA Consider omalizumab (in allergic patients)
	6	High-dose ICS + LABA + oral corticosteroid and consider omalizumab for patients with allergies (SABA as required in all earlier cases)

level should be increased by one step under close monitoring. For a child with poorly controlled asthma, the treatment may be raised by two steps.

SOME IMPORTANT FACTS ABOUT DIFFERENT DRUGS

Inhaled Corticosteroids

Daily inhaled corticosteroids (ICS) therapy is now the preferred first-line therapy for all patients with persistent asthma. It reduces asthma symptoms, improves pulmonary function, reduces airway hyper-responsiveness, and diminishes the need for use of quick-reliever inhaled β-agonists. It seems to even have some protective effect against death from asthma. Among different ICS preparations, fluticasone propionate, mometasone furoate and, to a lesser extent, budesonide are considered "second-generation" ICS, as they have greater anti-inflammatory potency and less systemic bioavailability for potential adverse effects. For dosage, side effects and other aspects of these drugs, *see* Section 4: "Pediatric Drug Formulary".

Leukotriene Receptor Antagonists (LTRAs)

Montelukast and zafirlukast have bronchodilator and targeted anti-inflammatory properties.

They are recommended as:
- An alternative controller drug in place of ICS in mild persistent asthma but are less beneficial.
- As an add-on drug to ICS in moderate and severe persistent asthma.
- To reduce exercise, aspirin, and allergen-induced bronchoconstriction.

Montelukast is approved for once-daily dose in children ≥1 year of age while zafirlukast is approved in twice-daily dose for children ≥5 years of age.

Long-acting Inhaled β-agonists (LABA)

Long-acting β-agonists (salmeterol, formoterol) are primarily used as an "add on" controller drugs, in addition to ICS to achieve better control of symptoms in moderate and severe persistent asthma. While formoterol has an onset of action within 5-10 minutes, salmeterol takes about 1 hour to achieve its maximal effect. The duration of effect of both drugs is about 12 hours and hence are well suited for cases with nocturnal asthma.

It is important to bear in mind that LABA must not be used alone, without concomitant use of ICS, in management of persistent asthma.

Theophylline

Besides acting as a bronchodilator, it has anti-inflammatory properties as a phosphodiesterase inhibitor. It is used in combination with ICS in management of moderate and severe persistent asthma in children above 5 years of age. As it has a narrow therapeutic window and its overdosage can cause several adverse effects (such as, headache, vomiting, cardiac arrhythmias, seizures, and even death), serum theophylline levels should be regularly monitored.

Nonsteroidal Anti-inflammatory Drugs (NSAIDs)—Cromolyn and Nedocromil

They inhibit exercise-induced bronchospasm and can be used in place of SABAs, or in addition to SABAs for the prevention/control of exercise-induced bronchospasm.

Anti-immunoglobulin E (Omalizumab)

It is useful as an "add on" therapy in selected cases of moderate and severe asthma with documented hypersensitivity to a perennial aeroallergen, and inadequate control with inhaled/oral corticosteroids in patients above 12 years of age. It is administered every 2-4 weeks subcutaneously. Extreme caution must be employed during its use as it can cause life-threatening anaphylactic reaction.

Short-acting Inhaled β-agonists (SABA)

Salbutamol, Levosalbutamol, Terbutaline, and Pirbuterol

These bronchodilator drugs are employed for quick relief during acute exacerbation of all types of asthma and for preventing exercise-induced bronchospasm. Levosalbutamol causes less headache, tachycardia, agitation, and tremors than salbutamol.

It is important that symptoms in a child with persistent asthma are kept under control through judicious regular use of "controller" drugs and use of the SABA drugs is kept to the minimum possible. Overuse of these drugs has been found to be associated with increased risk of death or near-death situations in asthma.

Systemic Corticosteroids

The use of oral corticosteroids (OCSs) is restricted primarily to assist in management of acute severe asthma exacerbations (described in next section). Rarely, when high-dose inhaled corticosteroids in combination with other bronchodilators, fail to maintain control in a child with severe persistent asthma, OCSs (prednisone, prednisolone, or methylprednisolone) may need to be administered for sometime (step 6 of stepwise management). Rarely, children with persistent severe asthma may need long-term use of oral corticosteroids. In these cases, any comorbid condition should be properly dealt with and dose of OCS kept at or below 20 mg/day. The dose should be gradually tapered over a period of several weeks while keeping close watch on control of asthma. Long-term use of high-dose corticosteroids is liable to cause growth suppression, osteoporosis, and cataracts.

Note: For information regarding dosage, precautions, and side effects of the various aforesaid drugs, *see* Section 4: "Pediatric Drug Formulary".

MANAGEMENT OF SEVERE ASTHMA EXACERBATION (STATUS ASTHMATICUS)

Goals of Therapy

The primary goals are: (1) correction of hypoxemia, (2) rapid reversal of airflow obstruction, and (3) prevention of progression or recurrence of symptoms.

MEASURES FOR CONTROL

- *Oxygen administration*: Humidified oxygen through mask/nasal cannula to maintain oxygen saturation above 92%.
- *Inhaled short-acting bronchodilators*:
  - *Salbutamol*: Nebulized @ 0.15 mg/kg (minimum 2.5 mg) q 20 minutes × 3 times as needed, then 0.15–0.3 mg/kg up to 10 mg q 1–4 hours or up to 0.5 mg/kg/h by continuous nebulization.
    Or
  - Salbutamol MDI (100 mg/puff) 2–8 puffs q 20 minutes × 3 times as needed; and then if needed, q 1–4 hours.
    Or
  - *Levalbuterol nebulized*: 0.075 mg/kg (minimum 1.25 mg) q 20 minutes × 3 times; and then 0.075 mg – 0.15 mg/kg up to 5 mg q 1–4 hr as needed.
- *Systemic corticosteroids*:
  - *Prednisolone oral*: 0.5–1 mg/kg q 6–12 hours for 48 hours
    Or
  - *Prednisolone intramuscular (IM)/intravenous (IV)*: 1–2 mg/kg/day divided q OD/BID.
- *Ipratropium*: If no response to above, add ipratropium by nebulization 250–500 µg/dose q 20 minutes × 3 doses.

Assess status after 1 hour

If no improvement:
- Continue oxygen
- *Salbutamol nebulization*: 0.15–0.3 mg/kg (maximum 10 mg) q 20 minutes or by continuous nebulization 0.3–0.5 mg/kg/h.
- *Prednisolone (oral/IV)*: 0.5–1 mg/kg/dose q 6 hours × 48 hours and then 1–2 mg/kg/day divided q BID (maximum 60 mg/day) × 3–5 days (up to total 7 days).
- *Ipratropium inhalation*: 250 µg/dose q 6 hours.
- *Adrenaline injection subcutaneous (SC)/IM*: If no response to above: 0.01 mg/kg (maximum 0.5 mg).
- *Magnesium sulfate 50% IV*: 25–75 mg/kg (maximum dose 2.5 g) diluted in 30 mL normal saline/5% dextrose over 30 minutes.
- *If life-threatening situation*:
  - *Terbutaline IV*: 2–10 µg/kg loading dose followed by continuous infusion @ 0.1–0.4 µg/kg/min.
  - *Aminophylline IV*: 5 mg/kg bolus over 20 minutes followed by 0.9 mg/kg/h infusion.
    Caution: Cardiovascular and drugs serum level monitoring must be closely maintained following use of terbutaline and aminophylline.
- If no improvement and evidence of respiratory failure, shift patients to intensive care unit (ICU) for intubation and mechanical ventilation.

When to discharge the patient?

If during the course of treatment, patient meets the following parameters, consider discharge with proper follow-up advice: Oxygen saturation above 92% in room air, able to feed and speak well, peak expiratory flow rate (PEFR) more than 70% of predicted, and need for bronchodilator 4–6 hourly.

Instructions on discharge:
- Inhaled salbutamol q 4–8 hours as required.
- Continue prednisolone 1–2 mg/kg/day divided q BID (maximum 60 mg/day) to total period of 5–7 days. Stop use thereafter; no need to taper dose.

15: Drug Therapy in Epilepsy and Neonatal Seizures

GUIDELINES FOR THERAPY

- *First establish the exact type of patients' seizure* [on basis of clinical features and electroencephalogram (EEG) findings].
- *Begin monotherapy with drug of choice* for that particular type of seizure (the best combination of high efficacy and low toxicity). If a patient has more than one type of seizure, begin with the drug of choice for the combination of seizure types present (Table 15.1).
- Starting with the average dose of chosen antiepileptic drug, *push up the dose* until the seizures are controlled

Table 15.1: Antiepileptic drugs of choice.

Types of seizure	Drugs of choice
Generalized Tonic-clonic	• Carbamazepine • Phenobarbitone (in 1st year of life) • Phenytoin • Topiramate • Valproate • Lamotrigine
Partial-onset	• Oxcarbazepine • Carbamazepine • Phenobarbitone • Phenytoin • Topiramate • Valproate • Vigabatrin • Lamotrigine

Contd....

Contd...

Types of seizure	Drugs of choice
Absence	• Ethosuximide • Valproate • Lamotrigine
Juvenile myoclonic	• Valproate • Lamotrigine • Topiramate • Levetiracetam
Infantile spasms	• Adrenocorticotropic hormone (ACTH) • Vigabatrin • Benzodiazepines • Topiramate • Valproate • Zonisamide/lamotrigine

Lennox–Gastaut syndrome	• *For drop attack*:
	  – Valproate
	  – Lamotrigine
	  – Clobazam
	  – Rufinamide (as add on)
	  – Topiramate
	• *For atypical absence seizures*:
	  – Lamotrigine
	  – Ethosuximide

Benign childhood epilepsy with centrotemporal spikes (BCECTS)	• Carbamazepine • Valproic acid • Levetiracetam • Lamotrigine • Oxcarbazepine

Note 1: Neurologists vary in their choice of antiepileptic drugs for different types of epilepsy. The earlier table largely reflects the recommendations of ILAE Subcommission on AED Guidelines. Epilepsia. 2013;54(3):551-63, and NICE, National Institute for Clinical Excellence, 2012.

Note 2: For dosage of various drugs, their side effects, etc. see under Section 4: Pediatric Drug Formulary.

or until side effects prevent further increase in dosage. Monotherapy is preferable to polytherapy.
- Therapy with more than one drug (polytherapy) exposes the child to several unnecessary risks including added toxic effects of more than one drug, drug allergy, drug

interactions, exacerbation of seizures, and the inability to evaluate the effectiveness of individual drugs. *Better increase the dosage of the first drug rather than add a more toxic second drug.*
- The drug plasma concentrations should be determined if a patient's seizures are not controlled by average or high drug dosage (short of causing toxicity).
- When a therapeutic plasma concentration of the second drug is obtained (in a child on two drugs), *try to taper the patient off the first drug* because of the many hazards of chronic polytherapy.
- A third drug should not be added until you are sure that seizures cannot be controlled with maximum tolerated doses of the first two drugs tried.

IMPORTANT CONSIDERATIONS DURING ANTICONVULSANT DRUG THERAPY

- Valproate may be combined with lamotrigine for control of refractory generalized, absence, myoclonic, and partial epilepsies. This combination, however, results in elevated serum level of lamotrigine. As such, the dose of lamotrigine should be cut down to almost half of its usual dose. For refractory absence seizures, valproate along with ethosuximide constitutes a good effective combination.
- It should be well borne in mind that *an inappropriate antiepileptic drug or occasional paradoxical effect of a usually effective drug may exacerbate some types of seizures* instead of controlling them.
    - Lamotrigine may precipitate myoclonic seizures in Dravet syndrome.
    - Carbamazepine may exacerbate absence seizures.
- Better avoid phenytoin and carbamazepine combination because both have similar mechanism of action.
- Use of phenobarbitone in children should be avoided due to cognitive function disturbances and compromised school performance often reported following its use.

- While phenytoin is a drug of choice for generalized tonic-clonic and partial seizures, close observation must be maintained for its possible acute toxic effects (e.g. ataxia, nystagmus) and chronic adverse effects (e.g. coarsening of facies, hirsutism, gingival hyperplasia and rickets) following prolonged use.
- Valproate is contraindicated in patients with hepatic disease/significant hepatic dysfunction. Considering highest risk of fatal hepatotoxicity in children below 2 years, valproate therapy may be avoided in this age group, if this is possible.
- Use of topiramate can cause cognitive dysfunction, renal calculi, glaucoma, paresthesias, and these possible adverse effects must be kept under watch.
- Vigabatrin is a good effective drug for infantile spasms. It however, carries a significant risk of causing irreversible impairment of visual fields following prolonged use. In otherwise refractory cases of infantile spasms (and partial epilepsies), it may be employed for short-term use restricted to a few months.
- Felbamate can cause life-threatening aplastic anemia and hepatotoxicity, hence its use should be limited to severe drug-resistant epilepsies under close monitoring.
- Clobazam, an otherwise effective drug in difficult cases, suffers from a major drawback of rapid development of tolerance. It loses its initial effectiveness within a few weeks or months.
- The use of benzodiazepines as a chronic treatment for epilepsy should be conducted with great caution as withdrawal of these drugs may lead to withdrawal seizures.

INDICATIONS FOR OBTAINING BLOOD LEVELS

- Persistence of seizures despite a correctly prescribed therapy.
- Occurrence of toxic effects of an antiepileptic drug.
- Before changing to another drug when the prescribed drug proves to be ineffective.

- For patients on polytherapy, especially valproic acid, phenobarbitone, and lamotrigine because of drug interactions.
- For patients with hepatic or renal disease.
- In cases with mixed seizure disorders.

DURATION OF TREATMENT AND RISK FOR RELAPSE

A minimum of two seizure-free years is an adequate and safe period of treatment for a patient with no risk factors. Anticonvulsant drugs should be weaned gradually over a period of 3–6 months, as abrupt withdrawal may cause status epilepticus. Chances of recurrence on rapid withdrawal are more in cases of phenobarbital and benzodiazepines.

Risk factors requiring longer duration of therapy and with higher chances of recurrence of seizures after drug withdrawal include: (1) age >12 years at onset, (2) numerous seizures before achievement of control, (3) presence of neurologic dysfunction/multiple seizure types, (4) need to use more than one antiepileptic drug for control, (5) abnormal EEG before medication is discontinued, and (6) children with remote symptomatic epilepsy.

MANAGEMENT OF STATUS EPILEPTICUS

Status epilepticus is defined as continuous seizure activity or recurrent seizure activity without regaining of consciousness lasting for more than 30 minutes. But for operational purposes, persistent repetitive seizure activity lasting for more than 5 minutes without recovery of consciousness in between episodes is considered to be status epilepticus. So, any child who is brought to the emergency room in a convulsive state should be treated as status epilepticus. Central nervous system (CNS) infections (meningitis, meningoencephalitis), febrile convulsions, vascular episodes, trauma, metabolic causes, and poisoning are prominent causes of status epilepticus in children younger than 2 years. Among older children, majority have a past history of seizures or have neurologic abnormality. Status epilepticus may be the first manifestation of epilepsy in some children.

Management Goals

- Stabilization of airway, breathing, and circulation for adequate brain oxygenation and cardiorespiratory function.
- Expeditious termination of clinical and electrical seizure activity.
- Identification and correction of precipitating factors (such as hypoglycemia, infection, electrolyte imbalance, fever, and withdrawal of anticonvulsant).
- Diagnosis of cause of status epilepticus and initiation of its therapy.

Step 1: Assessment of Vitals, Immediate Care, and Blood Sampling

- Establish airway, 100% oxygen; collect blood sample for complete blood count, sodium, potassium, calcium, glucose, arterial blood gas analysis, anticonvulsant levels (if child earlier on anticonvulsants), and toxicology studies (if suspected). Lumber puncture if indicated (when safe)
- *Monitoring*: Cardiovascular system (CVS), respiration, temperature, oxygenation, electrolytes, and metabolic status (with necessary corrective steps).

Step 2: Termination of Seizures

- *Intravenous (IV) lorazepam or IV diazepam or IV midazolam:*
  - *Lorazepam*: 0.05–0.1 mg/kg (maximum 4 mg/dose) IV bolus over 2–5 minutes; may repeat once after 5 minutes if seizures not controlled—0.05 mg/kg IV slowly.

Or
- *Diazepam*: 0.1–0.3 mg/kg (maximum 5 mg/dose in < 5 years, maximum 10 mg/dose in > 5 years) IV bolus @ 1 mg/min; may repeat once after 5 minutes.
  Or
- *Midazolam*: 0.15–0.2 mg/kg (maximum 5 mg dose) IV.

If IV access not available (as well as prior to reaching hospital):
- Buccal midazolam 0.5 mg/kg (maximum 10 mg)
  Or
- Rectal diazepam 2-5 yr: 0.5 mg/kg; 6–11 yr: 0.3 mg/kg; ≥ 12 yr: 0.2 mg/kg (maximum 10 mg)
  Or
- IM midazolam 0.2 mg/kg (maximum 10 mg)
  Or
- Intranasal midazolam 0.2 mg/kg (maximum 10 mg).
- Administer phenytoin or better fosphenytoin to sustain prolonged action of benzodiazepine.
  - *Intravenous phenytoin*: 20 mg/kg diluted in N/2 or normal saline IV @ 0.5–1.0 mg/kg/min (maximum 50 mg/min). Its administration at a higher rate is liable to cause hypotension and cardiac arrhythmia. It should not be administered in glucose solution as phenytoin may get precipitated.
  - *Intravenous fosphenytoin*: 20 mg PE (phenytoin equivalent/kg IV in NS/or D5W @ 3 mg PE/kg/min up to maximum rate of 150 PE/min.
- If seizures still uncontrolled even after 10 minutes, give:
  - Intravenous valproate 20 mg/kg @ 5 mg/kg/min.
    Or
  - Intravenous phenobarbitone 5–20 mg/kg in normal saline @ 1.5 mg/kg/min.
    Or
  - Intravenous levetiracetam 20–60 mg/kg @ 5 mg/kg/min infusion, in NS or D5W
- *For persistent seizures*: Shift to pediatric intensive care unit (PICU).
  - *Administer midazolam*: 0.2 mg/kg IV bolus then infusion @ 1 µg/kg/min increasing 1 µg/kg/min, every

5–10 minutes till seizures stop, up to a maximum of 12 µg/kg/min (some go up to 30 µg/kg/min); start tapering 24–48 hours after seizure stops @ 1 µg/kg/min every 3–4 hours.
- *If seizures continue after midazolam infusion*:
  - *Injection thiopentone*: Loading dose 5 mg/kg IV bolus followed by 3–5 mg/kg/h infusion to achieve burst suppression pattern on EEG. Start tapering after 24-hour seizure period.
  - *Propofol infusion*: Initial bolus of 1–2 mg/kg followed by continuous infusion of 1–2 mg/kg/h (maximum 5 mg/kg/h). To be given for maximum period of 48 hours.
  - *Phenobarbitone high dose*: Boluses of 5–10 mg/kg every 30 minutes up to 80 mg/kg in a 24-hour period; usual maintenance is 40 mg/kg/day.

MANAGEMENT OF NEONATAL SEIZURES

Seizures in the newborn constitute a medical emergency which must be quickly and properly tackled to prevent neonatal death/neurologic impairment and epilepsy disorders in later life. In India, hypoxic–ischemic encephalopathy, metabolic disturbances (hypoglycemia and hypocalcemia), and meningitis are the most common among many varied causes of neonatal seizures.

Step 1: Initial Urgent Medical Management

Following quick assessment of the character of seizures and baby's general condition, urgent steps should be taken to ensure clear airway, breathing, and circulation. Oxygen should be started, IV access secured, and blood samples be collected for estimation of glucose, calcium, magnesium, sodium, potassium, arterial blood gas, hematocrit, and septic screen. A brief relevant history should be obtained and quick clinical examination should be performed within 2–5 minutes.

Step 2: Pharmacotherapy

If glucostix shows hypoglycemia (blood sugar below 40 mg/dL) or if there is no facility for immediate testing of blood glucose, administer 2 mL/kg of 10% dextrose as bolus followed by a continuous infusion of 6–8 mg/kg/min.

If seizures persist, administer 2 mL/kg of 10% calcium gluconate IV over 10 minutes under strict cardiac monitoring. If blood report indicates hypocalcemia, give the baby calcium gluconate @ 8 mL/kg/day for 3 days. If seizures continue despite correction of hypocalcemia, administer 0.25 mL/kg of 50% magnesium sulfate IM every 12 hour × three doses.

In the event of continuation of seizures, administer phenobarbitone 20 mg/kg IV diluted in 1:10 dilution with normal saline slowly over 20 minutes. If seizures persist, repeat phenobarbitone 10 mg/kg/dose every 20–30 minutes until a dose of 40 mg/kg has been given. Following cessation of seizures, maintenance dose of phenobarbitone should be started 24 hours after the loading dose @ 3–5 mg/kg/day in one to two divided doses IV/IM/PO.

On the other hand, if seizures continue, administer phenytoin 15–20/mg/kg/IV diluted in normal saline (not in dextrose solution as it may get precipitated in it). The rate of administration should not exceed 1 mg/kg/min under cardiac monitoring. If seizures persist, repeat a dose of 10 mg/kg. If seizures get controlled, IV maintenance dose should be administered 3–5 mg/kg/day (maximum 8 mg/kg/day) in two to four divided doses. In view of unreliable, erratic absorption of oral phenytoin, its use for maintenance purpose should be avoided. IV administration of this drug should preferably be discontinued before discharge.

If available, fosphenytoin is preferable over phenytoin, as it is less liable to cause hypotension or cardiac arrhythmias. Its usual loading dose is 15–20 PE/kg administered over 30 minutes and maintenance dose is 4–8 PE/kg/day. PE stands for phenytoin equivalent (1.5 mg/kg of fosphenytoin is equivalent to 1 mg/kg of phenytoin). This drug can be administered IM.

If seizures continue, administer lorazepam or midazolam.

Lorazepam dose: 0.05 mg/kg (range 0.02–0.10 mg/kg) IV bolus over 2–5 minutes; it may be repeated every 4–8 hours.

Midazolam: 0.05–0.1 mg/kg IV bolus followed by infusion @ 0.05–1 µg/min, that can be titrated every 5 min to max 33 µg/kg/min (2 mg/kg/hr)

Drugs Sometimes Employed for Still Persistent Seizures

- *Lidocaine*: Bolus dose 4 mg/kg IV followed by infusion @ 2 mg/kg/h.
  It should not be administered with phenytoin. Watch for arrhythmias, hypotension, and seizure.
- *Topiramate*: 20 mg/kg/day.
- *Levetiracetam*: Loading dose 30–60 mg/kg IV @ 5 mg/kg/min, maintenance dose 10 mg/kg/dose q 8–12 hours IV/PO.
- *Pyridoxine*: This drug should be employed as a last resort in refractory seizures. Since its suitable IV preparation is not available, neurobion IM injection (which contains 50 mg pyridoxine in 1 mL) can be used. *Dose*: 1 mL each on both sides in anterolateral aspect of thigh.

FEBRILE SEIZURES

Seizures that occur in children between the age of 6 months and 5 years during a febrile episode in the absence of CNS infection or any metabolic imbalance, in a neurologically normal child, are termed as febrile seizures.

The seizures can be of simple or complex nature (Table 15.2).

Table 15.2: Types of febrile seizure.

Type of seizure	Duration	Recurrence within 24 hours	Types of convulsion
Simple	<15 minutes	No	Generalized; tonic–clonic
Complex	>15 minutes	Yes	Focal

Chapter 15: Drug Therapy in Epilepsy and Neonatal ...

Assessment

- *Quick clinical assessment*: Relevant history, general and neurologic examination.
- Lumber puncture to be done in following situations:
  - Infants younger than 6 months of age.
  - Infants between 6 months and 1 year of age who are not immunized/unsure about immunization with *Haemophilus influenzae* type b (Hib) and pneumococcal vaccine.
  - If meningitis is suspected.
- Electroencephalogram, CT, and MRI are not indicated in simple febrile seizure cases; to be considered in complex febrile seizure cases and those with neurological abnormality.

Management

- Ensure maintenance of airway, breathing, and circulation.
- Reduce body temperature with antipyretics/hydrotherapy.
- If seizures last for longer than 5 minutes, follow management guidelines as described earlier for termination of seizures (step 2) in cases of status epilepticus, through use of diazepam, lorazepam, or midazolam.
- Buccal or intranasal midazolam can sometimes be employed to control seizures in outdoor emergency situations following appropriate training; for dosage, see section 4: Pediatric Drug Formulary.

Prophylaxis

- *Intermittent prophylaxis*: In cases with frequent episodes of febrile seizures, and especially in those with anxious parents, following medication is recommended to prevent seizures during febrile episode (besides the use of antipyretics and hydrotherapy)
  - Oral diazepam 0.33 mg/kg or rectal diazepam 0.5 mg/kg every 8 hours
    Or
  - Oral clobazam 0.25–0.33 mg/kg every 8 hours or clonazepam 0.33 mg/kg every 8 hours.

- *Continuous prophylaxis*: It may be undertaken in cases of failure of intermittent prophylaxis and recurrent atypical seizures, especially in those where caretakers are unable to detect fever in initial stages.
    - *Sodium valproate*: 20–30 mg/kg/day divided q 8–12 hours
      Or
    - *Phenobarbitone*: 4–5 mg/kg/day divided q 12–24 hours.

***Note*:**
- Carbamazepine and phenytoin are ineffective for this purpose.
- Duration of therapy varies between 1 year and 5 years. It is desirable to avoid continuous prophylaxis due to risk of side effects of drugs and doubtful long-term benefits.

16 Pharmacotherapy in Congestive Heart Failure

In order to choose and employ appropriate drugs for the management of patients suffering from congestive heart failure (CHF), it is important to understand the basics about its development.

PATHOPHYSIOLOGY OF CONGESTIVE HEART FAILURE

Heart failure occurs when the heart is unable to deliver adequate cardiac output to meet the metabolic needs of the body. Cardiac output is a product of heart rate and stroke volume. The stroke volume is determined by—(1) contractility (myocardial function), (2) preload (ventricular end-diastolic volume), and (3) afterload (peripheral resistance). Within limits, increase in preload enhances cardiac output. On the other hand, cardiac output is inversely proportional to the resistance against which heart pumps (afterload). Heart failure develops when the demand for cardiac output exceeds the ability of the heart of fulfill it. The presence of a lesion causing increased preload (e.g. valvular insufficiency or left-to-right shunt) limits the capacity for further increase in ventricular end-diastolic volume and enhancement of cardiac output. Lesions, such as, aortic or pulmonary stenosis and coarctation of aorta impede cardiac output. Myocarditis and cardiomyopathy result in reduced myocardial contractility with propensity to development of heart failure. In cases with tachyarrhythmias reduced ventricular filling (due to shortened diastolic period) and the markedly slow heart rate in children with bradyarrhythmia result in reduced cardiac output.

At the advent of heart failure, compensatory reflex stimulation of sympathetic nervous system induces regional vasoconstriction along with augmentation of myocardial contractility in an effort to maintain blood pressure and to boost falling cardiac output. Simultaneous renin-angiotensin-aldosterone system stimulates renal fluid retention to expand vascular volume in order to enhance cardiac preload with the same objective of improving cardiac output. However, in the long-term, due to worsening myocardial function, severe vasoconstriction (postload) and hypervolemia (preload) not only fail to enhance cardiac output but also become counterproductive. Chronic volume expansion leads to peripheral edema, pulmonary edema, pulmonary hypertension, and respiratory insufficiency. Chronic elevation in filling pressure results in ventricular remodeling and increased diastolic capacitance at the expense of elevated systolic wall stress and myocardial oxygen consumption.

Congenital cardiac lesions are the preponderant cause of heart failure manifesting before the end of 1st year of life. Obstructive and duct-dependent lesions of different types present with heart failure or circulatory shock. Heart failure due to left-to-right shunts generally develops following fall in pulmonary vascular resistance at 4–6 weeks.

Acute rheumatic fever with carditis, decompensated chronic rheumatic heart disease, myocarditis, cardiomyopathies, and palliated congenital heart disease (CHD) are major causes of CHF in older children (usually beyond 2 years).

MANAGEMENT OF CONGESTIVE HEART FAILURE

For successful treatment of CHF in a child, it is important to understand the nature and physiological consequences of the specific cardiac defect leading to the failure, as well as, to recognize any associated or aggravating condition that may be the precipitating cause of the heart failure (e.g. severe anemia, dysrhythmia). Surgical correction of the causative anatomic cardiac lesion, if any, and where feasible, remains

Chapter 16: Pharmacotherapy in Congestive Heart Failure

the first choice. In such cases, medical management is done in preoperative and postoperative period. For example, in a newborn with heart failure due to duct-dependent systemic circulation (critical coarctation and aortic stenosis), prostaglandin is administered to keep the ductus open pending surgical correction of the anatomic defect.

For medical management, an appropriate combination of drugs is employed for correction of the disturbed physiological condition in a particular case.

Diuretics are employed to bring about reduction in hypervolemia for control of symptoms and effects of pulmonary and peripheral venous congestion. Inotropic agents such as digoxin, beta-adrenergic agonists, and phosphodiesterase inhibitors are useful in augmenting myocardial contractility and enhancing cardiac output. Angiotensin-converting enzyme (ACE) inhibitors bring about increase in cardiac output by lowering afterload, preload, and systolic wall stress. When ACE inhibitors cause troublesome cough in some children, angiotensin-receptor blockers (ARB) like losartan, are instead employed for this purpose. An aldosterone-blocking agent is usually added in patients with dilated cardiomyopathy. If there is severe dysfunction or symptoms persist, beta-blocking drugs are used.

Drugs Employed in CHF

A summary of different drugs used in the management of CHF—their mode of action and usage—is given below. For details regarding drug dosage, side effects, contraindications, etc. see under individual drug in Section 4: Pediatric Drug Formulary.

Diuretics

Diuretics are the first line of management in patients with CHF. By promoting water and sodium excretion by kidneys, diuretics reduce pulmonary fluid overload and ventricular preload in these cases. Diuretics are often used in conjunction with digoxin/ACE inhibitors.

These are classified into three categories according to the site and mode of action on the kidney.

- *Loop diuretics*: Furosemide, torsemide, and ethacrynic acid.

   These act on distal tubules and ascending loop of Henle; induce sodium (Na), potassium (K^+), chloride, and water excretion.

- *Thiazides*: Chlorothiazide and hydrochlorothiazide.

   Through action at distal convoluted tubule, these promote sodium, potassium, and chloride excretion.

- *Aldosterone antagonists*: Spironolactone and eplerenone.

   These compete for aldosterone receptors in the distal tubule; enhance sodium and water excretion while potassium excretion is spared.

Furosemide is the most commonly used diuretic, both in acute and chronic stages of CHF. It has rapid onset of action, high efficacy, and is effective even at low-glomerular filtration rate. Hypokalemia caused by furosemide may increase chances of digoxin toxicity. Instead of using potassium supplements, it should be used in combination with a potassium-sparing diuretic such as, spironolactone. Chronic administration of furosemide may cause contraction of extracellular compartment resulting in "contraction alkalosis".

Chlorothiazide is a mild diuretic and only occasionally used in children with less severe chronic CHF along with oral potassium supplements.

Spironolactone, an aldosterone inhibitor, is a potassium-sparing diuretic often used in conjunction with furosemide in management of CHF.

Afterload Reducing Agents

Angiotensin-converting inhibitor (ACE inhibitors)
Angiotensin-II receptor blockers (ARBs).

ACE inhibitors (captopril, enalapril):

- Very useful agents in management of CHF
- Improve cardiac output by—(1) reducing preload through suppression of renin-angiotensin-aldosterone system resulting in reduction in circulating blood volume, (2)

Chapter 16: Pharmacotherapy in Congestive Heart Failure

by reducing overload through induction of arteriolar vasodilation, and (3) by diminishing systolic wall stress.
- By suppressing catecholamines, these drugs prevent arrhythmias and their other adverse effects on myocardium.
- Currently recommended by many cardiologists as the first-line treatment of CHF in combination with diuretics. These can be combined with digoxin for synergistic effect.
- Especially useful in CHF secondary to L-R shunts.
- To be avoided in patients of aortic stenosis/other obstructive lesions, as might interfere with compensatory ventricular hypertrophy. In cases where ACE inhibitors cause persistent cough, angiotensin-II receptor blockers (ARBs) like losartan are employed.

Digitalis (digoxin):
- Inotrope; increases force of ventricular contraction
- Now less used by cardiologists due to potential toxicities
- Can be combined with ACE inhibitors for synergistic effect
- Particularly useful in cases with atrial fibrillation, atrial flutter, and supraventricular tachycardia, as it slows down ventricular rate
- Requires careful monitoring of serum electrolytes (K^+, Ca^{++}, Mg^{++}) and ECG during its use (risk of digoxin toxicity—cardiac arrhythmias)
- It should be used with caution in premature babies, those with renal decompensated state and heart failure due to myocarditis
- Its role in heart failure secondary to left-to-right shunt lesions where systolic function of the myocardium is preserved, is not well defined
- It is routinely administered orally. Rapid digitalization can be done in indoor patients intravenously.

Beta-blockers (metoprolol, bisoprolol, and carvedilol):
- Beta-blockers counteract the deleterious effects of activation of sympathetic nervous system and increased level of circulating catecholamines occurring in cases of CHF. These are useful in chronic management of mild

or moderate heart failure, especially in cases of dilated cardiomyopathy during tachycardia. Starting with low dose, carvedilol dose should be gradually titrated up every 2 weeks or so.
- Not to be used in acute phase of heart failure

Nondigitalis inotropic agents:
Adrenergic agonists (dopamine, dobutamine):
These drugs are employed in acute intensive care setting under expert hemodynamic control. Long-term use may be harmful in some cases.

Dopamine:
- Induces increased myocardial contractility with little peripheral vasoconstriction in low dose of 2–10 µg/kg/min
- Causes selective renal vasodilatation resulting in natriuresis
- Especially useful when compromised renal function with low-cardiac output (low blood pressure or patient in shock)
- Strict hemodynamic control required during its use.

Dobutamine:
- Direct cardiac inotropic effect
- Mild decrease in peripheral vascular resistance (at low dose)
- May use as adjunct to dopamine in low-cardiac output failure in patients in intensive care unit (ICU) set up
- In patients with dilated cardiomyopathy, dobutamine is used as 24-hour infusion once or twice a week.

Isoproterenol:
- Pure beta adrenergic with marked chronotropic effect
- Effective in patients of CHF with bradycardia; avoid if pre-existing significant tachycardia
- Monitor closely for arrhythmia.

Epinephrine:
- Mixed alpha and beta-adrenergic receptor agonist
- Reserved for patients with cardiogenic shock with low-arterial blood pressure.

Phosphodiesterase inhibitors:
Milrinone:
- Potent inotrope and peripheral vasodilator; useful in refractory low-output CHF as adjunct to dopamine/dobutamine in ICU.

Amrinone:
- Same mode of action as milrinone but less potent
- Extremely careful monitoring required.

Note: Clinical use of milrinone and amrinone restricted due to suspected implication in high patient mortality.

17 Pharmacotherapy in Hypertension and Hypertensive Emergencies

CLASSIFICATION OF HYPERTENSION

- Essential (primary)
- Secondary (to an underlying disease process; e.g. renal parenchymal, renovascular, endocrine, or cardiovascular).

DEFINITION AND STAGES OF HYPERTENSION

Prehypertension

It is a state wherein systolic or diastolic blood pressure is between the 90th and 95th percentile. However, adolescents having blood pressure above 120/80 mm Hg are classified in this category, even though it is below the 95th percentile.

Hypertension

Systolic or diastolic blood pressure above the 95th percentile for age, gender, and height, on at least three separate occasions, 1–3 weeks apart denotes hypertension.

Stage I Hypertension

Systolic or diastolic pressure values exceeding the 95th percentile and up to 5 mm above the 99th percentile, measured at least twice in the next 1–3 weeks are graded as stage-I hypertension.

Stage II Hypertension

Systolic or diastolic pressure 5 mm or more above the 99th percentile, confirmed on repeat measurement at the same visit, means hypertension stage II.

Figures 17.1 and 17.2 depict staging of hypertension in boys and girls respectively at the 50th percentile for the height for age. Blood pressure values are typically 3–5 mm Hg lower in subjects with height at the 10th percentile, and 3–5 mm Hg higher in those with height at the 95th percentile.

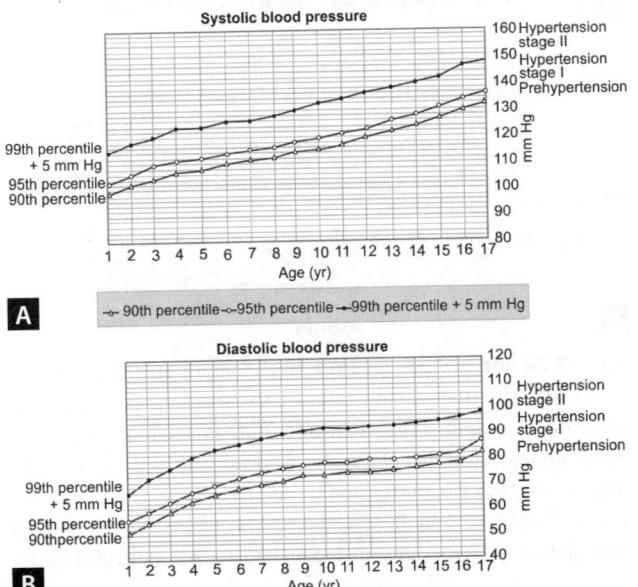

Figs. 17.1A and B: Staging of hypertension in boys. Blood pressure levels for boys at 50th percentile for height. Chart depicting 90th, 95th and 99th + 5 mm Hg percentile values for (A) Systolic and (B) Diastolic blood pressures, representing cutoff values for the diagnosis of prehypertension, stage I and stage II hypertension respectively in boys.
Source: Bagga A, Jain R, Vijayakumar M, et al. Evaluation and management of hypertension. Indian Pediatr. 2007;44:109-10.

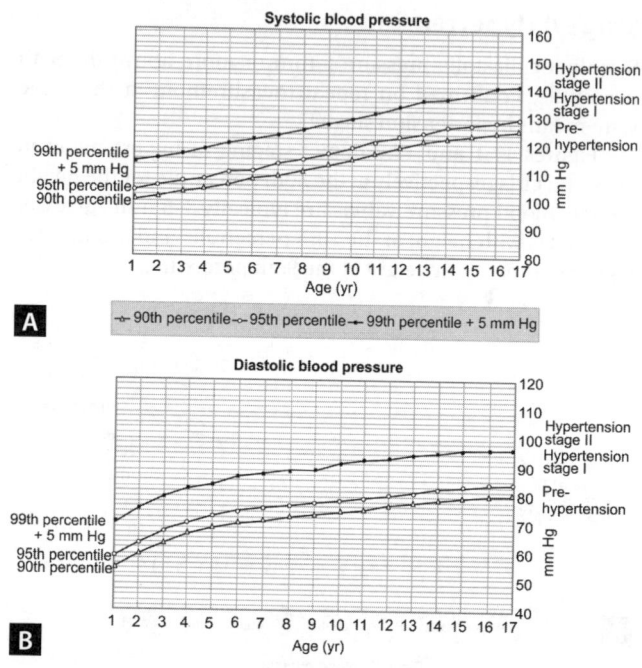

Figs. 17.2A and B: Blood pressure levels for girls at 50th percentile for height. Chart depicting 90th, 95th, and 99th + 5 mm Hg percentile values for (A) Systolic and (B) Diastolic blood pressure, representing cutoff values for the diagnosis of prehypertension, stage I and stage II hypertension respectively in girls.
Source: Bagga A, Jain R, Vijayakumar M, et al. Evaluation and management of hypertension. Indian Pediatr. 2007;44:109-10.

DRUG THERAPY

Indications

- Hypertension with complications
- Secondary hypertension
- Stage II hypertension

- Stage I hypertension persisting despite lifestyle modifications (weight reduction, dietary changes, and increased physical activity) over a period of 6 months
- Stage I hypertension with comorbid conditions (diabetes, chronic kidney disease, or dyslipidemia).

Antihypertensive Drugs

Classes, Mode of Action, and Usage.

ACE Inhibitors

(Captopril, enalapril/enalaprilat, lisinopril, ramipril, benazepril, fosinopril, quinapril)

- Block conversion of angiotensin-I to vasoconstrictor angiotensin-II
- *Major indications*:
    - High renin hypertension (secondary to renovascular or renal parenchymal disease and high renin essential hypertension)
    - Children with diabetes and microalbuminuria
- Useful in neonatal hypertension secondary to renal vessel partial occlusion by thrombus (angiotensin level high)
- If renal function impaired prescribe in low doses
- *Contraindicated* in second and third trimesters of pregnancy (risk of severe potentially fatal fetal abnormalities)
- Bilateral renal artery stenosis is a contraindication [relaxation of efferent arterioles causes severe reduction in glomerular filtration rate (GFR)].

Angiotensin Receptor Blockers (ARBs)

(Losartan, candesartan, olmesartan, valsartan)

These drugs block the action of angiotensin, which is responsible for causing hypertension. Their mode of action and indications for usage are same as that of ACE inhibitors. In cases where ACE inhibitors cause troublesome cough, angiotensin receptor blockers are instead employed.

Calcium Channel Blockers

(Nifedipine, nicardipine, amlodipine, isradipine, felodipine)
- Induce reduction in intracellular calcium in cardiac muscle and vascular smooth muscle, which leads to vasodilation and reduced peripheral vascular resistance without significant reflex tachycardia.
- Nifedipine primary drug of this group for use as an antihypertensive.
  - Its effect more on peripheral vasculature than on cardiac muscle as compared to diltiazem or verapamil
  - Nifedipine dosage unaffected by renal impairment.

Diuretics

- **Thiazides:** Chlorothiazide, hydrochlorothiazide
- **Loop diuretics** (e.g. furosemide, torsemide, ethacrynic acid)
- **Potassium-sparing diuretics (spironolactone, eplerenone):**
  - Enhance sodium excretion, which leads to decrease in extracellular fluid volume
  - May be effective as single agent in mild hypertension
  - Helpful in management of hypertension secondary to renal disease
  - As ancillary drug, enhance effectiveness of other antihypertensives
  - Thiazide diuretics effective only with renal function more than 50% of normal, and prolonged thiazide therapy leads to increase in serum triglyceride levels
  - Loop diuretics effective even with poor renal function.

Adrenergic Blocking Agents

- *Nonselective β-1 (and β-2 blocker) (Propranolol)*:
  - Induces β-1 receptor blockage, decrease in heart rate, cardiac output, and elevated blood pressure
  - Contraindicated in uncontrolled congestive heart failure (CHF) (due to negative chronotropic and inotropic effects)

- Avoid in patients with reactive airway disease (its blockage of β-2 receptors in bronchial smooth muscle may lead to bronchoconstriction).
- *Cardioselective β-1 blockers* (Atenolol, metoprolol):
  - *Effects*: Decrease heart rate, decrease cardiac output, and decrease in elevated blood pressure (BP)
  - Much less effect on bronchial smooth muscle and peripheral vasculature (when given in moderate doses)
  - β-adrenergic blockers nonselective and cardioselective especially useful in patients with left ventricular hypertrophy or a hyperdynamic state (with tachycardia).
- *α-1 and β-nonselective adrenergic blocker* (Labetalol, carvedilol):
  - Reduces peripheral vascular resistance and heart rate
  - A good drug for use in hypertensive emergencies
- *α-1 blockers* (Prazosin, phentolamine, phenoxybenzamine, terazosin):
  - These agents block vasoconstriction
  - Phentolamine and phenoxybenzamine, especially useful in hypertension due to pheochromocytoma (wherein levels of catecholamines are high).

Vasodilators

(Hydralazine, diazoxide, nitroprusside, minoxidil)
- Direct vasodilating effect on arterial smooth muscle
- Very potent, primarily used in hypertensive emergencies
- In chronic hypertension, reserved for refractory cases requiring triple drug therapy.

Sympatholytic Agents

- *Methyldopa* (α-2 adrenergic agonist):
  - Little used now due to its serious side effects (e.g. hepatitis, Coombs test positive hemolytic anemia).
- *Clonidine* (centrally acting α-2 adrenergic agonist):
  - Stimulates α-2 receptors in brain stem → decreased sympathetic tone and reduced peripheral vascular resistance

- Fairly effective but has several side effects (including risk of rebound hypertension).

GUIDELINES FOR THERAPY

Goal of Treatment

To reduce blood pressure less than 95th percentile level under ordinary circumstances. However, if there is evidence of target organ damage or there are coexisting morbid conditions such as diabetes or chronic kidney disease, aim of treatment is to reduce blood pressure to less than 90th percentile.

Choice of Drugs in Hypertension

Antihypertensive drugs preferred for management of hypertension in different disease entities are indicated in Table 17.1.

The recommended initial and maximum doses of various antihypertensive drugs along with other salient facts have been described under 'Antihypertensive Drugs' in the Pediatric Drug Formulary section.

Contraindications of various antihypertensive drugs are given in Table 17.2.

Stepwise Approach

- *Step 1*: Begin with the recommended initial dose of preferred medication in the light of nature and cause of hypertension.
- *Step 2*: If the desired BP control is not achieved, increase dose until desired BP target is achieved or maximum dose in reached.
- *Step 3*: If BP control is still not achieved, add a second antihypertensive drug with a complementary mechanism of action.
- *Step 4*: If BP control is still not achieved, add a third antihypertensive drug of a different class. Placed below are examples of some useful combinations:

Chapter 17: Pharmacotherapy in Hypertension...

Table 17.1: Disease entity with hypertension and preferred antihypertensive drug.	
Disease entity with hypertension	Preferred antihypertensive drug
Acute glomerulonephritis	Diuretics, ACE inhibitors, vasodilators (as adjunct)
Chronic renal parenchymal disease (e.g. chronic pyelonephritis, diabetic nephropathy, chronic glomerulonephritis, reflux nephropathy)	ACE inhibitors*, diuretics** Angiotensin receptor blockers
Renovascular hypertension	Calcium channel blocker or/and β-blocker
Unilateral renal artery stenosis	ACE inhibitors*, diuretics**
Essential hypertension	ACE inhibitors, calcium channel blockers, diuretics, β-blockers
Hypertension with CHF	ACE inhibitors, vasodilators (as adjuncts), diuretics
Neonatal hypertension	ACE inhibitors, vasodilators (in refractory cases)
Cyclosporine induced hypertension in post-transplant patients	Calcium channel blockers, diuretics
Pheochromocytoma	α-1 adrenergic blockers (phentolamine, phenoxybenzamine)
Hypertension with asthma	Calcium channel blockers
Athletes with hypertension	α-blockers

(ACE: angiotensin-converting enzyme; CHF: congestive heart failure)
Note:
*If impaired renal function, use ACE inhibitor in low dose. In cases with advanced (stage IV-V) chronic kidney disease, use calcium channel blocker (CCB) or a β-blocker instead of ACE inhibitor.
**In cases with severe renal impairment, use loop diuretics (e.g. furosemide) since thiazides would be ineffective.

- ACE inhibitor + calcium channel blocker or a thiazide diuretic
- Vasodilator + diuretic or β-blocker.

Table 17.2: Contraindications of antihypertensive drugs.	
Antihypertensive drug	Contraindicated in
ACE inhibitors	Bilateral[†] renal artery stenosis; post-transplant hypertension, patients with single kidney, second or third trimester of pregnancy[‡]
Calcium channel blockers	CHF
β-blockers	CHF, asthma, diabetes, Raynaud disease, hypertensive young athletes
Diuretics	Athletes

(ACE: angiotensin-converting enzyme; CHF: congestive heart failure)

Note:

[†]ACE inhibitors may cause severe reduction in glomerular filtration rate (GFR) because the efferent arterioles relax.

[‡]ACE inhibitors have been incriminated in causing fatal pulmonary hypoplasia, renal tubular dysplasia, hypocalvaria, neonatal hypotension, and anuria when administered to mothers during second or third trimester of pregnancy.

DRUG THERAPY IN HYPERTENSIVE EMERGENCY

Hypertensive Urgency

It refers to significant acute elevation in blood pressure (more than 95th percentile for age) without evidence of accompanying end-organ damage (e.g. to brain, eyes, heart, or kidneys). Symptoms include headache, nausea, and blurred vision.

Hypertensive Emergency

It is defined as elevation of both systolic and diastolic blood pressure with acute end-organ damage (e.g. hypertensive encephalopathy, cerebral hemorrhage, seizures, retinal hemorrhage, pulmonary edema, and renal failure). Hypertensive emergency can be life-threatening, if management is delayed.

The rapidity of rise of blood pressure and end-organ damage are more important than the absolute level of blood pressure alone. Clinical differentiation between hypertensive urgency and emergency is based on end-organ damage rather than the level of blood pressure.

Management

Treatment should be started promptly after establishment of diagnosis. Do not delay it while clinical assessment and diagnostic tests are being done to evaluate the underlying etiology [renal parenchymal, cardiovascular, renovascular, endocrine, central nervous system (CNS), corticosteroid therapy, etc.] and the extent and severity of end-organ damage.

The primary goal in a child with hypertensive emergency is to lower BP promptly to prevent target organ damage due to severe hypertension. This must, however, be done gradually in a controlled stepwise manner. Too rapid reduction may cause ischemic organ damage, especially in patients with long-standing severe hypertension. The aim should be to lower blood pressure by about one-third of the planned reduction, [the difference between the observed and desired (95th percentile) blood pressure], over first 6 hours, an additional one-third over the next 24 hours and the remaining over the next 48 hours. The final maintenance blood pressure (95th percentile for age) should be achieved in 48–72 hours.

Various drugs that are employed in the management of hypertensive emergency along with their dose and salient features are placed in Table 17.3.

Intravenous nitroprusside or labetalol and sublingual nifedipine are drugs of choice for management of hypertensive emergency. Intravenous (IV) infusion of nitroprusside and labetalol (which have short duration of action) permits controlled lowering of blood pressure with careful titration. Other parenteral preparations, such as diazoxide, enalaprilat, hydralazine, and esmolol, have to be administered at intervals of several hours and may not achieve the desired gradual fall of blood pressure.

Table 17.3: Drugs for hypertensive emergency.

Drug	Dose	Onset	Duration	Interval to repeat or increase dose	Comments
Nitroprusside IV infusion (*Arteriolar and venodilator*)	Initial 0.3–0.5 μg/kg/min (maximum 8 μg/kg/min); titrate with blood pressure response	<30 seconds	With infusion	30–60 minutes	Administer in ICU under continuous CVS monitoring, monitor cyanide, if prolonged use/in patients with renal failure
Labetalol IV bolus/infusion (*α- and β-blocker*)	Initial 0.2–1 mg/kg/dose bolus (maximum 20 mg/dose) q 10 minutes PRN followed by 0.25–3 mg/kg/h infusion	IV bolus onset: 2–5 minutes	With infusion	10 minutes	Careful monitoring required. C.I.: CHF, asthma, diabetes mellitus
Nifedipine PO or sublingual (*calcium channel blocker*)	0.25–0.5 mg/kg/dose; maximum dose 10 mg/dose (1–2 mg/kg/day)	Sublingual: 1–5 minutes oral (immediate release cap): 20–30 minutes	4–8 hours	Repeat q 4–6 hours PRN	Unpredictable hypotension, do frequent monitoring for timing of repeat doses, avoid or use very cautiously in CHF

Contd...

Contd...

Drug	Dose	Onset	Duration	Interval to repeat or increase dose	Comments
Hydralazine IV (*Arteriolar dilator*)	0.2–0.6 mg/kg/dose	5–20 minutes	2–6 hours	4–6 hours	May cause reflex tachycardia, prolonged hypotension, nausea C.I.: CHF
Enalaprilat IV (*ACE inhibitor*)	5–10 µg/kg/dose Up to 1.25 mg/dose	15 minutes (IV)	12–24 hours	8–24 hours	May cause prolonged hypotension and acute renal failure, hyperkalemia, angioedema, cough
Minoxidil PO (*arteriolar dilator*)	Initial 0.1–0.2 mg/kg/dose (maximum 10 mg/dose)	Onset 30 minutes (maximum effect: 2–8 hours)	Variable 12–24 hours (up to 5 days)	4–8 hours	Fluid retention Contraindicated in pheochromocytoma

(CHF: congestive heart failure; CVS: cardiovascular system; ICU: intensive care unit; IV: intravenous; PO: per oral)

Note: For other drugs, see under individual drug in Section 4 "Pediatric Drug Formulary"

Table 17.4: Other useful drugs and measures.		
Drug	Dose	Comments
Furosemide IV/IM (*Diuretic*)	1–2 mg/kg/dose IV/IM (maximum 6 mg/kg/24 hour)	Useful adjunct to other antihypertensives; especially in cases of hypertension associated with acute renal failure
Morphine (*Narcotic*)	0.1–02 mg/kg IM	For use, if pulmonary edema present

Note: For details regarding dose, mode of use, side effects, etc. of various drugs, see under Section 4 "Pediatric Drug Formulary".

Following control of severe hypertension with IV nitroprusside/labetalol, oral antihypertensive therapy should be instituted within 6–12 hours of parenteral therapy and IV infusion be slowly weaned off over the next 12–24 hours. The choice of appropriate drugs for management of different hypertensive states has been stated earlier in Table 17.1.

In cases of hypertensive urgency, you should aim to lower blood pressure by 20% over 1 hour and return to baseline level over 24–48 hours. Labetalol, clonidine and captopril, are most commonly used drugs for its management.

Guidelines for Management of Cardiac Arrhythmias

Note: For dosage and other information about drugs, *see* under Section 4: Pediatric Drug Formulary.

SUPRAVENTRICULAR TACHYCARDIA

Termination of Attack

Steps

- Vagal stimulation (Ice bag over face in infant/young child; Valsalva maneuver in older child)
- Adenosine intravenous (IV) push
- *In a child with supraventricular tachycardia with poor perfusion, if no response to vagal stimulation and adenosine IV push*: Direct current (DC) cardioversion 0.5–1 J/kg (may ↑ up to 2 J/kg).

Maintenance Therapy after Conversion to Sinus Rhythm

- Digoxin (but not in Wolff–Parkinson–White syndrome where it is contraindicated), or
- Propranolol or other beta-blockers
- *For resistant cases*: Flecainide, propafenone, sotalol, amiodarone (singly or in combination)
- If poor arrhythmia control or intolerable side effects: radiofrequency ablation/surgical ablation of bypass tracts.

POSTOPERATIVE JUNCTIONAL ECTOPIC TACHYCARDIA

Intravenous amiodarone followed by oral amiodarone or sotalol.

ATRIAL FLUTTER

- Vagal stimulation or adenosine IV for temporary slowing of heart rate
- *DC cardioversion*: Treatment of choice for conversion to sinus rhythm
- For maintenance of sinus rhythm, alternatives are propafenone, amiodarone and sotalol
- *Refractory cases*: Radiofrequency ablation.

ATRIAL FIBRILLATION

- *Initial*: Slow heart rate with calcium channel blockers. Digoxin not to be used in Wolff–Parkinson–White syndrome
- *Later for conversion to sinus rhythm*: Amiodarone IV, procainamide or DC conversion
  - *Precaution*: Give anticoagulants, e.g. warfarin for 3-4 weeks prior to pharmacologic or DC conversion
- In cases with chronic atrial fibrillation, warfarin anticoagulant to prevent thromboembolism and stroke.

VENTRICULAR TACHYCARDIA

- *Initial*
  - *Hemodynamically stable patient*: IV lidocaine
    - Alternative drugs for stable patients: IV amiodarone, procainamide
  - *Hemodynamically unstable*: DC cardioversion immediate. Consider alternative medications (amiodarone, procainamide, or lidocaine IV). Correct aggravating factors, e.g. electrolyte imbalance, hypoxia, acidosis.

VENTRICULAR FIBRILLATION

- *Immediate*: Thump on chest, external cardiac massage with artificial ventilation
- DC defibrillation (up to 3 times, if needed) 2–4 J/kg
- If defibrillation ineffective or fibrillation recurs, give IV amiodarone or lidocaine and repeat defibrillation.
- After recovery, look for underlying cause of ventricular fibrillation and manage in consultation with a pediatric cardiologist.

LONG QT SYNDROME

- Propranolol or other beta-blockers
- Cardiac pacing (for drug-induced profound bradycardia)
- Automatic implantable cardioverter defibrillator for refractory cases.

COMPLETE HEART BLOCK (THIRD-DEGREE ATRIOVENTRICULAR BLOCK)

Cardiac pacemaker implantation (if pauses >3 sec, progressive cardiac enlargement, awake heart rate <40/min in older children and <50/min in neonates).

SICK SINUS SYNDROME

Demand ventricular pacemaker + drug therapy (propranolol/quinidine/procainamide).

19. Pediatric Life Support Algorithms and Emergency Drugs

LIFE SUPPORT ALGORITHMS

- Pediatric Basic Life Support (Flowchart 19.1)
- Algorithm for Resuscitation of the Newly Born Infant (Flowchart 19.2)
- Pediatric Advanced Life Support (PALS) Bradycardia Algorithm (Flowchart 19.3)
- PALS Pulseless Arrest Algorithm (Flowchart 19.4)
- PALS Tachycardia Algorithm (for children with poor perfusion)(Flowchart 19.5).

EMERGENCY DRUGS FOR RESUSCITATION OF A CRITICALLY ILL CHILD

The emergency drugs employed for resuscitation in a critically ill child are outlined in Table 19.1.

Chapter 19: Pediatric Life Support...

Flowchart 19.1: Pediatric basic life support algorithm.

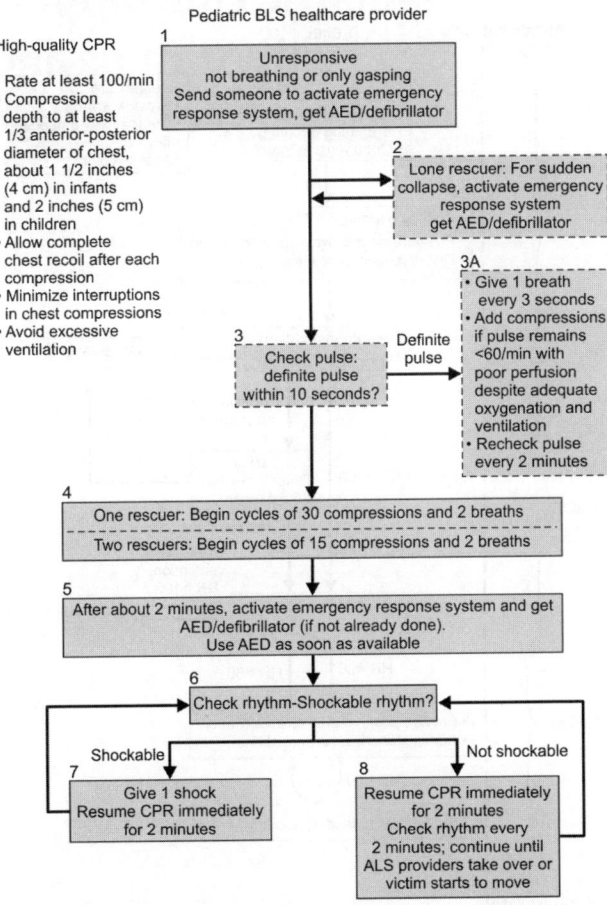

(AED: automated external defibrillator; ALS: advanced life support; BLS: basic life support; CPR: cardiopulmonary resuscitation)

Note: The boxes bordered with dashed lines are performed by healthcare providers and not by rescuers.

Source: From Berg MD, Schexnayder SM, Chameides L, et al. American Heart Association guidelines for cardiopulmonary resuscitation and emergency cardiovascular care, part 13. Circulation. 2010;122(Suppl 3):S862-75.

Flowchart 19.2: Neonatal resuscitation algorithm.

```
Approximate time
                           Birth
                             │
                             ▼
                  • Term gestation?           Routine care
                  • Amniotic fluid clear?     • Provide warmth
                  • Breathing or crying? ─Yes→ • Clear airway if needed
                  • Good muscle tone?         • Dry
                             │                • Assess color
30 sec                       │No
                             ▼
                  • Provide warmth
                  • Position, clear airway¹ (as necessary)
                  • Dry, stimulate, reposition
                             │
                             ▼
                  Evaluate respirations,   Breathing
                  heart rate, and color ── HR >100 ──→ Observational
                             │            and pink        care
                             │                             ▲
                             │ Breathing HR >100           │
                             │ but cyanotic               Pink
                             ▼
                        Give
                        supplementary
                        oxygen
                             │
                             │ Persistent cyanosis
         Apneic or HR <100   │                Effective
                             ▼                ventilation,
                  Provide positive-pressure   HR >100      Postresuscitation
                  ventilation¹          ──── and pink ───→ care
                             │
                    HR <60   │   HR >60
                             ▼
30 sec            • Provide positive-pressure ventilation¹
                  • Administer chest compressions
                             │
                    HR <60   │
                             ▼
                  Administer epinephrine and/or volume¹
```

(HR: heart rate)

Note: ¹Endotracheal intubation may be considered at several steps.
Source: Adapted from American Heart Association Emergency Cardiovascular Care Committee. 2005 American Heart Association (AHA) Guidelines for Cardiopulmonary Resuscitation (CPR) and Emergency Cardiovascular Care (ECC). Circulation. 2005;112(24 Suppl):IV1-169.

Flowchart 19.3: Pediatric bradycardia advanced life support algorithm.

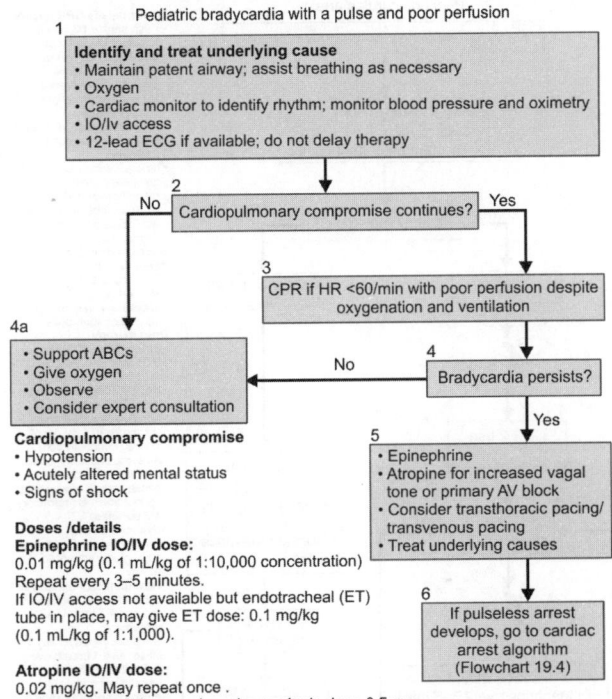

(ABCs: airway, breathing, and circulation; AV: atrioventricular (conductor); ECG: electrocardiogram; HR: heart rate).

Source: Adapted from Kleinman ME, Chameides L, Schexnayder SM, et al. 2010 American Heart Association guidelines for cardiopulmonary resuscitation and emergency cardiovascular care, part 14. Circulation. 2010;122(Suppl 3):S876-S908, Fig. 2, p. S887.

Note: A child is considered to have bradycardia when the heart rate is slower than the normal for age. It becomes clinically significant when the heart rate is slow and there are signs of systemic hypoperfusion.

During its management the common 6 factors responsible for its causation, referred to collectively as the 6 Hs [hypoxia, hypovolemia, hydrogen ions (acidosis), hypo- or hyperkalemia, hypoglycemia, hypothermia] should be carefully assessed and promptly treated.

Flowchart 19.4: Pediatric pulseless cardiac arrest advanced life support algorithm.

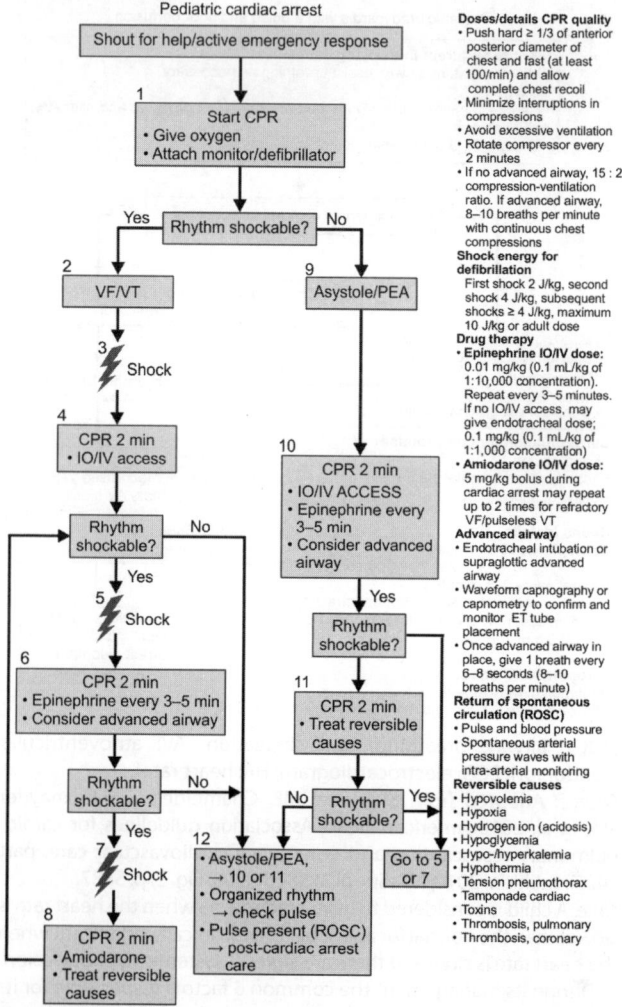

(CPR: cardiopulmonary resuscitation; PEA: pulseless electrical activity)
Source: Same as described in Flowchart 19.3; Circulation. 2010;122(Suppl 3):S876-S908, Fig. 1, p. S885.

Chapter 19: Pediatric Life Support... 155

Flowchart 19.5: Pediatric tachycardia advanced life support algorithm.

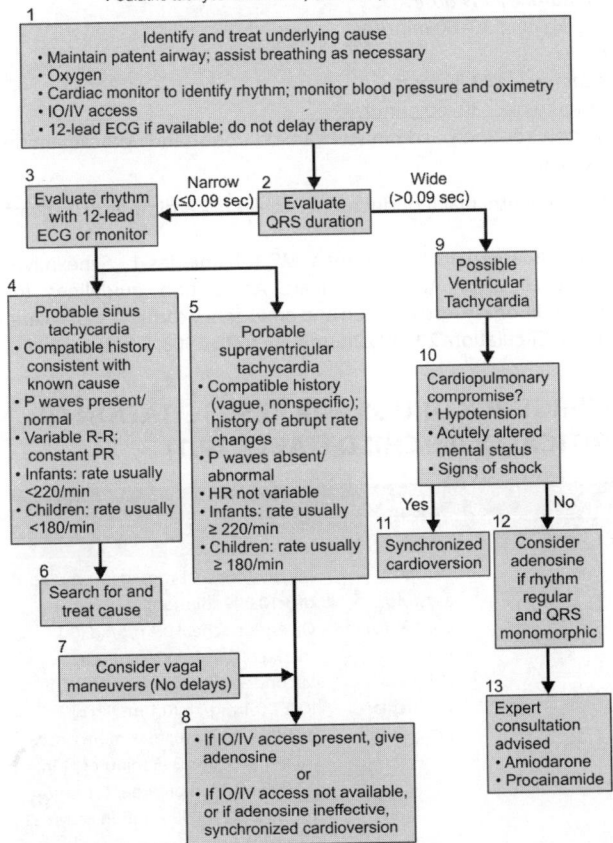

Doses/details

Synchronized cardioversion:
Begin with 0.5–1 J/kg; if not effective, increase to 2 J/kg. Sedate, if needed, but do not delay cardioversion.

Adenosine IO/IV dose:
First dose: 0.1 mg/kg rapid bolus (maximum: 6 mg)
Second dose: 0.2 mg/kg rapid bolus (maximum second dose 12 mg)

Contd...

Contd...

Amiodarone IO/IV dose:
5 mg/kg over 30–60 minutes
Or
Procainamide IO/IV dose:
15 mg/kg over 30–60 minutes
Do not routinely administer amiodarone and procainamide together.

[AV: atrioventricular (conductor); ECG: electrocardiogram; HR: heart rate]

Source: Adapted from Kleinman ME, Chameides L, Schexnayer SM, et al. 2010 American Heart Association guidelines for cardiopulmonary resuscitation and emergency cardiovascular care, part 14. Circulation. 2010;122(Suppl 3): S876-S908, Fig. 3, p. S888.

EMERGENCY DRUGS FOR RESUSCITATION OF CRITICALLY ILL CHILD (TABLE 19.1)

Table 19.1: Emergency drugs.

Drug	Indications	Dosage
Epinephrine	• Cardiac asystole • Ventricular fibrillation • Pulseless ventricular tachycardia	Initial IV/IO: 0.01 mg/kg (0.1 mL/kg of 1:10,000 solution) Or, endotracheal 0.1 mg/kg (0.1 mL/kg of 1 in 1,000 solution) Second and subsequent doses IV/IO/ET 0.1 mg/kg (0.1 mL/kg of 1 in 1,000 solution); maximum dose 10 mg; repeat q 3–5 minutes (1 in 10,000 solution provides 0.1 mg/mL and 1 in 1,000 solution provides 1 mg/mL)
Lidocaine	Ventricular fibrillation pulseless Ventricular tachycardia	1 mg/kg IV/IO bolus; follow with lidocaine infusion 20–50 µg/kg/min

Contd...

Contd...

Drug	Indications	Dosage
Bretylium	• Ventricular fibrillation • Ventricular tachycardia	5 mg/kg IV first dose, repeat q 10 min PRN (10 mg/kg IV second dose)
Atropine	Asystole, severe bradycardia	0.02 mg/kg/dose IV/IO/ET (minimum dose 0.1 mg; maximum dose 0.5 mg) may repeat q 5 min × once (maximum total dose 1 mg)
Adenosine	Supraventricular tachycardia	Initial 0.1 mg/kg IV push, (maximum 6 mg) Repeat dose 0.2 mg/kg (maximum 12 mg/dose)
Amiodarone	Pulseless VF/VT For perfusing tachycardias	5 mg/kg IV rapid bolus; may repeat up to 15 mg/kg, maximum 300 mg Loading dose 5 mg/kg over 1 hour, then continuous infusion at the rate of 5–10 µg/kg/min; maximum 15 mg/kg/day
Procainamide	Perfusing tachycardias (SVT, VT)	Loading dose 15 mg/kg over 30–60 min; stop IV infusion, if hypotension or QRS widens by > 50% of baseline
Sodium bicarbonate	Prolonged cardiac arrest with severe metabolic acidosis	1–2 mEq/kg dose (1–2 mL/kg 7.5% solution) after establishment of effective ventilation
Calcium chloride 10%	• Bradycardia • Hypotension • Hyperkalemia	0.2 mL/kg/dose IV (maximum 10 mL/dose) (20 mg/kg/dose)
Dopamine	Hypotension	5–15 µg/kg/min IV infusion
Dobutamine	• Hypotension • Low cardiac output CHF	2–20 µg/kg/min IV infusion (start at lower end, titrate upwards)

Contd...

Contd...

Drug	Indications	Dosage
Isoproterenol	• Bradycardia • Hypotension	0.1–2.0 µg/kg/min IV infusion
Furosemide	• Acute pulmonary edema • Hypertensive emergency	1–2 mg/kg/dose IV/IM q 6–24 hr
Naloxone	Opiate overdose	0.1 mg/kg/dose IV/IM/SC/ET, maximum 2 mg/dose. May repeat q 2–3 min till desired effect (maximum total dose 10 mg)

20 CHAPTER

Understanding and Management of Shock

INTRODUCTION

Shock is a clinical syndrome that results from an acute circulatory dysfunction leading to inadequate cellular perfusion with insufficient delivery of oxygen and nutrients to tissues. Anaerobic cellular and subcellular metabolism develops with accumulation of lactic acid.

Initially, a number of compensatory mechanisms act to maintain blood pressure and adequate oxygen supply to various vital organs. This is the state of compensated shock. Later, it may progress to an uncompensated state. Compensated and early uncompensated shock are treatable. Advanced uncompensated state leads to widespread irreversible cellular damage, multiple organ failure (irreversible shock) and death.

ETIOLOGY, PATHOPHYSIOLOGY AND CLINICAL FEATURES

Shock may result from (i) deficient functioning of the cardiac pump (*cardiogenic*), (ii) rapid loss of fluid with acute reduction in blood volume (*hypovolemic*), (iii) maldistribution of blood in different tissues (*distributive*), (iv) obstruction to blood flow (*obstructive*); and (v) *septic shock*—it involves a complex interaction of distributive, hypovolemic and cardiogenic shock.

Table 20.1 sums up in brief common causes and pathophysiology of different types of shock. Table 20.2 provides clinical features in different stages of shock.

Table 20.1: Common causes and pathophysiology of different types of shock.

Type of shock	Common causes	Pathophysiology	Clinical features
Hypovolemic	Diarrhea, vomiting, hemorrhage, pathologic renal loss, capillary leak syndrome, peritonitis	Circulating blood volume ↓ Cardiac output ↓ Compensatory vasoconstriction ++ CVP ↓ ↓ ↓ Wedge pressure ↓ ↓ ↓	Heart rate ↑ BP ↓
Distributive	Sepsis, anaphylaxis, CNS or spinal injury, drugs/toxins	Regional blood flow maldistribution *Early septic shock:* Systemic vascular resistance ↓ ↓ ↓ Preload ↓, Cardiac output ↑ CVP N or ↓ Wedge pressure N or ↓ *Late stage:**	*Variable:* Can present as any type of shock *Early: Compensated, warm shock* (bouncing peripheral pulses, warm extremities, due to peripheral vasodilation), *Late uncompensated "Cold Shock"**

Contd...

Chapter 20: Understanding and Management of Shock 161

Contd...

Type of shock	Common causes	Pathophysiology	Clinical features
Cardiogenic	Myocardial insufficiency, myocarditis, cardiomyopathy, dysrhythmia, congenital or acquired heart disease	Myocardial contractility ↓ Cardiac output ↓ ↓ ↓ Systemic vascular resistance ↑ ↑ CVP ↑ ↑ Wedge pressure ↑ ↑	Gallop rhythm/Arrhythmia, Signs of congestive heart failure
Obstructive	Cardiac tamponade, pneumopericardium, tension pneumothorax, pulmonary embolism	Cardiac output ↓ myocardial contractility N Intravascular volume N CVP ↑	Narrow pulse pressure Low voltage ECG

*"Cold shock": In late stage of septic shock (and advanced, uncompensated stage of all types of shock)—cardiac output ↓↓, BP ↓↓↓, systemic vascular resistance ↑, CVP ↑ or N, wedge pressure ↑; severe acidosis, hypoxemia and hypoxia. Skin cold and cyanotic.
Note: In children with shock due to sepsis, "warm shock" is not as commonly observed as in adults.
(BP: blood pressure; CNS: central nervous system; CVP: central venous pressure; ECG: electrocardiography)

Table 20.2: Clinical features in different stages of shock.			
Clinical features	Compensated	Uncompensated	Irreversible
Mental status	Anxiety/confusion	Drowsiness	Coma
Heart rate	↑	↑↑	↓
Blood pressure	N***	↓	↓↓↓/Unrecordable
Respiration	N/↑	↑, acidosis	↑↑, acidosis++/apnea
Capillary refill time*	↑ (>3 sec)	↑↑	↑↑↑
Skin	Cold**	Cold, mottling	Cold and cyanotic
Urinary output	N	↓/Anurea	Anurea
Vital organs function	N	Impaired	Irreversibly damaged

*Capillary refill time is measured after blanching pressure on skin for 5 seconds (sternum or a digit held at the level of the heart).
**Cold: Core/toe temperature difference of >2°C is a sign of poor skin perfusion.
*** Blood pressure is normal in compensated stage of shock

MANAGEMENT

i. Early Recognition of Shock

It is vital that shock is recognized at an early stage when it is amenable to successful reversal with vigorous treatment. *Bear in mind that hypotension**** (Table 20.2) *is not an essential component of shock.* It is absent in early compensated stage and is a late bad sign. One should stay alert for any early symptoms or signs of shock (Table 20.2).

ii. Steps of Therapy

Oxygen administration: Initially, administer oxygen at maximum concentration to achieve an arterial oxygen saturation of 90% or more. After stabilization, reduce oxygen concentration to a level below 60%; persistent high levels cause pulmonary oxygen toxicity.

Fluid therapy: Administration of fluids for effective restoration of circulatory volume is the key initial step in management of shock, *except* for patients with signs that heart failure is their primary pathology.

Choice of fluids

Crystalloids (normal saline, Ringer's lactate) are the initial fluid of choice for shock of undetermined etiology, hypovolemic shock (e.g. due to diarrhea, vomiting and burns) and in cases of septic and distributive shock.

Colloids (albumin, dextran) are combined with crystalloids in case of refractory hypovolemic shock. Colloids are, however, contraindicated in patients with severe capillary leak states, as occurs during first few hours of severe burn injuries and late shock. If administered, it would lead to obligatory water shift into interstitial space. Administration of albumin and plasma protein fractions is appropriate in situations of plasma losses due to inflammatory processes, such as, peritonitis and pancreatitis.

Blood products (whole blood, plasma, packed red blood cells) are used in cases of hemorrhage and trauma.

Administration

Initially, Ringer's lactate solution or normal saline* is given in a bolus of 20 mL/kg over 10–15 minutes. This may be repeated up to 60–80 mL/kg, carefully titrated to normalize heart rate (as per child's age), urine output (to 1 mL/kg/hr), capillary refill time (to <2 sec) and child's mental status.

If there is no satisfactory response to initial fluid therapy,** central venous pressure (CVP) should be measured. If the CVP is less than 10 cm of water, another fluid bolus of 10–20 mL/kg should be administered. It is desirable to maintain CVP between 10 cm and 15 cm of water. Persistent hypotension despite adequate volume replacement is an indication for institution of drug therapy with catecholamines (dopamine/epinephrine/norepinephrine). Rapidly rising sustained CVP or CVP greater than 15 cm of water suggests either fluid overload, myocardial dysfunction or increased right ventricular afterload. In such situation, further fluid administration may lead to pulmonary edema.

Patients with cardiogenic shock have poor cardiac output, often with a compensatory elevation in systemic vascular resistance (SVR). These should be given only small boluses of fluid (5–10 mL/kg) cautiously to replace deficits and maintain preload. Larger volumes are liable to cause cardiac decompensation.

If in a case of gastroenteritis the child is still in shock after two boluses of crystalloid, give third bolus as colloid (human albumin 5% or plasma) and also exclude the possibility of an alternative diagnosis (volvulus, intussusception, peritonitis) or coexisting septicemia.

In case of hypovolemia due to bleeding or loss of protein rich fluid, begin prompt replacement with whole blood, packed red blood cells, fresh frozen plasma or albumin. *In case of persistent hypovolemia due to hemorrhage, give more blood and undertake surgery to stop bleeding.*

DRUG THERAPY

The chief aims of drug therapy are two fold—(1) optimizing cardiac pump function (contractility); and (2) ensuring proper peripheral distribution of blood.

 i. Inotropic drugs may be required when shock persists despite significant fluid replacement. Patients in septic shock commonly demonstrate poor myocardial contractility and concurrent low systemic vascular resistance (SVR) in the presence of metabolic acidosis and endothelial injury. These children benefit from agents producing strong inotropy and peripheral vasoconstriction. Dopamine is widely used as the first-line drug followed by epinephrine/norepinephrine.
 ii. Afterload can be too great or too low to allow normal delivery of blood to the tissues. In vasodilated child such as in sepsis, norepinephrine provides vasoconstriction to improve SVR and reduce maldistribution.
iii. In a child with cardiogenic shock, epinephrine, dopamine or milrinone should be administered to boost cardiac output. Milrinone has the advantage of improving systolic cardiac function as well as decreasing SVR and

enhancing cardiac relaxation. Norepinephrine and vasopressin which boost blood pressure by enhancing SVR should be avoided in patients with cardiogenic shock, as these may cause decompensation.

When afterload is high in a child with cardiogenic shock, use of dobutamine and vasodilators such as nitroprusside may be considered.

Table 20.3 provides a list of commonly used inotrope, vasopressor and vasodilator drugs along with their mode of action and indications for use.

In some cases, a combination of inotropic agents is employed to manage hypotension. Combinations of low dose dopamine with epinephrine, dobutamine with norepinephrine, or dopamine with dobutamine are commonly used.

Table 20.3: Cardiovascular drugs for shock.

Drug	Action	Indications for use
Dopamine 5–15 µg/kg/min	Strengthens myocardial contraction. At high dose (>15 mg/kg/min) risk of arrhythmias and increased peripheral vasoconstriction	First choice for fluid refractory hypotensive shock. Preferred drug for cardiogenic shock
Dobutamine 2–20 µg/kg/min	Inotrope; little effect on heart rate; peripheral vasodilator especially kidney and other viscera; reduces afterload	Good drug for cardiogenic shock. Preferred agent for low output state with adequate BP
Epinephrine 0.05–3 µg/kg/min	Inotrope, chronotrope and potent vasoconstrictor. High risk of arrhythmias; may reduce renal perfusion	Drug of choice in anaphylactic shock. Employed for dopamine resistant low cardiac output cold shock
Norepinephrine 0.05–1.5 µg/kg/min	Strong vasoconstrictor, poor inotrope. Useful when systemic vascular resistance low. Induces short run rise in blood pressure	Used for dopamine resistant warm shock cases (with high cardiac output and low systemic vascular resistance)

Contd...

Contd...

Drug	Action	Indications for use
Phenylephrine 0.5–2 µg/kg/min	Same mode of action as norepinephrine; can cause sudden hypertension. Increases oxygen consumption	*Selected cases*
Isoproterenol 0.05–2 µg/kg/min	Potent chronotrope, weak inotrope. Risk of causing arrhythmias	*Selected cases*
Amrinone Load with bolus over 20 min 1.5–5 mg/kg and then 5–10 µg/kg/min	Strong inotrope and chronotrope. Peripheral vasodilator, ↓ afterload	*Employed in fluid refractory, dopamine resistant "cold shock" with normal BP (seen in cases of sepsis with low cardiac output and high vascular resistance). Beneficial in advanced treatment of cardiogenic shock*

Note: For mode of use, side effects and other information about individual drugs, see under Section 4 Pediatric Drug Formulary.

- Fluid therapy and drug intervention in septic shock (Flowchart 20.1)

Other Therapeutic Measures

- ***Correction of acidosis:*** Partially correct severe metabolic acidosis (arterial pH <7.15) by administration of sodium bicarbonate. Initial dose: 1–2 mEq/kg. Dose subsequently: Body weight kg × base deficit × 0.3 = mEq of $NaHCO_3$. Avoid overcorrection as this may cause paradoxical CNS acidosis.
- ***Correct hypocalcemia:*** If serum ionized calcium below 3 mg/dL: Administer 1–2 mL/kg of 10% calcium gluconate by slow IV infusion under close cardiac monitoring.
- ***Maintain adequate hematocrit:*** Use packed red cells as and when required to maintain hematocrit between 35–40%.

- ***Prevent and manage complications***
  - H_2 receptors and antacids to prevent gastrointestinal bleeding
  - Low dose dopamine (besides volume resuscitation) to prevent acute renal failure. Peritoneal dialysis or hemodialysis for established acute renal failure.

Flowchart 20.1: Fluid therapy and drug intervention in septic shock.

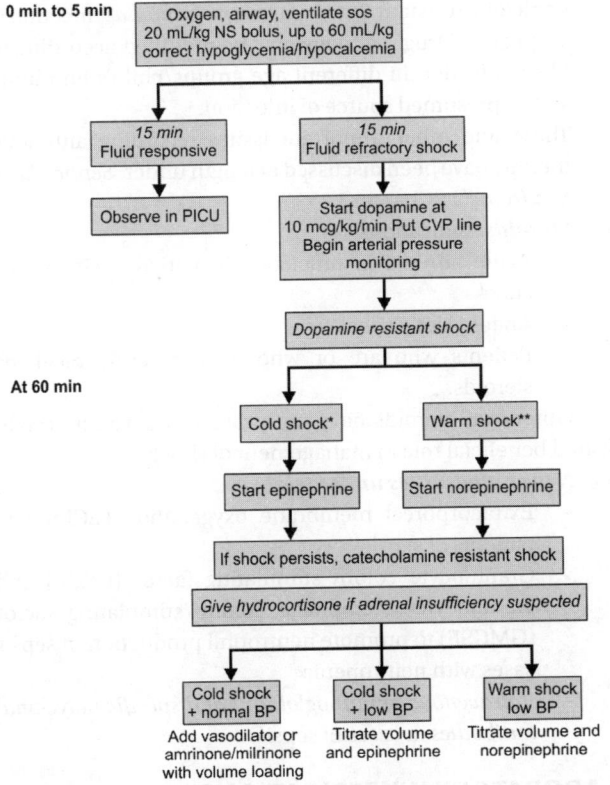

*"Cold shock": Extremities cold-cardiac output ↓, SVR ↑, BP ↓↓↓
**"Warm shock": Extremities feel warm-cardiac output ↑, SVR ↓ (vasodilatation)

- For coagulopathy, such as disseminated intravascular coagulation (DIC): Vitamin K, fresh frozen plasma and platelets
- *Antibiotics:* In cases of septic shock: Initially—a broad-spectrum antibiotic cover (e.g. combination of ceftriaxone and aminoglycoside) on empirical basis for effectiveness against most gram-positive and gram-negative organisms. Add vancomycin if coagulase-negative staphylococci or penicillin-resistant *Streptococcus pneumoniae* infection is suspected. Drug regimens may be modified according to likely infection in different age groups/child's immunity status/presumed source of infection.

  These and other important issues regarding antibiotic therapy have been discussed at length under *'Septic Shock Syndrome'* in Chapter 1.
- *Steroids:* Indications:
  - Acute adrenal insufficiency in patients with septic shock
  - Anaphylactic shock
  - Patients who are or who were recently receiving steroids.

  Otherwise, steroids have not proven to have any established beneficial role in management of shock.
- ***Newer modalities under trial***
  - Extracorporeal membrane oxygenation (ECMO) in patients of sepsis
  - Granulocyte colony-stimulating factor (GCSF) and granulocyte-macrophage colony stimulating factor (GMCSF) to promote neutrophil production in sepsis cases with neutropenia
  - *Intravenous immunoglobulin and specific polyclonal antibodies* in cases of sepsis.

LABORATORY INVESTIGATIONS

- *Blood*: Complete blood count, platelet count, serum electrolytes (Na^+, K^+, Ca^{++}) glucose, urea, creatinine,

arterial blood gas, coagulation screen, serum proteins, liver function tests and blood culture
- *Urine*: Specific gravity, protein, sugar, sediment, M/E (culture sos)
- *X-ray chest, ECG*
- *Other specialized tests,* e.g. echocardiography, wedge pressure measurement, as and when required.

MONITORING

Clinical:
- Pulse (rate, rhythm and character), respiration (rate and character), blood pressure, sensorium, skin color, capillary refill time, temperature (skin and core), hourly urinary output, general condition.
- For hemodynamic assessment—CVP, invasive blood pressure and pulmonary artery wedge pressure monitoring.

SHOCK IN SPECIAL SITUATIONS

Anaphylactic Shock

Anaphylactic reaction in a child can lead to two life-threatening complications—(1) acute airway obstruction due to laryngeal edema and severe bronchospasm; and (2) shock due to acute vasodilatation and fluid loss from the intravascular space caused by increased capillary permeability.

The management of anaphylactic shock consists of—(1) good airway management; (2) administration of epinephrine; and (3) aggressive fluid resuscitation.

Various drugs and measures employed in management of anaphylactic reaction are described in a separate section—"Drug Therapy in Anaphylaxis."

Cardiogenic Shock

Its management is guided by measures to tackle the underlying pathologic process—impaired myocardial contractility, arrhythmia, congenital/acquired valvular/anatomic defect or outflow obstruction to blood flow. The assistance of a pediatric cardiologist should be promptly obtained.

Dengue Shock Syndrome

The mechanisms underlying dengue shock syndrome are complex. This condition requires rigorous monitoring and aggressive regulated therapy. It is described in separate section on "Dengue Hemorrhagic Fever and Dengue Shock Syndrome".

CHAPTER 21

Management of Dengue

DENGUE—MILD

In this condition caused by dengue virus infection, the child generally has acute biphasic fever with headache, myalgias, arthralgias, erythematous rash over extremities, leukopenia, and lymphadenopathy. Platelet counts are normal and tourniquet test only infrequently positive. Patients do not show any evidence of plasma leak from capillaries in the form of rise in hematocrit or accumulation of fluid in serous cavities (pleural effusion/ascites).

Management

It comprises bedrest, control of pyrexia through judicious use of paracetamol, avoidance of aspirin and nonsteroidal anti-inflammatory drugs (NSAIDs) (↑gastritis, bleeding), adequate diet, and plenty of oral fluids. Administration of low-osmolar WHO oral rehydration solution is recommended to treat dehydration, if present. Before sending the child home, parents should be advised, to take the child to hospital, if he develops warning symptoms, such as abdominal pain, persistent vomiting, lethargy, bleeding from nose or any other site.

DENGUE—MODERATE

Children having dengue infection with warning symptoms and signs such as abdominal pain, persistent vomiting, lethargy, bleeding tendencies, hepatomegaly, pleural effusion/ascites, or CNS (central nervous system) involvement; platelet count less than 50,000/mm^3, hematocrit more than or equal to

20%, or having a comorbid condition (such as renal disease, diabetes, hepatitis, heart disease, hypertension) and infants with this infection are considered to be having moderate dengue. They need hospitalization and proper care with monitoring of vitals and for signs of bleeding, dehydration/fluid overload as well as frequent estimation of hematocrit and platelets. Management of a child with moderate dengue is depicted in Flowchart 21.1.

Flowchart 21.1: Management of moderate dengue.

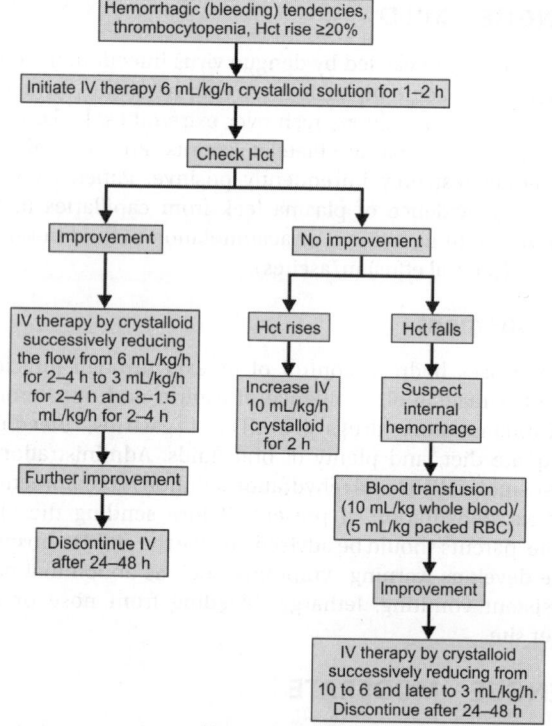

(Hct: hematocrit; RBC: red blood cell)
Source: WHO. 2015 National guidelines for clinical management of dengue fever. [online] Available from http:nvbdcp.gov.in/Doc/Dengue-National-Guidelines-2014.pdf. [Accessed October, 2018].

Estimation of Change in Hematocrit Level

In cases where hematocrit has not been monitored from an early stage of the disease, expected normal value of hematocrit in children of the same age group may be considered as baseline value. An anemic child will have lower hematocrit to begin with.

DENGUE–SEVERE

Cases of dengue showing evidence of severe bleeding; shock or severe liver, CNS or cardiac dysfunction are considered to be suffering from severe dengue. They need hospitalization and intensive care with close clinical monitoring, regular hematocrit, and platelet studies and other appropriate investigations when necessary, such as LFT (liver function tests), CXR (chest X-ray) and serum electrolytes. Children with compensated shock have low-systolic blood pressure, narrow pulse pressure (<20 mm Hg), and rise in hematocrit above 20%. The plan for their management is placed in Flowchart 21.2.

On the other hand, some severe dengue cases develop signs of profound shock with unrecordable blood pressure. Their management is outlined in Flowchart 21.3.

SOME IMPORTANT RELEVANT ISSUES

Role of Platelet Transfusion

These should not be used prophylactically. Their use should be restricted to cases with severe bleeding or in those with platelet count less than 10,000/mm^3. However, there is not much evidence of their conferring any significant benefit. Platelets obtained by single donor apheresis are better than random donor platelets.

Fluid Overload

It may develop due to excessive administration of IV fluids, especially hypotonic fluids, or their inappropriate use at the

Flowchart 21.2: Algorithm for fluid management in compensated shock.

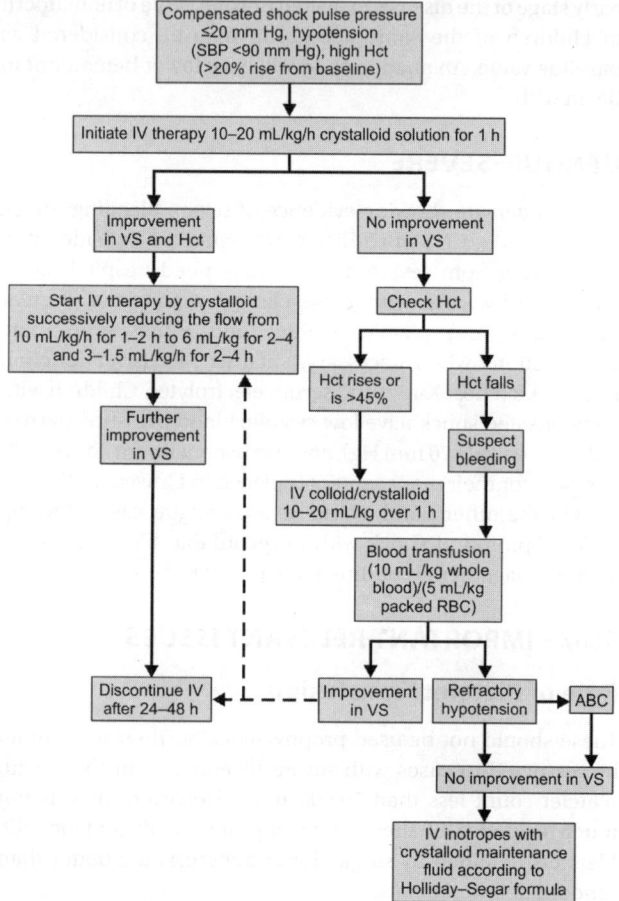

(SBP: systolic blood pressure; VS: vital signs; Hct: hematocrit; RBC: red blood cell; ABC: airway, breathing, and circulation)
Source: WHO. 2015 National guidelines for clinical management of dengue fever. [online] Available from http:nvbdcp.gov.in/Doc/Dengue-National-Guidelines-2014.pdf. [Accessed October, 2018].

Flowchart 21.3: Algorithm for fluid management in hypotensive decompensated shock.

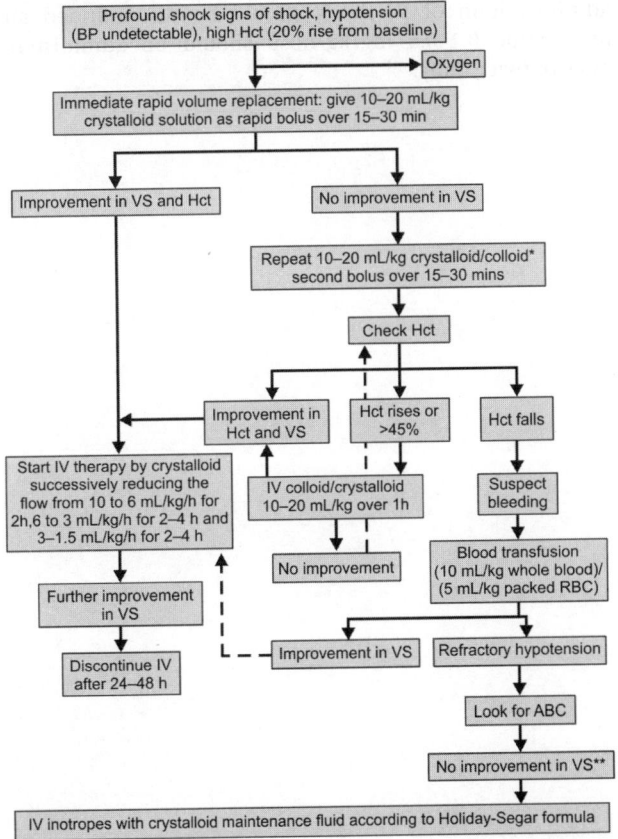

Source: WHO (2015). National guidelines for clinical management of dengue fever. [online] Available from http:nvbdcp.gov.in/Doc/Dengue-National-Guidelines-2014.pdf. [Accessed October, 2018].

*Colloid (hydroxyethyl starch)–Hetastarch (e.g. Hespan infusion).

**Note:* If the child still shows no improvement, exclude presence of disseminated intravascular coagulation, continuing severe blood loss, acidosis and cardiac dysfunction and act accordingly.

Infusion of fresh frozen plasma and platelet concentrates may be beneficial in cases of DIC with severe bleeding.

time of patient's recovery. It may manifest as pulmonary edema or congestive heart failure. In this situation, administration of IV fluids should be discontinued and furosemide 0.1–0.5 mg/kg/dose should be administered once or twice daily.

22. "Blue Spells" in Tetralogy of Fallot: Management and Prevention

MANAGEMENT OF HYPERCYANOTIC ATTACKS ("BLUE" OR "TET" SPELLS) IN TETRALOGY OF FALLOT (TABLE 22.1)

Table 22.1: Management of hypercyanotic attacks in tetralogy of Fallot.

Steps of action	Effect
Place infant on abdomen in knee-chest position or squatting position	Decreases venous return and increases systemic resistance
Administer oxygen	Some reduction in hypoxemia; limited effectiveness
Morphine IV/subcutaneous Inj. (0.1–0.2 mg/kg)	Depresses respiratory center, reduces harmful hyperpnea
Normal saline 10–20 mL/kg by IV push	Augments preload
For resistant cases: Phenylephrine IV (5–20 µg/kg) or norepinephrine infusion 0.05–2 µg/kg/min	Increases systemic resistance and decreases right to left shunt
Propranolol IV (0.1–0.2 mg/kg slow push)	Negative inotropic effect on right ventricular infundibular myocardium Increase in pulmonary blood flow
Sodium bicarbonate IV (1 mEq/kg)	If cyanotic spell severe, prolonged and has not responded to above therapy; to rapidly correct resultant metabolic acidosis

PREVENTION OR REDUCTION IN FREQUENCY AND SEVERITY OF "BLUE" SPELLS

- *Propranolol oral*: 0.5–1 mg/kg/dose q 6 h
- *Iron oral*: To maintain red cell indices in normocytic range
- *Prevention and prompt treatment of dehydration*: To avoid hemoconcentration and thereby reduce risk of thrombotic episodes
- *Avoid exposure to cold*: Cold increases oxygen consumption
- *Ensure adequate glucose intake*: Cyanotic infants prone to develop hypoglycemia.

23. Management of Childhood Type I Diabetes and Diabetic Ketoacidosis

INSULIN MANAGEMENT OF CHILDHOOD TYPE I DIABETES

Routine insulin management of diabetes, in combination with other measures, is aimed at:
- Achieving good 24-hour glucose control
- Avoiding hypoglycemia
- Preventing ketoacidosis
- Eliminating polyuria and nocturia
- Allowing normal growth and development of the child with maintenance of his fairly normal lifestyle.

Most diabetic children need administration of 0.5–1.0 unit/kg/day of insulin. The optimum dose in an individual child is initially generally determined with frequent monitoring of blood glucose (and urine glucose) levels, and close watch on symptoms of hypoglycemia, while he is administered regular insulin thrice a day, before breakfast, lunch and evening meal. After assessment of daily insulin needs of the child, he is put on a combination of short-acting regular/lispro insulin and an intermediate/long-acting insulin. The recent availability of several types of insulins now provide several alternatives to the clinician to employ a combination most suited to a particular child and his family. Table 23.1 provides information about the characteristics of different types of insulin.

Table 23.1: Types of insulin and their characteristics.			
Insulin	Onset (hr)	Peak (hr)	Duration (hr)
Rapid acting			
Lispro	0.25	0.5–2.5	3–5
Aspart	10–20 min	1–3	3–5
Glulisine	5–15 min	1–3	3–5
Short acting			
Regular	0.5–1	1–5	6–10
Intermediate acting			
Neutral pH protamine—NPH (human)	2–4	6–8	12–16
Long acting			
Glargine	3–4	–	20–24

Alternative Regimens of Insulin Therapy

Twice-daily Injections

A combination of intermediate or neutral protamine Hagedorn (NPH) with short-acting regular or rapid-acting lispro/aspart insulin.

In this regime, two-thirds of the total daily required dose is given before breakfast and one-third before the evening meal. For example, if the daily requirement is 30 units, 20 units are given before breakfast and 10 units before evening meal.

The insulin in each injection is split between intermediate and short-acting insulin in the ratio of 2:1 to 3:1. In the above case, morning dose of 20 units would thus consist of 14 units of NPH + 6 units of regular; and evening dose of 10 units would comprise 6 units of NPH + 4 units of regular insulin.

If the child develops hyperglycemia or glycosuria during mid-morning to noon, the dose of short-acting insulin is increased by 10–15%; but if he develops hypoglycemia during this period, the dose is reduced by 10–15%. On the other hand, development of hyperglycemia during late afternoon or evening demands enhancement of the morning dose of NPH insulin by 10–15% and development of hypoglycemia during this period, reduction of its dose by 10–15%. Similar adjustments have to be made in the evening doses of regular and NPH insulin depending upon glucose levels shortly or long after their administration. Through such stepwise changes, optimum dose of both types of insulin in proper combination are arrived at. Lispro, glulisine and aspart insulins are better than regular insulin because of their quick, short-term peak effects and short tail effects. These provide better control of postmeal glucose rise and less between-meal and nocturnal hypoglycemia.

Four Times Daily Injections

Three bolus doses of short-acting or rapid-acting insulin before meals + a single dose of glargine insulin at bedtime.

In this regime, the component of glargine insulin is around 25–30% of the total dose in toddlers and 45% in older children. The balance is split equally as short-acting insulin boluses before breakfast, lunch and evening meal. This plan provides good glycemic control but suffers from serious drawback of requiring four daily injections, which becomes practically difficult for many families and unacceptable by many diabetic children.

MANAGEMENT OF DIABETIC KETOACIDOSIS

Diagnostic features of diabetic ketoacidosis: Hyperglycemia, ketonemia, ketonuria and metabolic acidosis (pH < 7.30, bicarbonate < 15 mEq/L).

Step I: Clinical Assessment and Baseline Investigations

- *History*: Symptoms suggestive of diabetes, precipitating infection/missed insulin dosage, vomiting, abdominal pain, neurologic symptoms, etc.

- *Physical examination*: Hemodynamic and respiration status (especially for tachycardia, hypotension, Kussmaul's breathing, tachypnea, fruity breath), degree of dehydration, and mental status.
- *Laboratory evaluation*: Blood glucose, electrolytes, gasometry, pH, bicarbonate, complete blood counts, urea, creatinine, urine examination for glucose and ketone.

Step II: Therapeutic Measures and Monitoring

A. *Treatment*
  i. *1st hr*: 10–20 ml/kg IV bolus of N. saline or Ringer's lactate. (Note: Do not give Ringer's lactate if hyperkalemia, urine not passed). Follow up with insulin drip @ 0.1U/kg/hr.
  ii. *2nd hr onward*: 0.45% saline drip with insulin 0.05 to 0.1 U/kg/hr.
      - Add potassium @40 mEq/L after urine flow is established and serum potassium is below 5.5 mEq/L. A combination of 20 mEq/L of K phosphate and 20 mEq/L of K acetate is better than use of 40 mEq/L potassium chloride. *Fluid volume* and rate: 85 mL/kg deficit + 24 hrs maintenance fluid – bolus should be given over next 23 hrs; divided uniformly over each hour (For maintenance requirement calculation: for first 10 kg @ 100 mL/kg; for next 10 kg @ 50 mL/kg and next 10 kg @ 20 mL/kg).
  iii. *When blood glucose falls to 250–300 mg/dL:* Replace 0.45% saline by 1/2 saline in 5% dextrose. May reduce insulin infusion rate in decrements of 0.02 U/kg/hr if blood glucose level drops to 150 mg/dL.
  iv. As therapy progresses, there occurs steady rise in pH and bicarbonate level. If acidosis persists, check for inadequate insulin and fluid therapy, infection and for rare presence of lactic acidosis. Serum sodium level should increase by about 1.6 m mol/L (28.5 mg/dL) for each 100 mg/dL decline in blood glucose level. Declining sodium level during therapy suggests excess

free water accumulation with risk of development of cerebral edema. Persistence of ketonuria in the presence of other parameters of clinical improvement should not be interpreted as evidence of therapeutic failure.

  v. *When pH > 7.30 or sodium bicarbonate > 20 mEq/L, normal electrolytes, no ketosis, no emesis*: Children with mild DKA recover in about 10-12 hrs and those with more severe DKA take 30-36 hrs for recovery.
     - Known diabetic child: Restart old insulin regimen.
     - New established diabetic: Begin with 0.1-0.25 U/kg q 6-8 hrs SC to establish daily insulin needs; switch later to combination insulin regimen.

Regarding sodium bicarbonate administration: The routine administration of $NaHCO_3$ is not recommended. It enhances risk of development of hypokalemia and serious cerebral edema. It may be rarely necessary if there is extreme acidosis (pH < 7.10) and it needs very cautious administration.

B. *Monitoring*

Regular monitoring and recording on a flow sheet.
- *Laboratory investigations*: Blood glucose—hourly at first, then 2 hourly. Electrolytes, pH, blood gases—2 hourly, later 3-4 hourly. Urine for glucose and ketones—each voided sample. Watch serum sodium level closely. It should rise with decline in blood glucose level.
- *Regular ECG monitoring for evidence of hypokalemia.*
- *Clinical*: Close monitoring of hemodynamic status, urinary output and for signs of raised intracranial pressure (altered consciousness, depressed respiration, increasing headache, bradycardia, hypertension, apnea, pupillary changes, papilledema, and seizures).
- If raised intracranial pressure suspected, immediately give 20% mannitol IV 1 g/kg and closely follow-up.

24. Drug Therapy in Anaphylaxis

Anaphylaxis is a serious allergic reaction that is rapid in onset and may cause death.

PATHOGENESIS AND CLINICAL FEATURES

Severe allergic reaction to a variety of allergens results in sudden release of potent biologically active mediators from mast cells and basophils leading to varied clinical manifestations such as the following:

- *Cutaneous*: Urticaria, angioedema, flushing
- *Respiratory*: Bronchospasm, laryngeal edema
- *Cardiovascular*: Hypotension, dysrhythmias, myocardial ischemia
- *Gastrointestinal*: Nausea, colicky abdominal pain, vomiting.

ETIOLOGY

Food allergy to a variety of items (such as peanuts, eggs, fish, shell fish); allergy to some drugs (penicillins, cephalosporins, sulfonamides, nonsteroidal anti-inflammatory drugs, others), hymenoptera stings and to allergen immunotherapy are among many agents that can induce anaphylactic reaction in a particular sensitive individual.

MANAGEMENT

Immediate Management

- Epinephrine 0.01 mL of 1 in 1,000 solution/kg IM stat; max dose 0.3 mL

- Antihistaminic PO/IV
  - Cetirizine 0.25 mg/kg up to 10 mg PO, or
  - Diphenhydramine 1.25 mg/kg up to 50 mg PO or 1–2 mg/kg IV slowly/IM, or
  - Pheniramine maleate 0.15 mg/kg PO/IV.

Hospital or Emergency Management

- Supplemental oxygen and airway management
- *Epinephrine:*
  - 0.01 mL/kg of 1:1000 solution up to 0.3 mL IM; may repeat 2 times or 3 times at interval of 5–15 minutes, if symptoms persist.
  - Alternatively, 0.01 mL/kg/dose of 1 in 10,000 slow IV push
- *In case of circulatory failure:*
  - Intravenous normal saline or Ringer's lactate 30 mL/kg in first hour
  - Follow-up by IV colloids/vasopressor dopamine infusion SOS
    Dopamine 5–15 µg/kg/min (max. 20 µg/kg/min)
  For details, see Chapter 20 (Understanding and Management of Shock)
- *Bronchodilator inhalation* by nebulization (salbutamol/terbutaline)—for dosage, see section 4: "Pediatric Drug Formulary".
- *Corticosteroids* administration:*
  - Methylprednisolone IV: 1–2 mg/kg up to 125 mg, or IM: 1 mg/kg up to 80 mg
  - Prednisone 1 mg/kg up to 75 mg PO
- *Histamine 2 receptor antagonist:*
  - Ranitidine 1 mg/kg IV (max 50 mg), or
  - Cimetidine 4 mg/kg IV (max 200 mg)

---

*Note: Corticosteroids do not have significant role in the immediate management of life-threatening complications in anaphylaxis because of delay of several hours in the onset of their therapeutic effect. These may, however, prevent/alleviate late-phase reactions (recurrence of urticaria, bronchospasm or hypotension).

- If severe refractory airway obstruction:
  - Intubation or tracheostomy or cricothyroidotomy, as required.

Post-emergency Management

- H_1 antagonist—cetirizine, fexofenadine or loratadine for 3 days
- Oral prednisone 1 mg/kg/day div q 8 h ×3 days
- Evaluate etiology. Educate patient/parents regarding prevention, early recognition of anaphylaxis symptoms and keeping essential drugs readily available for early treatment.

25 Management of Intracranial Hypertension

Intracranial pressure (ICP) is the sum total of pressure exerted by the brain 80%, blood 10% and cerebrospinal fluid (CSF) 10%, in the noncompliant intracranial vault. It is 1.5–6 mm Hg in infants, 3–7 mm Hg in young children and 10–15 mg Hg in older children and adults. Cerebral perfusion pressure (CPP) is the difference between arterial pressure and ICP. It is the CPP at which brain is perfused with blood.

Intracranial pressure may rise abnormally due to:
- Cerebral edema—in cases of meningitis, encephalitis, head injury, hypertensive, hepatic and toxic encephalopathy
- Intracranial space-occupying lesions—such as hematoma, tumor, and abscess.

In such situation, the effective CPP gets diminished resulting in deleterious cerebral ischemia and neuronal injury. If unchecked, intracranial hypertension may progress into herniation syndrome and death.

Intracranial hypertension manifests in awake patients as headaches, vomiting, confusion, irritability, squint, neck retraction and decreased alertness. Tense fontanelle in infants and papilledema suggest raised ICP. Abnormal posturing, abnormal pupillary dilatation, hypertension, bradycardia, irregular breathing, sixth nerve palsy and papilledema indicate severe intracranial hypertension and impending brain herniation.

MANAGEMENT

Intracranial pressure more than 20 mm Hg is considered to be intracranial hypertension that requires treatment.

- *Airway, breathing and circulation:* To begin with, airway, breathing and circulation status should be quickly assessed and necessary corrective steps be initiated. 100% oxygen should be started with nonbreathing mask and if needed, bag and mask ventilation undertaken to ensure adequate oxygenation (PaO_2 should be maintained above 60 mm Hg and oxygen saturation above 92%). Endotracheal intubation may be necessary to ensure adequate oxygenation and ventilation. Blood pressure must be maintained at level appropriate for age to achieve adequate CPP. In a hypotensive, neurologically injured child, administration of a bolus of normal saline 20 mL/kg or a vasopressor agent (dopamine/norepinephrine) may be required.
- *Head position:* The patient's head should be kept elevated 30° in midline. It allows optimum blood drainage from brain via external regular vein with some help in reducing ICP. If head is hyperflexed/hyperextended/turned sideways, venous outflow from cranium gets reduced resulting in elevation of ICP. However, the child must be euvolemic prior to head elevation to avoid orthostatic hypotension.
- *Deep sedation and analgesia:* The child should be deeply sedated and given adequate analgesia to minimize movement and allay pain and anxiety, both of which promote rise in ICP. Midazolam 1–3 µg/kg/min IV infusion or morphine 0.1 mg/kg/dose SC/IM q 6 h may be employed for this purpose.
- The following to be considered:
  - *(i) Mannitol:* It is a useful drug for treatment of acute intracranial hypertension (e.g. in cases of bacterial meningitis, viral encephalitis). The increased osmolality produced by IV administration of 20% mannitol induces shift of fluid from brain (intracellular space) to the intravascular space

resulting in reduction of ICP. Initial dose of 0.5–1 g/kg followed by 0.25–0.5 g/kg/dose every 4–6 hr IV. Its use should be limited to 48–72 hrs and the dose should be tapered before its discontinuation to prevent rebound of ICP. Mannitol is contraindicated in decompensated shock, oliguria, anuria and heart failure.

- *(ii) Hypertonic saline:* Hypertonic saline is employed in children who are hypovolemic or hypotensive or show evidence of real failure. It exerts osmotic force which draws water from the interstitial space of brain parenchyma into intravascular space. Thereby, it promotes rapid CSF absorption, reduces ICP, expands intravascular volume, induces cardiac output and augments CPP. It is generally administered as a continuous infusion at 0.1–1 mL/kg/hr to target a serum sodium level of 144–155 mEq/L.

- *General measures:* Fluid therapy is done to maintain euvolemia largely through use of normal saline/Ringer lactate. Hypotonic fluids must be avoided.
  Blood glucose must be maintained between 80 mg/dL and 120 mg/dL and hyponatremia must be avoided. Hemoglobin should preferably be maintained around 10 g/dL. Temperature should be maintained in normal range. Anticonvulsants may be used prophylactically on short-term basis to prevent seizures.

- *Role of corticosteroids:* Dexamethasone 0.15 mg/kg/dose every 6 hrs (max 16 mg/day) is employed for reducing vasogenic edema in cases of brain tumor, abscess, inflammatory conditions and infections. These are not indicated in cases with diffuse traumatic brain injury and may be detrimental in cerebral malaria and intracranial hemorrhage.

- In hemodynamically stable patients wherein intracranial hypertension has failed to respond to various therapeutic measures explained above and where adequate ICU facilities are available—(i) heavy sedation with use of morphine and midazolam; (ii) induction of barbiturate coma; and (iii) moderate hypothermia (32°C–34°C) may be employed.

- *Surgical procedures under special circumstances:* Cerebrospinal fluid drainage (intermittent or continuous) through external ventricular drainage or ventriculoperitoneal shunt effectively helps to lower ICP in cases of hydrocephalus. Surgical decompression and evacuation of extravasated blood under pressure is sometimes essential in cases of head trauma. Decompressive craniectomy has to be occasionally done to treat uncontrolled intracranial hypertension.

26. Management of Hemophilia

SOME BASIC FACTS

Hereditary deficiency of clotting factor VIII is present in patients of hemophilia A, that of factor IX or Christmas factor in hemophilia B and of Willebrand factor in cases with Von Willebrand disease. Besides them, some rare hereditary clotting disorders occur due to deficiency of factors II, V, VII, X and a few others.

The severity of disease in a hemophilia patient is determined largely by the level of clotting activity of factor VIII/factor IX present in his/her blood.

Clotting activity present in 1 mL of pooled plasma is deemed as one unit, and average normal activity of clotting factor in blood is considered as 100%.

Normal persons: Factor level (Above 50%)—No bleeding tendency

Mild hemophilia: Factor level (>5%)—Bleeding only during surgery/injury

Moderate hemophilia: Factor level (1–5%)—Bleeding after trauma

Severe hemophilia: Factor level (< 1%)—Spontaneous bleeding into muscles and joints, epistaxis, hematuria, may have life-threatening central nervous system or gastrointestinal bleeding.

In the event of bleeding in hemophilia cases, prompt adequate replacement therapy of the deficient factor must be done to raise it to a level which will achieve hemostasis and prompt arrest of bleeding. Adequate level should be

Table 26.1: World Federation of Hemophilia recommendations for desired factor level and duration in various bleeds.

Site of bleed	Hemophilia A		Hemophilia B	
	No resource constraints	Resource constrained	No resource constraints	Resource constrained
Joints	40–60% for 2 days	10–20% for 2 days	40–60% for 2 days	10–20% for 2 days
Superficial muscles	40–60% for 2–3 days	10–20% for 2–3 days	40–60% for 2–3 days	10–20% for 2–3 days
Iliopsoas/deep muscles; neurovascular compromise; significant blood loss	80–100% (days 1–2), 30–60% for days 3–5 or longer	20–40% initially, then 10–20% for days 3–5 or longer	60–80% (days 1–2), 30–60% for days 3–5 or longer	15–30% initially, then 10–20% for days 3–5 or longer
Brain, spine, head	80–100% (days 1–7); 50% (days 8–21)	50–80% (days 1–3); 30–50% (days 4–7); 20–40% (days 8–14)	60–80% (days 1–7); 30% (days 8–21)	50–80% (days 1–3); 30–50% (days 4–7); 20–40% (days 8–14)
Throat and neck	80–100% (days 1–7); 50% (days 8–14)	30–50% (days 1–3); 10–20% (days 4–7)	60–80% (days–7); 30% (days–14)	30–50% (days 1–3); 10–20% (days 4–7)
Gastrointestinal	80–100% initially, then 50% (total 7–14 days)	30–50% (days 1–3); 10–20% (days 4–7)	60–80% initially, then 30% (total 7–14 days)	30–50% (days 1–3); 10–20% (days 4–7)
Renal	50% for 3–5 days	20–40% for 3–5 days	40% for 3–5 days	20–40% for 3–5 days

Contd...

Contd...

Site of bleed	Hemophilia A		Hemophilia B	
	No resource constraints	Resource constrained	No resource constraints	Resource constrained
Deep laceration	50% for 5–7 days	20–40% for 5–7 days	40% for 5–7 days	20–40% for 5–7 days
Major surgery	80–100% pre-operatively; 60–80% (post-op days 1–3); 40–60% (days 4–6); 30–50% (days 7–14)	60–80% preoperatively; 30–40% (post-op day 1–3); 20–30% (days 4–6); 10–20% (days 7–14)	60–80% preoperatively; 40–60% (post-op day 1–3); 30–50% (days 4–6); 20–40% (days 7–14)	50–70% (pre-operatively; 30–40% (post-op days 1–3); 20–30% (days 4–6); 10–20% (days 7–14)
Minor surgery	50–80% preoperatively; 30–80% 1–5 post-op days (as required)	40–80% preoperatively; 20–50% 1–5 post-op days (as required)	50–80% preoperatively; 30–80% 1–5 post-op days (as required)	40–80% preoperatively; 20–50% 1–5 post-op days (as required)

Source: Consensus statement of the Indian Academy of Pediatrics in Diagnosis and Management of Hemophilia. Indian Pediatr. 2018;7: 582-90.

further maintained for a few days. Dose of factor varies with the type, site and severity of bleeding, the desired hemostatic factor level in the patient and ability of the concerned specific factor to achieve it. For example, 1 unit of factor VIII per kg of body weight will raise factor VIII level by 2% while 1 unit of factor IX per kg will raise it by 1%.

World Federation of Hemophilia Recommendations for desired factor level and duration in various bleeds in hemophilia cases in resource constrained areas (like India) and for those areas with no constraints on resources are placed in Table 26.1.

CALCULATION OF DOSE OF FACTORS

Calculation of the doses in individual bleeding episodes for different patients to achieve a desired factor level is based on the formula given below:
- Factor VIII (IU per dose) = U/dL desired rise (%) × body weight × 0.5
- Factor IX (IU per dose) = U/dL desired rise (%) × body weight × 1

(In case recombinant factor IX is used, its dose is 1.2 to 1.5 times that of therapeutic plasma-derived factor IX).

The frequency of dose administration in a patient should be 12 hourly in hemophilia A and 24-hourly in hemophilia B.

Ideally, the dosage of factors should be individualized on the basis of factor level studies performed prior to treatment and at regular intervals during treatment. However, in the absence of actual estimation, the patient's baseline antihemophilic factor in a case of severe hemophilia may be assumed as < 1% and calculation of the factor dose done on the basis of the desired increase in his blood factor level.

The use of factor concentrates is preferable to cryoprecipitate in cases of hemophilia A due to their risk of causing transfusion-transmitted infections. Desmopressin acetate given IV or SC can be used to increase plasma concentrations of factor VIII and VWF (and not factor IX). Tranexamic acid (an antifibrinolytic agent) is useful for bleeds in nasal and oral cavity. Information about these agents can be accessed in the pediatric drug formulary Section III.

Besides factor replacement, as soon as a patient perceives a joint bleed, he should be provided 'RICE' management comprising of Rest, Ice, compression and elevation. Ice pack (not is direct skin contact) should be applied for 20 minutes once in 4–6 hours.

Indian Academy of Pediatrics Hemophilia Group recommends a continuous primary prophylaxis in severe hemophilia cases (at least low-dose regimen of 10–12 IU/kg twice or thrice per week)

Considering the need for regular comprehensive care, hemophilia cases should ideally be managed in a specialized center by multispeciality team comprising of pediatric hematologist, laboratory hematologist, orthopedic surgeon, pain management expert, physiotherapist, dentist and social worker.

27
Blood Component Therapy

PACKED RED BLOOD CELL TRANSFUSION

Indications in Chronic Anemia

A. *Neonates and infants < 4 months:*
   - Hemoglobin (Hb) less than or equal to 7 g/dL (a) with symptomatic anemia, or (b) during postoperative period
   - Hb less than or equal to 10 g/dL (hematocrit < 30%) (a) with coexisting moderate pulmonary disease; and (b) preoperatively and during major surgery
   - Hb less than or equal to 12 g/dL and infant has severe pulmonary/cardiac disease.
B. *Children above 4 months of age and adolescents:*
   - Hb less than 7 g/dL with symptomatic chronic anemia/during perioperative period/marrow failure
   - Hb less than 12 g/dL and coexisting severe cardiopulmonary disease.

Note: Hematocrit level is approximately estimated at Hb/dL × 3.

Indications during Acute Blood Loss

When loss is more than 25% of circulating blood volume (>15 mL/kg) and the patient's condition unstable:
Volume of packed red blood cells (RBCs) required for correction

Volume of packed RBCs (mL) =

$$\text{Estimated body blood volume (mL)} \times \frac{\text{Desired Hct} - \text{Actual Hct}}{\text{Hct of packed RBCs}}$$

where, Hct is hematocrit.

For example, infant's weight 10 kg; present hematocrit 30%, desired hematocrit 40%, estimated blood volume of baby 800 mL at the rate of 80 mL/kg, hematocrit of packed RBCs 60%.

Required volume of packed RBCs (mL) would be

$$= 800 \text{ mL} \times \frac{40 - 30}{60}$$

$$= 133.3 \text{ mL (i.e. 13 mL/kg approx)}.$$

Usual dose and rate of administration: 10–15 mL/kg at the rate of 2–3 mL/kg/hr (generally 10 mL/kg aliquots over 4 hrs).

In severe compensated anemia, say with Hb 5 g/dL, transfuse smaller aliquot at a time, about 5 mL/kg over 4 hrs, and say 6.5 mL/kg over 4 hrs when Hb is 6.5 g/dL.

PLATELET TRANSFUSION

Indications

A. *Neonates and infants ≤ 4 months:*
   - Platelet count less than or equal to 100,000/mm^3 and baby bleeding or clinically unstable or major surgery planned
   - Platelet count less than or equal to 50,000/mm^3 and minor invasive procedure planned/clinically unstable and/or bleeding
   - Platelet count less than 20,000/mm^3 and clinically stable
   - Any platelet count, if platelet dysfunction + bleeding or invasive procedure planned.

B. *Children (above 4 months) and adolescents:*
   - Platelet count less than or equal to 50,000/mm^3 and child bleeding or major invasive procedure planned
   - Platelet count less than or equal to 20,000/mm^3 and marrow failure with coexisting risk factors for hemorrhage (e.g. infection, clotting abnormalities, anemia, organ failure)

- Platelet count less than or equal to 10,000/mm^3 and marrow failure without hemorrhagic risk factors
- Any platelet count, if platelet dysfunction + bleeding or invasive procedure planned.

It is generally attempted to ideally raise the platelet count to greater than 50,000/mm^3 in children and greater than 100,000/mm^3 in neonates.

Usual Dose and Mode of Administration

- *For children < 30 kg:* 5–10 mL/kg of standard unmodified platelet concentrate (obtained either from whole blood units or by plateletpheresis). It raises platelet count by about 50,000/mm^3.
- *For older children >30 kg:* 4–6 pooled whole blood-derived platelet units (or 1 apheresis unit).

Rate of transfusion of platelets: As rapidly as patient's condition permits, maximum within 2 hours. Peak post-transfusion platelet concentration is reached 45–60 minutes after transfusion.

PLASMA TRANSFUSION

Plasma is separated from single units of whole blood by heavy spin or obtained from plasmapheresis and then frozen. The volume from a single donation is about 200 mL. Each bag of fresh frozen plasma (FFP) (200 mL approx.) contains 180–200 units of factor VIII and IX, factors II, V, VII, IX, X, XII and XIII.

Indications for Use

- Disseminated intravascular coagulation (DIC); with bleeding
- Bleeding due to rare inherited deficiency of factors II, V, X and XI. Plasma is the only available treatment in these cases.
- Mild bleeding* due to inherited deficiency of following hemostatic factors, when specific concentrate preparations are not available.

Hemophilia A and B, von Willebrand disease, deficiency of factors VII, X, fibrinogen and prothrombin and antithrombin deficiency.
- Severe liver disease—prophylaxis or control of bleeding
- Emergency reversal of warfarin effect
- Massive transfusion causing dilutional coagulopathy and bleeding
- Hemorrhage secondary to vitamin K deficiency in neonates.

*Large volumes of FFP needed to provide the required large amount of deficient factor VIII/IX in cases of severe bleeding in hemophilia A and B cannot be infused for fear of circulatory overload. In these cases, safer factors VIII, IX concentrates should be employed.

Dose and Mode of Administration

Usual dose: 10–15 mL/kg (in a single dose) at a rate not exceeding 10 mL/min.

CRYOPRECIPITATE

It is a protein precipitate obtained by freezing plasma fast and then thawing it at 4°C–6°C for 18–24 hours. Subsequently, plasma is separated by rapid centrifugation to form the precipitate which is refrozen and stored.

A single donor bag (10–15 mL approx.) contains about 80 units of factor VIII, von Willebrand factor, 200–250 mg of fibrinogen and fibronectin.

Indications for Use

- Hemophilia A and von Willebrand disease in the absence of factor VIII concentrates
- Dysfibrinogenemia, hypofibrinogenemia and consumptive coagulopathies.

- Congenital factor XIII deficiency
- Also useful in DIC with bleeding.

Note:
1. Children with severe hemophilia A and B and factor VII deficiency are ideally managed with specific factors VIII, IX and VII concentrates
2. Mild cases of hemophilia A and some cases of von Willebrand disease can be managed by administration of desmopressin.

Section 2

Immunization and Immunoprophylaxis

28: Active Immunization

ACTIVE IMMUNIZATION

In this process, an individual's immunity system is actively stimulated to produce antibodies and cellular responses through administration of a vaccine/toxoid, which will subsequently protect him against the respective infectious agent.

Vaccines Employed for Routine Immunization

Bacillus Calmette-Guérin (BCG), polio, hepatitis B, rotavirus, diphtheria, pertussis, and tetanus (DPT), *Haemophilus influenzae* type B (Hib), pneumococcal, measles, mumps, and rubella (MMR), hepatitis A, varicella, typhoid, and human papillomavirus (HPV).

Vaccines for Special Situations

Japanese encephalitis, influenza, meningococcal, rabies, and cholera.

IMMUNIZATION SCHEDULE

The routine immunization schedule recommended by Indian Academy of Pediatrics (IAP) 2014 is placed in Table 28.1.

Important Notes:
Polio Vaccine
- All doses of IPV may be replaced by OPV if IPV not feasible
- Additional doses of OPV on all supplementary immunization activities (SIAs)

Table 28.1: Indian Academy of Pediatrics (IAP) immunization schedule, 2014.

Age (completed weeks/months/years)	Vaccines
Birth	BCG, OPV0, and Hep B1
6 weeks	IPV1, Hep B2, DTwP1, Hib1, rotavirus 1, and PCV1
10 weeks	IPV2, DTwP2, Hib2, rotavirus 2, and PCV2
14 weeks	IPV3, DTwP3, Hib3, rotavirus 3, and PCV3
6 months	OPV1, Hep B3
9 months	OPV2, MMR1
9–12 months	Typhoid conjugate vaccine
12 months	Hep A1†
15 months	MMR2, varicella 1, and PCV booster
16–18 months	DTwP/DTaP B1, IPVB1, and Hib B1
18 months	Hep A2†
2 years	Typhoid booster
4–6 years	DTwP/DTaP B2, OPV3, varicella 2, and MMR 3
10–12 years	Tdap/Td, HPV

(BCG: bacillus Calmette-Guérin; DTaP: diphtheria, tetanus, and acellular pertussis; DTwP: diphtheria, tetanus, and whole-cell pertussis; Hep A: hepatitis A; Hep B: hepatitis B; Hib: *Haemophilus influenzae* type B; HPV: human papillomavirus; IPV: inactivated poliovirus vaccine; MMR: measles, mumps, and rubella; OPV: oral poliovirus vaccine; PCV: pneumococcal conjugate vaccine)
† Indicate different no. of doses of hepatitis A vaccine (1 dose for live, 2 doses for killed) described in text later.

Immunization in Certain Special Situations

- **Preterm/low-birth weight infants:**
    - *Bacillus Calmette-Guérin vaccine (BCG) and birth dose of oral poliovirus vaccine (OPV):*
    - Better give after stabilization at the time of discharge.
    - *Hepatitis B vaccine:*
        □ *Baby weight ≥2 kg:* Any time after birth
        □ *Baby weight <2 kg:* Delay till 1 month of age
        □ *Baby weight <2 kg; mother hepatitis B positive:*
            « *Hepatitis B vaccine + hepatitis B immune globulin (HBIG):* Within 12 hours of birth +

three doses of hepatitis B vaccine at 1 month, 2 months, and 6 months.
  - *All other vaccines*: As per chronological age.
- **Children on corticosteroids:**
  - *Oral corticosteroids high doses (e.g. prednisolone > 2 mg/kg/day or more than 20 mg/day or its equivalent for more than 14 days)*:
    - *Live viral vaccines*: Contraindicated till 1 month after withdrawal
    - *Killed vaccines*: Safe but may be less effective.
  - *Topical or inhaled steroids or lesser doses of oral steroids*:
    - Immunization as usual.
- **Children with asplenia or hyposplenia:** Immunize with pneumococcal, Hib, meningococcal, and typhoid vaccines in addition to all routine vaccines.
- **Missed immunization:**
  - No need to restart the whole schedule for the concerned vaccine; complete the usual course.
- **Vaccines for travelers:**
  - *Indians traveling abroad*:
    - *For those going on a Haj pilgrimage*: Meningococcal vaccine
    - *For destinations in South America and Sub-Saharan Africa (except infants < 6 months and pregnant)*: Yellow fever vaccine.
  - *Incoming visitors from North America, West Europe*:
    - *Typhoid vaccine*: 1 week before departure (one dose)
    - Hepatitis A vaccine before departure (one dose).
- **Immunization of human immunodeficiency virus (HIV)-infected children.**

The IAP recommendations for vaccination of HIV-infected children are placed in Table 28.2.

VACCINES

Bacillus Calmette-Guérin Vaccine

Time of administration: At birth—2 weeks; alternatively, at 6 weeks with other vaccines (till the age of 5 years).

If missed earlier, give as soon as possible

Section 2: Immunization and Immunoprophylaxis

Table 28.2: IAP recommendations for immunization of HIV-infected children.

Vaccine	Asymptomatic	Symptomatic
BCG	Yes (at birth)	No
DTwP/DTaP/TT/Td/TdaP	Yes, as per routine schedule at 6, 10, 14 weeks 18 months and 5 years	
Polio vaccines	IPV at 6, 10, 14 weeks, 12–18 months and 5 years. If indicated IPV to household contacts. If IPV is not affordable, OPV should be given	
Measles	Yes, at 9 months	Yes, if CD4 + count >15%
MMR	Yes, at 15 months and 5 years	Yes, if CD4+ count >15%
Hepatitis B	Yes, at 0, 1 and 6 months	Yes, four doses, double dose, check for seroconversion and give regular boosters
Hib	Yes, as per routine schedule at 6w, 10w 14w and 12–18 months	
Pneumococcal vaccines (PCV and PPSV23)	*PCV:* Yes, as per routine schedule at 6w, 10w, 14w and 12–15 months. *PPSV23:* One dose 2 months after PCV. Second dose five years after first dose (not more than two doses)	
Inactivated influenza vaccine	Yes, as per routine schedule beginning at 6 months, revaccination every year	
Rotavirus vaccine	Insufficient data to recommend	
Hepatitis A vaccine	Yes	Yes, check for seroconversion, boosters if needed

Contd...

Contd...

Vaccine	Asymptomatic	Symptomatic
Varicella vaccine	Yes, two doses at 4–12 weeks interval	Yes, If CD4 count ≥15% Two doses at 4–12 weeks apart
Vi-typhoid/Vi-conjugate vaccine	Yes, as per routine schedule	
HPV vaccine	Yes (females only), as per routine schedule of 3 doses at 0, 1–2 and 6 months starting at 10 years of age	

Dose: 0.05–0.1 mL (as per manufacturer's recommendation) intradermal (over deltoid region of left shoulder).

Special considerations:
- Bacillus Calmette-Guérin vaccine should be avoided in immunocompromised children. However, may be given to asymptomatic HIV children at birth.
- There should be a gap of 4 weeks between measles/MMR vaccine and BCG vaccine.
- If there is no reaction/scar following BCG vaccination, it may be repeated once in children <5 years of age.

Precautions: Store at 2–8°C. Protect from light. Use within 4 hours after reconstitution of the freeze-dried vaccine with sterile normal saline.

S/E: Local ulceration, regional lymphadenitis (uncommon) without or with suppuration/sinus formation. For its management: Surgical removal of the nodes or repeated needle aspiration, antitubercular therapy is not recommended. (*Tubervac 1 mL inj*: dose for under one month—0.05 mL; for over one month—0.1 mL)

Polio Vaccines

- Oral poliovirus vaccine
- Inactivated poliovirus vaccine (IPV).

Schedule of Administration

- *As per recommendation of IAP Advisory Committee on Vaccines and Immunization Practices (ACVIP), 2014:*

- *At birth*: OPV0.
- *6 weeks, 10 weeks, and 14 weeks (primary doses)*: IPV1, IPV2, and IPV3
- *6 months and 9 months*: OPV1, OPV2
- *15–18 months*: IPV (booster dose)
- *5 years*: OPV3
- *Additional on all supplementary immunization days*: OPV.

- *Alternative schedule*: If IPV not feasible, all doses may be replaced by OPV; rest as earlier.
- Two doses of IPV instead of three for primary series if started at 8 weeks, and give 8 weeks interval between the two doses
- The Government of India has recently directed one dose of IPV to be given with third dose of OPV in general immunization program.

Note:
- *Minimum age for IPV*: 6 weeks
- *Inactivated poliovirus vaccine catch-up schedule for children <5 years of age who have completed primary immunization with OPV*: Give three doses of IPV; two doses at 2 months interval followed by a third dose after 6 months of last dose.
- IPV can be combined with diphtheria, tetanus, pertussis, Hib and Hepatitis B vaccines

Contraindications to Poliovirus Vaccine

- Severe immunodeficiency (leukemia, solid tumors, and long-term immunosuppressive therapy)
- Severe HIV infection.

Note: The World Health Organization (WHO) recommends administration of OPV to asymptomatic HIV children and to newborn babies of HIV positive and negative mothers in developing countries.

[OPV: by Haffkine, Panacea, Aventis, GlaxoSmithKline (GSK), BE].

(IPV: (i) Movax, Biopolio, Evapol 0.5 mL inj; (ii) IPV + DPT + Hepatitis B + Hib (Easy six; and Hexaxim) IM inj 6 weeks,

10 weeks, 14 weeks; (iii) IPV + DPT+ Hib (Pentaxim IM inj) 6 weeks 10 weeks 14 weeks

Hepatitis B Vaccine

(Purified Surface Antigen of hepatitis B Virus; Recombinant or Plasma-derived)

Schedule of Hepatitis B Immunization

For infants born to hepatitis B virus surface antigen-negative mothers:

  Recommended schedule: 0 week, 6 weeks, and 6 months.
- It is recommended that the first dose of monovalent hepatitis B vaccine should be given within 48 hours of birth.
- The final third/fourth dose in the hepatitis B series should be given no earlier than age 24 weeks and at least 16 weeks after the first dose whichever is later.

For infants born to mothers whose hepatitis B virus surface antigen status is unknown:
- Give first dose of hepatitis B vaccine within a few hours of birth (to prevent possible perinatal transmission, if mother is hepatitis B virus surface antigen (HBsAg) positive).
  Follow-up dose: At 6 weeks and 14 weeks or 6 weeks and 6 months.
- Send mother's blood sample for assessment of HBsAg status. If mother is HBsAg positive, follow procedure as given below.

For infants born to hepatitis B virus surface antigen-positive mothers:

  Recommended schedule by the IAPCOI 2013–2014
- *At birth (within 12 hours)*: Hepatitis B vaccine (first dose) + HBIG 0.5 mL.

  The two injections should be given simultaneously IM at two separate sites. If not feasible along with hepatitis B vaccine, HBIG should be administered as soon as possible but no later than age 1 week.

- *Second dose of hepatitis B vaccine*: At age 1 month/6 weeks and *third dose* at age 6 months (Do not use closely spaced schedule).

When HBIG is not available or is unaffordable:
Hepatitis B vaccine at 0 month, 1 month, and 2 months + additional dose between 9 months and 12 months.

Hepatitis B vaccine immunization in preterm infants:
- *Weight >2000 g*: As for full-term infants.
- *<2,000 g*:
  - *Mother HBsAg negative*: Dose one at 30 days of age, doses two and three as per schedule for full-term infants.
  - *Mother HBsAg positive*:
    - *Hepatitis B vaccine + HBIG*: Within 12 hours of birth. Additional series of three doses of hepatitis B vaccine beginning at 4–6 weeks of age as per full-term infants basis (total four doses).
    - Check anti-HBs and HBsAg 1 month after completion of vaccine session.

Dose: Hepatitis B vaccines marketed by different manufacturers do not have a uniform dosage schedule, it is important to check the products' literature prior to its use.

Vaccines:
- *Engerix B, GeneVac-B,* and *Shanvac-B*:
  - *Children and adolescents up to 19 years*: 10 µg/IM
  - *20 years and above*: 20 µg IM.
- *Revac-B*:
  - *Pediatric dose up to 10 years*: 10 µg IM
  - *Above 10 years*: 20 µg IM.

Site of injection: Infants and young children: anterolateral aspect of thigh; older children and adults: deltoid region; not to be given in gluteal region.

(Engerix B, Bevac, Euvax-B, Enivac HB, Hepashield, Shanvac-B, Revac-B

Pediatric: 10 µg–0.5 mL inj, adult 20 µg–1 mL inj and 10 mL multidose vial).

Rotavirus Vaccines

For prevention of diarrhea in children due to rotavirus infection.

Either monovalent RV1 or pentavalent RV5 live rotavirus vaccines may be employed.

Human Monovalent Rotavirus Live Vaccine RV1

Age of administration and dose schedule:
- *Two doses:*
  - *Dose one:* At 6 weeks or 10 weeks; preferably at 10 weeks but not later than 14 weeks 6 days.
  - *Dose two:* 4 weeks after the first dose, but not later than 32 weeks.

Human Bovine Pentavalent Rotavirus Live Vaccine RV5

- *Three-dose schedule:*
  - At 6 weeks, 10 weeks, and 14 weeks
  - First dose not later than 14 weeks 6 days
  - Last dose not later than 32 weeks.

Contraindications for both RV1 and RV5 vaccines:
- History of severe allergic reaction after a previous dose of vaccine or to any component of vaccine.
- History of intussusception in the past or presence of uncorrected congenital malformation (such as, Meckel's diverticulum) which would predispose to intussusception.

Precautions: Postpone in a child with acute severe febrile illness, diarrhea, or vomiting.

S/E: Irritability, diarrhea, vomiting, fever, crying, rarely upper respiratory infection, and otitis media.

Rotarix Vaccine (Monovalent): 1 mL Oral; RotaTeq (Pentavalent 2 mL Oral).

Diphtheria, Tetanus and Pertussis Vaccines

For Active Immunization against Diphtheria, Pertussis, and Tetanus

Two types of DTP vaccine are available:
1. Diphtheria, tetanus toxoid with inactivated whole-cell pertussis vaccine (DTwP)
2. Diphtheria, TT with acellular pertussis vaccine (DTaP).

Primary Immunization Regime

Three doses at an interval of 4–8 weeks intramuscular (IM) over anterolateral aspect of thigh as per IAP Immunization Time Table I (2014), to be given at the age of 6 weeks, 10 weeks, and 14 weeks (along with IPV/OPV).

Boosters: At the age of 15–18 months and 5 years (the first booster should be 12 months after the primary immunization).

Subsequently: A dose of Td/Tdap is recommended at 10 years and 16 years of age followed by TT boosters at 10-year intervals thereafter.

Contraindications:
- Anaphylactic reaction to a previous dose of vaccine
- Encephalopathy within 7 days of previous dose of DPT
- Evolving or changing neurological disorder.

Precautions:
- *Temperature of more than or equal to 40.5°C (105°F) within 48 hours of a previous dose*
- *Collapse or shock-like state (hypotonic-hyporesponsive state) within 48 hours of a previous dose*
- *Persistent inconsolable crying lasting more than or equal to 3 hours within 48 hour of a previous dose*
- *Seizures within 72 hours of receiving a previous dose*
- *Guillain-Barré syndrome within 6 weeks after a dose.*

The benefits and risks of administering the vaccine under the earlier circumstances should be carefully considered. If benefits are believed to outweigh the risks, and it is decided to use the vaccine, the whole situation should be carefully explained to the relatives and their prior consent taken. It may

Chapter 28: Active Immunization

be preferable to use DPT with acellular pertussis vaccine in these situations.

Note:
- Diphtheria, pertussis, and tetanus vaccine should not be used in children beyond their 7th birthday (i.e. only through 6 years of age). Instead Td should be used for older children. DTP vaccine should be given to even those who are recovering from diphtheria and pertussis as natural disease does not offer complete protection.
- Diphtheria, tetanus, and acellular pertussis vaccines are not more efficacious than DTwP vaccines but have fewer adverse effects. On the other hand, priming with wP is now considered more effective at sustained prevention of pertussis than aP vaccines.
- The IAP now recommends that wP vaccine (DTwP) should be used for primary series immunization and not aP (DTaP) vaccine. First and second boosters should preferably also be of DTwP.
- The aP vaccine may be preferred to wP vaccine in children with history of severe adverse effects to wP vaccine and in children with neurologic disorders, if resources permit.

S/E: Local pain, induration, redness, mild fever, and irritability; other rare S/E mentioned earlier.

- *Diphtheria and TT with inactivated whole-cell pertussis vaccine:* Contents of DTwP (pertussis whole-cell) vaccine: Diphtheria toxoid 25 Lf, TT 5 Lf, *Bordetella pertussis* 20,000 million killed bacteria in each 0.5 mL (one dose) adsorbed on aluminum phosphate.
  Triple antigen—Serum Institute, GSK, Haffkine 0.5 mL single dose/5 mL vial.
- *Diphtheria and TT with acellular pertussis vaccine:* 0.5 mL dose contains pertussis toxoid 10 mg, filamentous hemagglutinin (FHA) 5 µg, filamentous fimbria (FIM) 5 µg, PRN 3 µg, diphtheria toxoid more than or equal to 30 IU (15 Lf), TT more than or equal to 40 IU (5 Lf), and adjuvants *0.5 mL single dose vial.*
  [Tripacel (Aventis Pasteur); Infanrix (GSK) contains diphtheria toxoid 30 IU, TT 40 IU, pertussis toxoid 25 µg, and FHA 25 µg].

Tdap Vaccine

(Tetanus Toxoid with reduced dose of Diphtheria Toxoid and reduced dose of Acellular Pertussis Vaccine)
Indications:
- Recommended for administration in children who have missed the second booster dose of DTwP/DTaP and are >7 years of age. It should be followed by Td boosters every 10 years.
- According to the Indian Academy of Pediatrics Committee on Immunization (IAPCOI) recommendations 2013–2014, one dose of Tdap should be administered to all adolescents aged 11 years through 12 years. This recommendation has been made on the assumption that the incidence of pertussis among adolescents and adults in India is significant

(Boostrix GSK; Adacel: Sanofi Pasteur).

Diphtheria-Tetanus Toxoid Vaccine

For active immunization against diphtheria and tetanus infection in children up to the age of 7 years when use of pertussis vaccine is contraindicated.
Children ≤7 years:
Dose: 0.5 mL IM (anterolateral aspect of thigh).
For older children above 7 years: Use Td vaccine with reduced dose of diphtheria toxoid (*see* below).
Contraindication: Children above 7 years (risk of adverse reaction due to high dose of diphtheria toxoid).
[Dual antigen (Haffkine) 10 mL vial; Serum Institute: single-dose amp; constituents per dose: diphtheria toxoid 50 Lf/25 Lf, TT 10 Lf; aluminum phosphate 3 mg; and thiomersal 0.01%].

Td Vaccine

(Tetanus Toxoid with Reduced Dose of Diphtheria Toxoid)
Indication: For catch-up immunization against diphtheria and tetanus in children above 7 years of age (in place of Tdap vaccine). Subsequently, a dose of Td vaccine every 10 years.

Contents: TT 5 Lf, diphtheria toxoid 2 IU (instead of 25–30 IU in DPT).

Tetanus Toxoid

For active pre-exposure immunization against tetanus:
- *Initial*: As a constituent of DTP vaccine during routine immunization of infants and children up to 7 years of age. Subsequently, one dose of TT/Td at 10 years and 16 years and thereafter TT/Td every 10 years.

  It is now recommended that after two doses of Td/TT at 10 years and 16 years of age, booster doses of TT/Td should be given at 10 years intervals to maintain adequate levels of neutralizing antibody. More frequent administration can cause accentuated adverse reactions, such as Arthus reaction due to very high serum antitoxin levels.
- *Unimmunized persons ≥7 years*: 0.5 mL IM once followed by second dose 4–6 weeks after the first dose and the third dose 6–12 months after the 2nd dose.
- *For previously unimmunized pregnant woman*: Two doses of TT at least 1 month apart; the second dose at least 2 weeks before delivery.

For tetanus prophylaxis in wound management: The schedule for tetanus prophylaxis in case of wounds among children with varied history of prior receipt of tetanus toxoid is indicated in Table 28.3.

Haemophilus influenzae Type B Conjugate Vaccine

Immunization Schedule

Primary schedule: For infants below 6 months
At 6 weeks, 10 weeks, and 14 weeks of age.

Booster: At 15–18 months.

Contraindication: Age below 6 weeks.

Table 28.3: Tetanus prophylaxis in wound management.

Prior tetanus doses received	Clean, minor wounds		Other wounds†	
	Tetanus toxoid (TT)	Tetanus immune globulin (TIG)*	TT/Td	TIG
Three or more doses	No (Yes, if > 10 years since last dose)	No	No (Yes, if > 5 years since last dose)	No
Uncertain or < three doses	Yes	No	Yes	Yes

Adapted from IAP Guidebook on Immunization 2013–14.

*Dose of TIG: 250 U intramuscular (IM) once (500 U IM once for highly tetanus-prone wounds or more than 24-hour old wounds)

†Other wounds, such as, but not limited to wounds contaminated with dirt, feces, and saliva; puncture wounds; avulsions; and wounds resulting from missiles, crushing, burns, and frostbite.

Note: The dose of TT required for immunoprophylaxis at the time of wound management should be suitably replaced by Td or Tdap in children ≥7 years of age/adolescents, in the light of their previous/desired immunization status.

Dose: 0.5 mL IM (anterolateral thigh or deltoid; not in gluteal region).

Catch-up schedule for Hib immunization is placed in Table 28.4.

Haemophilus influenzae Type B + Diphtheria, Tetanus, and Pertussis Combined Vaccines

For use when simultaneous immunization with DTP and Hib vaccine is desired

Two types of combinations are available:
1. *Whole-cell pertussis containing DTwP + Hib vaccine*: (TETRAct-HIB, Tetramune, and Easy Four).
2. *Acellular pertussis containing DTaP + Hib vaccine*:
    i. Diphtheria, tetanus, and acellular pertussis vaccine (Tripacel-Aventis) can be combined in the same syringe with Hib vaccine (ActHIB-Aventis).

Table 28.4: Catch-up schedule for Hib immunization.		
Age at first immunization	Number of doses	Age at booster
2–6 months	Three (1–2 months apart)	15 months
>6–<12 months	Two (1–2 months apart)	15 months[#]
12–15 months	One	16–18 months
15 months–5 years	One	Nil
Above 5 years	Nil[†]	Nil

[#]*A single booster dose is given at 15 months of age or later but not <2 months after the first dose. Previously unvaccinated children 15 months to 5 years of age receive only a single dose of the vaccine.*
Haemophilus influenzae type B (Hib) vaccine is, however, recommended for all children, irrespective of age, in children with functional/anatomic hyposplenia and in patients with sickle cell disease.
(Hiberix, ActHIB: 0.5 mL/vial containing 10 mcg PRP antigen of Haemophilus influenzae type b conjugated with tetanus protein; Hib titer IM: 0.5 mL/vial containing 10 μg of Haemophilus influenzae B saccharide, 25 μg of diphtheria CRM 197 protein conjugate).
Source: Adapted form IAP Guidebook on Immunization 2013-14 pg. 170 Publisher IAP National Publication House, Gwalior, 2014.

ii. Diphtheria, tetanus, and acellular pertussis vaccine (Infanrix-GSK) can be combined with Hiberix vaccine (GSK) to provide simultaneous administration of these vaccines through a single injection.

Note: Diphtheria, tetanus, and acellular pertussis + Hib combinations should not be used for primary series ordinarily and preferred only in certain specific circumstances.

Combined Diphtheria, Tetanus, and Whole-cell Pertussis + Hepatitis B Vaccine

(DTwP + Hepatitis B vaccine)
Children ≤6 years: 0.5 mL/dose IM.
Schedule of administration: As for DTwP and hepatitis B vaccine when proposed to be given simultaneously in special situation.

Contraindications and S/E: As for DPT and hepatitis B vaccine. *(Tritanrix HB 0.5 mL vial).*

Combined Diphtheria, Tetanus, and Whole-cell Pertussis + Hepatitis B + Haemophilus influenzae Vaccine type B (DTP + Hep B + Hib)

i. *"Easyfive"* 0.5 mL (single dose vial) IM;
ii. *"Pentavac"* 0.5 mL (Serum institute)
iii. *"Hiberix"* (Hib vaccine–GSK) can be reconstituted with *"Tritanrix HB"* (combined DPT + Hepatitis B vaccine–GSK) and administered through a single IM injection.

For mode of reconstitution to prepare combined vaccine, follow manufacturer's instructions

i. (Easyfive vaccine 0.5 mL contains diphtheria toxoid 20 Lf, tetanus toxoid 7.5 Lf, inactivated whole-cell pertussis 12 OU–12,000 × 10^6 organisms, HBsAg 10 μg, and Haemophilus influenzae type B 10 μg).
ii. DTaP + Polio + Hib (Pentaxim vaccine)

Combination of DTP, Hep B, Polio, H. Influenzae B

i. Diphtheria, Tetanus, Pertussis (Whole cell), Hepatitis B; *H. influenzae b and polio vaccine (inactivated)* (Easy six) 0.5 mL inj IM
ii. Diphtheria, Tetanus, Pertussis (acellular), Hepatitis B, *H. influenzae* b and polio vaccine (inactivated) (Hexaxim) 0.5 mL inj IM

Note about various combination vaccines:

The indications, precautions, contraindications, side effects and mode of use of different components of the combination vaccines have been described individually separately and these should be carefully considered while employing the combination vaccines.

Pneumococcal Vaccine

A. *Pneumococcal conjugate vaccines (PCVs):* There are two types of pneumococcal conjugate vaccines for active immunization of children from 6 weeks to 5 years of age, for the prevention of pneumococcal disease—PCV10 and PCV13. While PCV 10 provides protection against infection by 10 serotypes of pneumococci, PCV13 provides coverage against 13 serotypes.

The schedule for both PCV10 and PCV13 vaccines is placed in Table 28.5.

Routine use of PCV10/13 is not recommended for healthy children aged >5 years while the minimum age for administering first dose is 6 weeks.

Minimum interval between two doses:
a. In children age <12 months: 4 weeks
b. In children age >12 months: 8 weeks

(Prevnar 13; Synflorix 10-valent pneumococcal vaccine)

B. *Pneumococcal polysaccharide vaccine (PPSV23):* It provides protection against invasive pneumococcal disease and pneumonia in healthy adults and it is not recommended for routine use in children. Children with chronic heart and lung disease, diabetes mellitus, sickle cell disease and other hemoglobinopathies, asplenia and

Table 28.5: Recommended schedule for use of PCV13/PCV10 among previously unvaccinated infants and children by age at time of first vaccination.

Age at first dose	Primary series		Booster dose	
	PCV13	PCV10	PCV13	PCV10
6 weeks– 6 months	3 doses	3 doses	1 dose at 12–15 months*	1 dose at 12–15 months*
7–11 months	2 doses	2 doses	1 dose during 2nd year	1 dose during 2nd year
12–23 months	2 doses#	2 doses#	NA	NA
24–59 months	1 dose	2 doses#	NA	NA

Abbreviation: NA = not applicable; *At least 6 months after the third dose; #At least 8 weeks apart.

immunocompromising conditions are recommended administration of 1 dose of PPSV23 at age ≥ 2 years and at least 8 weeks after the most recent dose of PCV (conjugate vaccine) (Pneumo23 0.5 mL inj; Pneumovax23)

Measles Vaccine

Live-attenuated measles virus (Edmonston-Zagreb strain or Schwartz strain) vaccine.

For Active Immunization against Measles

Dose: 0.5 mL subcutaneous (SC) at 9 months of age (or older) in upper arm or anterolateral aspect of thigh.

Note: In epidemic situation, this vaccine may be given earlier to as young as completed 6 months. In such an event, a second dose of this vaccine (as MMR vaccine) should be given at 12–15 months of age (at least 4 weeks after the previous dose) and another MMR dose at 4–6 years.

Precaution: Measles vaccine vial can get contaminated with bacterial infection when the cap is punctured. Staphylococcal contamination can cause toxic shock in the recipient. Besides proper care, multidose measles vaccine vial must be discarded 4–6 hours after reconstitution.

Contraindication: *See* under MMR vaccine.

S/E: Short duration fever with or without rash 6–14 days later in 2–5% of the vaccinees.

[MVAC (live Edmonston-Zagreb strain measles virus); and RIMEVAX (live Schwartz strain measles virus) single dose vials].

Measles, Mumps, and Rubella Vaccine

Schedule of Administration

- *Schedule A*:
  - *First dose*: 9 months (when measles vaccine not given earlier)

- *Second dose*: 15 months (dose must during 2nd year).
- Third dose: 5 years (4–6 years)
- *Schedule B*:
  - *First dose*: 12–18 months (when received measles vaccine at 9 months)
  - *Second dose*: At 4–6 years of age (school entry) or at any time (8 weeks) after the first dose.

Note: The IAPCOI (October, 2014) now prefers schedule A and omission of stand-alone measles vaccine.

Catch-up immunization with a total of two doses of MMR vaccine (with minimum interval of 4 weeks between two doses) is recommended for those children/adolescents (especially girls) who have not earlier received any dose of MMR vaccine. Give one dose, if child had previously received one dose of this vaccine.

Contraindications:
- *Pregnancy*: Females should avoid becoming pregnant for 3 months after receiving rubella-containing MMR vaccine.
- Long-term immunosuppressive therapy, severe HIV infection, long-term high-dose corticosteroid therapy, and other states of severe immunodeficiency.
- Anaphylactic reaction to neomycin or gelatin.
- Untreated tuberculosis.

Precautions:
- At least 3 months gap after measles vaccine.
- Recent (within 3–11 months) administration of immune globulin or blood product administration. Check details for each product.
- Thrombocytopenic or history of thrombocytopenic purpura.

S/E: Fever and rash 6–14 days following the day of vaccination, cervical and occipital lymph node enlargement, parotitis, and purpura.

(Tresivac, Morupar single dose vial, Trimovax 10 dose vial).

Typhoid Vaccines

Unconjugated Vi-capsular Polysaccharide Vaccine

Children ≥2 years: 0.5 mL (containing 25 µg of polysaccharide) IM/SC single dose.

For maintenance of protection, revaccination with a single dose is recommended every 3 years.

S/E: Pain and swelling at injection site.

(Typhim Vi, Biovac Typhoid, Vactyph, and Typhivax—single dose inj and multidose vial).

Typhoid Conjugate Vaccine–(Typbar–TCV*)

Age of administration: Between 9 months and 12 months (minimum age 6 months).

A booster may be given during second year of life.

Precaution: Maintain an interval of at least 4 weeks either from before or after measles vaccine.

[Typebar—typhoid conjugate vaccine (TCV) by Bharat Biotech; 0.5 mL and 2.5 mL multidose].

Hepatitis A Vaccine

Killed hepatitis A vaccine

Schedule of routine immunization
First dose: At 12 months
Second dose: 6–12 months after the first dose
Indication in older children and adults
i. Hepatitis A virus (HAV)–seronegative patients with chronic liver disease
ii. For catch-up immunization

Dose:
The pediatric and adult closes of inactivated vaccines marketed by different manufacturers are not uniform. The drug literature of individual product must be consulted prior to its use.

1. Havrix vaccine (GSK): Inactivated IM
   Age >1 yr–18 yr: 720 ELU: Two doses: Second dose 6–12 months after first

Age ≥19 yr: 1440 ELU: Two doses: Second dose 6–12 months after first
2. Avaxim vaccine (Aventis pasteur) IM
   Age 1–15 yr: 80 units: Two doses: Second dose 6–12 months after first
   Age >15 yr and adults: 160 units: Two doses: Second dose 6–12 months after first

Route and site of administration
Young children: IM; anterolateral aspect of thigh, not in gluteal region; older children and adults: IM; deltoid region, not in gluteal region

[Havrix 720 U (0.5 mL inj), 1,440 U (1 mL inj); Avaxim pediatric 80 U, adult 160 U (0.5 mL inj)].

Contraindication:
Anaphylactic reaction to alum or 2-phenoxyethanol

Note: Better check hepatitis antibody level in children older than 10 years. If antibody present, no need for vaccine administration.

Combined Hepatitis A and Hepatitis B Vaccine

Twinrix Junior vaccine 0.5 mL = Inactivated HAV 360 EL U + HBsAg 10 µg.
Twinrix Adult vaccine 1.0 mL = Inactivated HAV 720 EL U + HBsAg 20 µg.

Dose and immunization schedule: As per manufacturer—GSK.
- *≥1–15 years*: 0.5 mL (junior vaccine) three doses at 0–1 months–6 months
- *≥16 years–adults*: 1.0 mL (adult vaccine) three doses at 0–1 months–6 months.

Contraindication: As for hepatitis A and hepatitis B vaccines.
(Twinrix vaccine junior 0.5 mL, adult 1 mL).

Varicella Vaccine

Live-attenuated Oka strain of varicella-zoster virus vaccine.

Schedule of administration

Children; First dose at 15 months*, second dose at 4–6 years. Dose: 0.5 mL SC

- *For catch-up immunization:*
  - *<13 years*: Two doses 3 months apart
  - *≥13 years*: Two doses 4–8 weeks apart.

Indications: The IAPCOI 2013–2014 recommends immunization with this vaccine to all healthy children with no prior history of varicella, it suggests special emphasis in the following categories of individuals:

- Children with chronic lung/heart disease, humoral immunodeficiencies, HIV infection (but with CD4+ counts above 15% of the age-related norms), leukemia (but in remission for at least 1 year), those on long-term salicylates/high-dose oral steroids, and to household contacts of immunocompromised children. Salicylates should be avoided for at least 6 weeks after vaccination. In those on high-dose steroids (≥2 mg/kg) for 14 days or more, the vaccine should be given only 4 weeks after stopping steroids.
- For postexposure prophylaxis to normal children within 3–5 days of varicella exposure. It prevents or modifies disease (Refer to VZIG for its role in postexposure prophylaxis in the following section).
- Nonimmunized adolescents leaving home for studies in a residential school/college, and children attending creches and daycare centers.

Precautions:

- *While any other vaccine (including measles-containing vaccine) can be given at the same time as the varicella*

The Indian Academy of Pediatrics Committee of Immunization (2013–2014) recommends varicella vaccine administration after 15 months of age instead of 12 months (as per recommendation of AAP, USA) as breakthrough infections are expected to be less if given at later age.

The American Academy of Pediatrics recommends the administration of varicella vaccine at or after 12 months of age.

vaccine, it is recommended that if not given simultaneously, there should be an interval of at least 1 month between administration of measles-containing vaccine and varicella vaccine. This is advised since measles vaccination may lead to short-lived suppression of the cell-mediated immune response and a higher risk of breakthrough disease.
- Pregnancy should be avoided for at least 4 weeks after vaccination.

Contraindications:
- Cell-mediated immunodeficiency, long-term immunosuppressive therapy.
- Human immunodeficiency virus infection with evidence of severe immunosuppression (CD4+ count less than 15%).
- Anaphylactic reaction to neomycin or gelatin.
- Pregnancy.

(Varilrix 0.5 mL injection single dose, Okavax one vial + ID).

MMR + Varicella Vaccine

This combined preparation of MMR and Varicella vaccines can be used as a single injection, when it is proposed to administer MMR and Varicella vaccines simultaneously, for example, at 15 months and 5 years of age.

(Priorix-tetra vaccine 0.5 mL inj, GSK).

Human Papillomavirus Vaccine

- *Bivalent vaccine*: "Cervarix" (HPV serotypes 16 and 18)
- *Quadrivalent vaccine*: "Gardasil" (HPV serotypes 16, 18, 6, and 11).

Indications

- Both vaccines for the prevention of cervical cancer and precancerous lesions caused by HPV types 16 and 18.

- Quadrivalent vaccine, in addition protects against anogenital warts, in both sexes; and against vaginal and vulvar cancer in females which are caused by HPV types 6 and 11.
- *Sex and age of administration*: Females; at age 9–14 years; if needed, at 15–18 years, latest by 45 years.

  It is advisable that vaccination takes place before sexual debut since the rate of HPV infection acquisition is high shortly after onset of sexual activity and the vaccine is effective prior to occurrence of infection. However, females who are sexually active should also be vaccinated.

Dose and Schedule of Vaccination

- *For girls 9–14 years*: Two doses at interval of 6 months of either Cervarix or Gardasil vaccine.
  - *Cervarix*: Two doses of 0.5 mL IM into deltoid region; at 0–6 months (second dose after 6 months).
  - *Gardasil*: Two doses of 0.5 mL IM into deltoid region; at 0–6 months (second dose after 6 months).
- *For girls 15 years and older and immunocompromised*: Three doses. Cervarix vaccine: 0–1–6 months (0.5 mL in vial for inj) Gardasil vaccine: 0–2–6 months

  All three doses with both vaccines should be completed within a 12-month period. The third dose should be at least 24 weeks after the first dose.

Precautions

The vaccine should be administered in a sitting/lying down position and the patient observed for 15 minutes pastvaccination as a precaution against syncope following administration of any vaccine in adolescents.

Contraindications

- Hypersensitivity to any vaccine component
- Avoid administration in pregnancy.

  [Cervarix bivalent vaccine (GSK); Gardasil quadrivalent vaccine (Merck)]

Influenza Vaccine

Trivalent and Quadrivalent Inactivated Influenza Vaccines

According to Indian Academy of Pediatrics Advisory Committee on Immunization, seasonal influenza vaccine administration is recommended only for high-risk children 6 months and older. These include children with chronic pulmonary disease (excluding asthma), heart disease, diabetes mellitus, renal dysfunction, hemoglobinopathies, HIV infection, and other immunosuppressive disorders.

For primary immunization:
- *Trivalent inactivated vaccine and quadrivalent inactivated vaccine:*
  - *Children 6–35 months*: 0.25 mL/dose IM × two doses, at least 1 month apart
  - *3–8 years*: 0.5 mL/dose IM × two doses, at least 1 month apart
  - *9 years and older*: 0.5 mL/dose IM single dose.

Subsequently: Single-dose IM annually before onset of rainy season, i.e. before October in South India and in rest of India before June as soon as the vaccine is released.

Note: In view of changes in the composition of influenza virus vaccine every year, current guidelines regarding dosage and schedule issued for their use for that year should be followed. (*Trivalent Vaxigrip, Agrippal, Flurarix, and Influgen*). (*Quadrivalent: Flu-Quadri*).

Meningococcal Vaccines

Protective vaccines with variable immunogenicity and efficacy are now available against A, C, Y, and W135 serotypes of meningococcal infection. There is no vaccine against serogroup B infection.
- *Meningococcal polysaccharide vaccines*:
  - A bivalent A and C, and
  - Quadrivalent A, C, Y, and W135 vaccine.

These are effective in children above 2 years of age. The duration of protection may vary between 1 year and 5 years. It tends to be less when first given to children below 4 years of age.

- *Conjugate (polysaccharide-protein) meningococcal vaccines:*
  - A quadrivalent ACY and W135 conjugate vaccine*, and
  - A monovalent serogroup A conjugate vaccine*.

*The quadrivalent vaccine is recommended only for children above 2 years of age, while monovalent group A conjugate vaccine can be administered to children above 1 year of age.

Indications

- *For protection of children during epidemic due to meningococcus A, C, Y, or W135 infection.*
  Since majority of outbreaks of meningococcal infection in India are caused by meningococcus A, monovalent vaccine is appropriate for mass immunization during them.
- *Routine immunization of following types of high-risk children, 2 years or older, with quadrivalent vaccine A, C, Y and W135 is desirable:*
  - Children with functional or anatomic asplenia, sickle cell anemia, and prior to splenectomy.
  - Those with deficiency of terminal components of serum complement (C5–C8) and properdin.
  - Children with HIV infection.

Dose and Mode of Administration

- Quadrivalent polysaccharide vaccine (Mencevax GSK; Qudri Mening, Biomed) 0.5 mL SC or IM.
- Bivalent A + C polysaccharide vaccine (MPV A + C, GSK; Bi Meningo Biomed) 0.5 mL SC/IM.
- Quadrivalent A, C, Y and W-135 conjugate vaccine (Menactra, Sanofi Pasteur) 0.5 mL IM.
- Monovalent conjugate group A (Serum Institute of India Ltd.) 0.5 mL IM for age group 1–29 years.

Contraindications

- Acute infections disease.
- History of severe reaction to previous dose of vaccine or its components.
- Pregnancy—unless the risk of acquiring disease is substantial.

S/E: Localized erythema and induration, occasional transient fever.

Rabies Vaccine

- Human diploid cell vaccine (HDCV)
- Purified chick embryo cell vaccine (PCECV)
- Purified duck embryo vaccine (PDEV)
- Purified Vero cell rabies vaccine (PVRV).

For Postexposure Prophylaxis*

The World Health Organization (WHO) recommendations for immunoprophylaxis in case of suspected rabid animal bites are placed in Table 28.6.

Schedule of administration

Rabies vaccine: 5 doses on days 0, 3, 7, 14, and 28.

Dose of PVRV is 0.5 mL/dose and of HDCV, PCECV and PDEV vaccines 1 mL/dose IM.

A sixth optional dose may be given on day 90 in patients with immunosuppression/severe debility.

Site of administration: IM in deltoid region; in small children may be given in anterolateral thigh. Not to be given in gluteal region

Human rabies immunoglobulin (HRIG) should be given along with vaccine, besides proper local wound care in all category III bites cases. For details regarding HRIG see under Chapter 29 on post-exposure prophylaxis

The Directorate General of Health Services (DGHS), Government of India has recently approved intradermal administration of two specific vaccines at selected centers (having large intake of animal bite patients) on a trial basis. It is not yet recommended in individual practice.

Table 28.6: Categories of rabies exposure and recommended post-exposure prophylaxis.

Category	Type of contact	Type of exposure	Recommended post-exposure prophylaxis (PEP)
I	Touching or feeding of animals. Licks on intact skin.	None	None, if reliable case history is available
II	Nibbling of uncovered skin. Minor scratches or abrasions without bleeding.	Minor	Would management + Anti-rabies vaccine
III	Single or multiple transdermal bites or scratches, licks on broken skin. Contamination of mucous membrane with saliva (i.e. licks)	Severe	Wound management + Rabies immunoglobulin + Anti-rabies vaccine

NB: Bites from unidentified animal is classified as category III.

Pre-exposure Prophylaxis

For laboratory personnel working in rabies research centers, veterinarians, dog catchers, zoo keepers, and medical staff treating rabies patients.

Dose: 1 mL/dose IM (deltoid region) × three doses on days 0, 7, and 28.
Boosters: One after 1 year and then every 5 years.
Side effects:
- *With HDCV, PCECV, Verorab, and PDEV:* Allergic reaction, malaise, fever, and local pain.
- *With nerve tissue vaccine (not recommended but still used in Government hospitals):* Neurologic abnormalities.

Preparations:
- *Vero cell vaccines: Verorab, Verovax-R, Abhayrab,* injection single dose vials

- *Chick embryo cell vaccine*: Rabipur injection vial (1 mL) single dose vial.
- *Duck embryo vaccine*: Vaxirab-single dose vial
- *Human diploid cell vaccine*: Merieux MIRV-HDC—single dose vial.

Japanese Encephalitis Vaccines*

Three types of Japanese encephalitis (JE) vaccines are licensed in India.

Indications for Use

- Presently only for individuals living in the rural areas of endemic districts. 180 endemic districts identified. Administration of this vaccine now being included in Universal Immunization Programme (UIP) in these districts by Government of India.
- **Live attenuated, cell-culture derived SA-14-14-2:**
  - *Minimum age*: 8 months
  - *Schedule*: First dose at 9 months (along with measles vaccine)
  - Second dose at 15–18 months (along with DPT booster).
- **Inactivated vero cell culture-derived SA-14-14-2 (JEEV by BE India):**
  - *Minimum age*: 1 year [United States Food and Drug Administration (USFDA) 2 months]
  - *Primary schedule*: Age 1 to ≤3 years: Two doses of 0.25 mL IM at interval of 28 days
  - *Age >3 years–adults*: Two doses of 0.5 mL IM at interval of 28 days.
- **Inactivated Vero cell-derived JE vaccine (JENVAC by Bharat Biotech):**
  - *Primary immunization minimum age*: 1 year
  - *Schedule*: Two doses of 0.5 mL IM at 4 weeks interval.

Catch-up Vaccination

All susceptible children up to 15 years of age during/ahead of anticipated outbreak in campaigns.

Source of information: Vashishtha VM, Choudhary P, Bansal CP, et al. IAP Guidebook on Immunization 2013-14, 1st edition. Gwalior: National Publication House; 2014. p. 312.

Cholera Vaccine

Killed whole-cell *Vibrio cholerae* O1 (classical and El Tor) and *Vibrio cholerae* O139 oral vaccine.

Indications for use: To be used in special circumstances, such as, where there is a risk of an outbreak (e.g. in Kumbh Mela); travel to or residence in a highly endemic area.

Children age >1 year.

Dose: Two doses 2 weeks apart.

Note: Protection starts 2 weeks after receipt of the second dose.

Duration of efficacy: About 67% across all ages for up to 2 years after vaccination.

S/E: No significant adverse effects have been noted.

(Shanchol: mfr Shantha Biotech)

Pre- and Postexposure Prophylaxis

IMMUNIZATION AFTER EXPOSURE TO DISEASE (IMMUNOPROPHYLAXIS)

Diphtheria: Exposure to Household Case

a. *Indications for giving DPT (diphtheria, pertussis and tetanus)/DT (Diphtheria and tetanus) or/Td (Tetanus and low dose diphtheria) toxoids.*
   i. Unimmunized, under immunized or unknown immunization status: Administer primary schedule as per age
   ii. Immunized individuals who have not received diphtheria booster in last 5 years. Give booster dose of vaccine as per age.

   Type of vaccine to be administered:
   Child younger than 7 years: DPT or DT; age 7 years or more: Td/Tdap (Tetanus and low dose diphtheria toxoids without/or with acellular pertussis vaccine)
b. *In addition, provide antimicrobial prophylaxis with* Erythromycin 40–50 mg/kg/day × 7 days PO (maximum 2 g/day), or
   Benzathine penicillin G 600,000 units IM single dose for children <6 years; for children 6 years or more: 120,000 units IM single dose.

Measles: Household, School or Other Exposure

Prevention/attenuation
a. *Susceptible children 6 months of age or older; within 72 hr of exposure;* measles vaccine

b. *Susceptible children exposure more than 3 days but within 6 days*: Immune globulin 0.25 mL/kg/IM for immunocompetent children and 0.5 mL/kg for immunocompromised (max. dose 15 mL).

This should be followed by administration of measles/MMR vaccine after an interval of 6 months or more.

Varicella

Steps for Postexposure Prophylaxis

i. *Newborn whose mothers develop varicella 5 days before to 2 days after delivery*: Give varicella zoster immunoglobulin (VZIG) 125 units (1 vial) IM as soon as possible for those weighing > 2 kg and 0.5 mL for those ≤2 kg.
ii. *Susceptible healthy children*: Varicella vaccine within 3–5 days of exposure (prevents or modifies disease)
iii. *Immunocompromised children, pregnant women and newborn*: VZIG as soon as possible but may be efficacious up to 10 days after exposure.

Dose: 125 units (1 vial) for each 10 kg increment, maximum 625 units IM.

Child < 2 kg: 62.5 units IM
2–10 kg: 125 units IM
10.1–20 kg: 250 units IM
20.1–30 kg: 375 units IM
30.1–40 kg: 500 units IM
> 40 kg: 625 units (max)

Pertussis: Household, Other Close Contacts, Day Care

a. *Antimicrobial prophylaxis (Table 29.1)*:
b. *In addition, ensure prophylactic immunization for children < 7 years of age as follows*:
   i. *Unimmunized*: Administer DPT vaccine and complete course

Table 29.1: Antimicrobial prophylaxis of pertussis.

Age group	Primary agents		Alternatives	
		Erythromycin	Clarithromycin	Trimethoprim/sulfamethoxazole
				Contraindicated below 2 months (risk for kernicterus)
Age group < 1 month	Azithromycin 10 mg/kg OD × 5 days	• Not recommended • Use if azithromycin not available 40–50 mg/kg div QID × 14 days	Not recommended	
1–5 months	10 mg/kg OD × 5 days	40–50 mg/kg/day div QID × 14 days	15 mg/kg/day div q BID × 7 days	< 2 months: contraindicated ≥ 2 months: trimethoprim 8 mg/kg day + sulfamethoxazole 40 mg/kg/day div q BID × 14 days
Infants ≥ 6 months and children	10 mg/kg/day single dose—day 1 (max 500 mg) Then 5 mg/kg/day (max 250 mg) × days 2–5	As above (max 2 g/day) × 14 days	As above (max dose 1 g/day) × 7 days	Trimethoprim 8 mg/kg/day + sulfamethoxazole 40 mg/kg/day div q BID × 14 days

Note: Erythromycin/azithromycin must be given promptly to all household and other close contacts regardless of age, history of immunization, and symptoms.

Table 29.2: Prevention of tetanus.

Prior tetanus doses received	Clean, minor wounds		Tetanus-prone wounds	
	Tetanus toxoid	Tetanus immune globulin (TIG)	Tetanus toxoid	TIG*
3 or more	Yes, if > 10 years since last dose	No	Yes, if > 5 years since last dose	No
<3 or uncertain	Yes	No	Yes	Yes

*Dose of TIG: 250 U IM once (500 U IM once for highly tetanus-prone wounds or more than 24-hr-old wounds)

ii. *Three doses taken, with last dose > 6 months earlier, or 4 doses taken with the 4th dose 3 years or more before exposure*: Give DPT booster dose.

Tetanus

Prevention in cases of wounds or bites (Table 29.2):

For details regarding dose etc. of "Tetanus toxoid" and "Tetanus immune globulin" see in the section on "Vaccines and Immunoglobulins".

Hepatitis A

- *For postexposure prophylaxis (when future exposure also likely)*
  Age ≥ 2 years:
  - *2 weeks or less since exposure*: Immunoglobulin 0.02 mL/kg IM and hepatitis A virus (HAV) vaccine
  - *> 2 weeks since exposure*: HAV vaccine
- *For pre-exposure prophylaxis (Table 29.3):*

Hepatitis B

- *For infants of hepatitis B surface antigen (HBsAg)-positive mothers:*

Table 29.3: Hepatitis A pre-exposure prophylaxis (for travelers to India from nonendemic areas).

Age	Duration of stay	Agent recommended
Age < 1 year	Expected < 3 mo	Immunoglobulin (IG) 0.02 mL/kg
	Expected 3–5 mo	IG 0.06 mL/kg
	Expected long term	IG 0.06 mL/kg (at departure); repeat every 5 mo thereafter
Age ≥ 1 year	Expected < 3 mo	IG 0.02 mL/kg or hepatitis A virus (HAV) vaccine
	Expected 3–5 mo	IG 0.06 mL/kg or HAV vaccine
	Expected long term	HAV vaccine

First dose of hepatitis B vaccine (3-dose schedule) at birth + hepatitis B immune globulin (HBIG) 0.5 mL IM within 12 hr of birth at a separate site.

- *Exposure to acute hepatitis B virus infection in susceptible case*
    - *Intimate contact, accidental needle exposure, accidental mucocutaneous exposure to infected blood*: Hepatitis B vaccine: At exposure, 1 and 6 months + HBIG within 24 hr of exposure 0.06 mL/kg IM (min dose 0.5 mL, max dose 5 mL)
    - *Household contact*: Hepatitis B vaccine at exposure, 1 and 6 months
    - *Casual contact*: No vaccine, no HBIG.

Rabies

World Health Organization (WHO) recommendations for immunoprophylaxis in case of animal bites are listed in Table 29.4.

Table 29.4: World Health Organization (WHO) recommendations for immunoprophylaxis in case of animal bites.

Category	Type of contact with suspected or confirmed domestic or wild rabid animal or animal unavailable for observation	Recommended treatment
I	Touching or feeding of animals, licks on unbroken skin	None if reliable case history is available
II	Nibbling of uncovered skin, minor scratches or abrasions without bleeding, licks on broken skin	*Administer vaccine immediately.* Stop treatment if animal remains healthy throughout an observation period of 10 days, or, if the animal is euthanized and found to be negative for rabies by appropriate laboratory technique
III	Single or multiple transdermal bites or scratches, contamination of mucous membrane with saliva (i.e. licks)	*Administer rabies immunoglobulin and vaccine immediately*.* Stop treatment if animal remains healthy throughout an observation period of 10 days, or if the animal is euthanized and found to be negative for rabies by appropriate laboratory technique

*Both vaccine and rabies immunoglobulin (RIG) should be given as soon as possible after exposure but if neither is available immediately, both can be given any time after exposure. However, RIG if not given initially should be administered within 7 days of the first dose of vaccine and not later.

Note 1: The details about use of 'rabies vaccine' have been described in preceding chapter 28 and about 'rabies immunoglobulin' in latter part of this chapter.

Note 2: Important steps in management of exposure to rabies

i. Clean the wound thoroughly with soap and flush under running water for 10 minutes.

Contd...

Contd...

ii. Next irrigate the wound with 70% alcohol or povidone iodine or some other virucidal agents.
iii. In all categories 3 wounds, infiltrate RIG into and around the wound. The dose of human rabies immunoglobulin (HRIG) is 20 U/kg body weight, max dose 1500 IU and that of equine rabies immunoglobulin (ERIG)—40 U/Kg BW, max 3000 IU; HRIG is preferable.
Inject the remaining dose of RIG into the deltoid region or anterolateral aspect of thigh away from the site of vaccine administration to avoid vaccine neutralization
iv. If RIG could not be given at the same time as first dose of rabies vaccine, it should be administered as early as possible but no later than the seventh day after the first dose of vaccine.

Note 3: See under rabies immunoglobulin and rabies vaccine for more details.

IMMUNOGLOBULINS AND ANTITOXINS

Anti-RhD Immunoglobulin

Prevention of Rh sensitization of unsensitized Rh-negative mothers
Dose: 300 µg IM single dose
Give within 72 hours of delivery of an Rh-positive infant, abortion, CV biopsy, amniocentesis
CI: Rh-positive mothers, RhD-negative mothers already sensitized
(Rhogam, Matergam-P 300 µg Inj., Vinobulin 100 µg, 300 µg vials)

Diphtheria Antitoxin

Dose based on duration of illness and extent of disease, not age of the patient
Pharyngeal/laryngeal disease less than 48 hr duration: IV 20,000–40,000 IU single dose
Nasopharyngeal disease: IV 40,000–60,000 IU single dose
Diffuse swelling neck/extensive disease more than 3 days duration: IV 80,000–120,000 IU.

Note: Test for hypersensitivity before antitoxin administration. Also, give erythromycin, penicillin-G or procaine penicillin for 14 days for eradication of infection.
[Diphtheria antitoxin (Haffkine) 10,000 IU/vial]

Hepatitis B Immunoglobulin

For prevention of hepatitis B virus infection

- *Infants born to HBsAg-positive women:*
  IM preparation of HBIG (100 IU in 0.5 mL): *0.5 mL IM, preferably within 12 hr of birth*
  First dose of 3-dose schedule of hepatitis B vaccine should be given IM simultaneously with HBIG at a different site.
- *Infants born to mothers whose HbsAg status is unknown:*
  Give Hepatitis B vaccine first dose within 12 hr of birth. Test maternal blood for mother's HbsAg status; if the HbsAg test is positive, give HBIG as soon as possible but no later than 1 week of age
- *Intimate contact with acute hepatitis B virus infection, accidental needle exposure, or accidental mucocutaneous exposure to infected blood:*
  IM preparation: HBIG 0.06 mL/kg IM (min dose 0.5 mL, max dose 5 mL)
  It should be administered within 24 hours (preferably within 6 hours) after exposure. In addition, give first dose of hepatitis B vaccine 3 dose schedule at a separate site.
  CI: Intolerance to human immunoglobulin
  [Hepabig, Hepaglob 0.5 mL (100 IU), 1 mL (200 IU) vials for IM use; Hepatect 2 mL amp (100 IU)]

Intravenous Immunoglobulin

Immunodeficiency Syndrome

100–400 mg/kg/dose every 2–4 weeks IV

Idiopathic Thrombocytopenic Purpura

800–1000 mg/kg/dose for 1–2 days for induction of response, maintenance dose 400–800 mg/kg/dose once every 4–6 weeks PRN IV

Kawasaki Disease

2 g/kg single dose over 10–12 hr IV or 400 mg/kg OD × 4 days.

Important: Follow scrupulously the instructions for administration as given in package insert for the specific product being used.

S/E: Fever, chills, hypotension, hypersensitivity reactions, anaphylaxis

(Sandoglobulin 3 g, 6 g, vials; Venimmun 500 mg vial; inj. 2.5 g, 5 g, 10 g Gamma IV 0.5 g, 2.5 g, 5 g vials; IV globulin 0.5 g, 1 g, 2 g)

Human Normal Immunoglobulin (Intramuscular)

i. For Measles Prophylaxis

The details regarding use of immunoglobulin and measles vaccine for measles prophylaxis have been given earlier in this chapter.

ii. For Hepatitis A Pre- and Postexposure Prophylaxis

The details regarding its use given earlier in this chapter.

iii. For Immunodeficiency

The use of intravenous immunoglobulin is recommended in this condition (see under intravenous immunoglobulin described earlier). If IM immunoglobulin is employed, its initial dose will be 1.2 mL/kg. Maintenance: 0.6 mL/kg q 2–4 weeks.

Important: Follow scrupulously the instructions for administration as given in package insert for the specific product being used

(Human normal immunoglobulin-Bharglob 10%, 16.5% solution Inj.; Intraglobulin F 5% solution 10 mL, 50 mL, 100 mL)

Rabies Immunoglobulin

Postexposure prophylaxis against rabies (in all cases of WHO category III bites*)

- *Human rabies immunoglobulin (HRIG)*
  Dose: 20 IU/kg: Infiltrate as much as possible of the full dose in the area around and into the wound. Inject remaining volume with a separate syringe and needle IM at a site distant from that of vaccine administration.
- *Equine rabies immunoglobulin (if HRIG not available)*
  Dose: 40 IU/kg: Administer as per procedure described earlier for HRIG

Note: Also see 'Rabies vaccine' (Chapter 28)

Precaution: Since equine rabies immunoglobulin can rarely cause anaphylaxis, test for patient's hypersensitivity before its administration.

- *Human rabies immunoglobulin:* Berirab P 300 IU (2 mL inj.), 750 IU (5 mL inj.); Imogam rabies 300 IU (2 mL vial)
- *Equine antirabies immunoglobulin:* Imorab 1000 IU (5 mL vial), Pars more than 1,000 IU (5 mL inj.)

Monoclonal Antibody against Respiratory Syncytial Virus

For protection of selected high risk children from serious respiratory syncytial virus (RSV) disease

- 115 mg/kg IM once a month (from just prior to and during RSV season)
- *CI*: Cyanotic congenital heart disease.

Tetanus Immunoglobulin

- *As a preventive measure after trauma:*
  - For contaminated wounds: 250 U/IM
  - If wound is highly tetanus prone or wound more than 24 hours old: 500 IU/IM.

---

*For information regarding category III bites and indications for use of rabies vaccine and rabies immunoglobulin see under 'Rabies' in section on 'Immunoprophylaxis'

- *As a part of treatment of tetanus*:
  Five hundred units of tetanus immunoglobulin (TIG) IM single dose (to neutralize tetanus toxin that is released from the wound into circulation before it binds at distant muscle groups): In case of severe disease, total dose up to 3,000–6,000 IU.
  [Tetglob (Human tetanus hyperimmunoglobulin) 250 IU, 500 IU, 1000 IU vials; Immunotetan 250 IU, 500 IU inj.]

Varicella Zoster Immunoglobulin

For prophylaxis against varicella in newborn, whose mothers develop varicella 5 days prior to and up to 2 days after delivery, postexposure prophylaxis, in immunocompromised children and pregnant women, and susceptible healthy children (Please see indications for postexposure prophylaxis under section on "Varicella" in this chapter).

Section 3

Poisoning

30 Nontoxic Household Products and Pharmaceuticals

NONTOXIC PRODUCTS

The following household products and drugs in common use are nontoxic. If ingested in small quantity, these do not cause any significant harm. They do not need any kind of treatment beyond observation for a few hours.

Pharmaceuticals

Antacids, antibiotics, oral contraceptives, corticosteroids, laxatives, and mercury of thermometer.

Cosmetics

Baby products, hair dye, hair oil, cologne, deodorants, eye makeup, mascara, lipstick, perfumes, and hand lotion.

Soaps, Detergents, and Others

Toilet soap, bath foam, bubble bath, hand and dish washing soap, shampoo, toothpaste, and shaving cream.

Household Products

Lead pencils, crayons, chalk, clay, ballpoint pen ink, fountain pen ink (blue, black), water colors, paint (without lead), matches, cigarettes, candles, household bleach, deodorizers, dehumidifying packets, shoe polish, artificial sweeteners, lubricating oil, silica gel, greases, adhesives, newspaper, toy pistol "caps", and house lizards discovered in food.

MODERATELY TOXIC

Nail polish and its remover (acetone), depilators, after shave lotion (alcohol), and skin lighteners (hydroquinone).

31 CHAPTER

Antidotes for Common Poisoning

ACETAMINOPHEN POISONING

Antidote: N-acetylcysteine

Children/adults: *PO*: Loading dose 140 mg/kg, followed by 70 mg/kg/dose q 4 hours for 17 doses.

Note: Give oral acetylcysteine solution diluted 1:4 in a soft drink or juice orally or through nasogastric tube.

Intravenous (IV): If patient cannot tolerate enteral therapy or if it is contraindicated [gastrointestinal (GI) bleed, bowel obstruction], give the drug by IV route.

Loading dose: 150 mg/kg (diluted in 5% dextrose) IV over 1 hour; *followed by* 50 mg/kg IV infusion over 4 hours, and then 100 mg/kg IV infusion over 16 hours (total dose 300 mg/kg over 20 hours).

S/E: Nausea, vomiting.
(Mucomix 20% solution: 1 mL, 2 mL, and 5 mL amp; Antifen 20% solution: 1 mL, 5 mL, and 10 ml amp).

ANTICHOLINERGICS POISONING/TOXICITY (ANTISPASMODICS, ANTIHISTAMINES, "DATURA", ETC.)

Antidote: Physostigmine

0.02 mg/kg/dose (maximum dose 0.5 mg) by slow IV push/intramuscular (IM) q 10 minutes until a therapeutic effect is seen (maximum total dose 2 mg).

S/E: May cause excess cholinergic effects; if so, control with atropine 0.5 mg subcutaneous (SC) for each mg of physostigmine just given.

ARSENIC* AND MERCURY POISONING

Drugs for Chelation

- *For parenteral therapy*: British anti-Lewisite (BAL) (for critically ill patients who cannot tolerate oral therapy).
- *For oral chelation therapy, 2,3-dimercaptosuccinic acid (DMSA) (succimer)*—When patient is stable enough to tolerate oral therapy and prolonged chelation is necessary.

British anti-Lewisite (Dimercaprol)

- *For mild/moderate arsenic poisoning*: 2.5 mg/kg/dose q 6 hours IM × 2 days; then 2.5 mg/kg/dose q 12 hours IM 1 day; and then 2.5 mg/kg/dose q OD IM × 10 days.
- *For severe arsenic poisoning*: 3 mg/kg/dose q 4 hours IM × 2 days; then 3 mg/kg/dose q 6 hours IM × 1 day; and then 3 mg/kg/dose q 12 hours IM × 10 days.

  Continue chelation therapy till 24-hour urinary arsenic levels falls to less than 50 µg/L. Give a gap of 5 days between courses of chelation.

- *For inorganic mercury poisoning*: 5 mg/kg IM × 1 day, then 2.5 mg/kg IM q 12–24 hours × 10 days.

  Continue chelation therapy till urinary mercury level falls below 20 µg/L. A gap of 5 days is recommended between two courses of chelation therapy.

2,3-Dimercaptosuccinic Acid; Also Known as Succimer and DMSA

10 mg/kg/dose q 8 hours PO × 5 days, then 10 mg/kg/dose q 12 hours PO × 14 days.

Continue chelation therapy till 24-hour urinary mercury level falls below 20 µg/L and urinary arsenic level falls below 50 µg/L. A period of 2 weeks between courses of chelation is recommended.

---

*Inorganic arsenic is present in pesticides, herbicides, dyes, and certain folk remedies.

Note:
- Oral (DMSA) may be used in addition to BAL or instead of BAL when prolonged chelation is indicated and patient is able to tolerate oral therapy.
- Supportive care is important in the management of arsenic and mercury intoxication besides chelation therapy. Emesis is not recommended after ingestion of inorganic arsenic and mercury salts. The use of activated charcoal may be of some help.

BENZODIAZEPINES POISONING

Antidote: Flumazenil

Initial dose: 0.01 mg/kg (maximum 0.2 mg) IV; over 15 seconds then 0.01 mg/kg (maximum dose 0.2 mg) IV every 1 minute to a maximum total dose of 1 mg or 0.05 mg/kg whichever is lower.

Caution: Avoid its use to counteract sedative effect of benzodiazepines employed for control of serious conditions like status epilepticus and intracranial hypertension as it may precipitate seizures.

β-BLOCKERS (PROPRANOLOL, ATENOLOL, AND OTHERS) POISONING

Antidote: Glucagon

Initial: 0.15 mg/kg bolus IV followed by 0.05 mg/kg/h infusion

S/E: Hyperglycemia, nausea, and vomiting.
(Inj. glucagon 1 mg, 10 mg/vial).

CALCIUM CHANNEL BLOCKERS (e.g. NIFEDIPINE, VERAPAMIL) POISONING

Antidote 1: Calcium Salts

Calcium chloride 10%: 0.2 mL/kg IV bolus.

Or

Calcium gluconate 10%: 0.6 mL/kg IV; repeat doses and IV infusion may be required.

Antidote 2: Insulin

Dose: 1 unit/kg bolus followed by infusion of 0.5–1 unit/kg/h IV.

CARBON MONOXIDE POISONING

Antidote: High Concentration Oxygen

100% oxygen till carboxyhemoglobin (COHb) levels fall below 10%.

CYANIDE POISONING

Antidotes: Amyl Nitrite, Sodium Nitrite, and Sodium Thiosulfate

- Amyl nitrite (crushable ampoule) or pearls to be inhaled for 15–30 seconds, then 30 seconds of each min.
- Sodium nitrite 3% solution 0.33 mL/kg IV over no less than 5 min, or slower if hypotension develops followed by
- Sodium thiosulfate 25% solution 1.6 mL/kg IV over 15 minutes. Sodium thiosulfate may be repeated every 30–60 minutes to a maximum of 50 mL.

DIGITALIS POISONING

Antidote: Digoxin-specific Fab Antibodies (Digibind)

Dose: One vial IV for each 0.6 mg of digitalis glycoside ingested (ingested dose may be estimated from serum level). As a rough measure, 10 vials if acute overdose, five vials if chronic overdose.

(Digibind 40 mg vial)

ETHYLENE GLYCOL AND METHANOL (ALCOHOL) POISONING

Antidote: Fomepizole

15 mg/kg load IV; followed by 10 mg/kg q 12 hours × 4 doses; then 15 mg/kg q 12 hours until ethylene glycol or methanol

level is less than 20 mg/dL. Dialysis is recommended if methanol level more than 50 mg/dL, acidosis, severe electrolyte disturbances; kidney failure; fomepizole is given q 4 hr during dialysis to prevent washout.

Monitor: Blood alcohol and glucose level. Maintain adequate urine output.

S/E: Nausea, vomiting, and sedation.

HEPARIN POISONING

Antidote: Protamine Sulfate

Potency as antidote: 1 mg protamine sulfate will neutralize 115 IU of porcine/90 IU beef lung heparin.

Dose to be administered:
- *Protamine administration soon after heparin*: 1.5 times the neutralizing dose indicated earlier.
- *Protamine administration within 0.5–1 hour*: One-half of earlier stated dose.
- *Protamine administration after 2 hours*: One-fourth of earlier stated dose.

Maximum dose: 50 mg IV, slowly over 1–2 minutes.

Monitor: Activated partial thromboplastin time (APTT).

S/E: Hypotension, hypersensitivity, and dyspnea.
(Inj protamine sulfate 1%—BE, Gland Pharma—5 mL amp; 10 mg/mL).

IRON POISONING

Iron Poisoning (Acute)

Antidote: Deferoxamine Mesylate (Desferal)

- *For severe cases (presence of significant clinical symptoms):* IV 15 mg/kg/h continuous infusion (maximum 6 g/24 h).
- *For mild cases:* IM 90 mg/kg/dose every 8 hours (maximum 6 g/24 h).

Ingestion of elemental iron more than 20 mg/kg produces gastrointestinal toxicity while more than 60 mg/kg induces systemic toxicity. For severe cases, continuous IV infusion should be continued until the patient is symptom free, signs of toxicity have resolved, and 24 hours after reddish color (vine rose) in urine disappears. Urine color change occurs due to deferoxamine-iron complex being excreted in the urine. It is, however, an unreliable indication of iron excretion

CI: Acute renal failure, primary hemochromatosis.

S/E of deferoxamine mesylate: Allergic reactions (including hypotension, rashes, itching, and flushing), abdominal pain, diarrhea, muscle cramps, fever, and dysuria. Lens and retinal changes on repeated use.

Chronic Iron Overload

(as with multiple, prolonged transfusions in Thalassemia major).

Antidote: Deferoxamine Mesylate (Desferal)

Subcutaneous: 20–40 mg/kg/dose (maximum 2 g/dose); as subcutaneous infusion over 8–12 hours (or 24 hours) × 5–6 nights/week. The infusion is given via portable battery operated infusion device.

Intravenous: 15 mg/kg/h infusion (maximum 6 g/24 h).

Note:
- Therapeutic index calculation prevents underdosing or overdosing with Desferal. It should be kept less than 0.025 at all times.

$$\text{Therapeutic index} = \frac{\text{Mean daily dose (mg/kg)}}{\text{Ferritin (µg/L)}}$$

- Give vitamin C 2–3 mg/kg PO at the time of Desferal infusion. It increases iron excretion by increasing availability of chelatable iron.

CI: Acute renal failure, primary hemochromatosis.

S/E: Local skin reactions at site of infusion, hypersensitivity (rare—fall in BP, flushing, and urticaria), ophthalmic toxicity, ototoxicity, pseudorickets type skeletal changes, platyspondylosis of the spine, and tendency to *Yersinia* spp. septicemia.

Antidote: Deferiprone

PO: 75–100 mg/kg/day divided q BID/TID/QID (100 mg/kg/day for gross iron overload).

S/E: Nausea, vomiting, arthropathy, neutropenia followed by agranulocytosis (reversible on discontinuation of therapy), and liver fibrosis after prolonged use (does not occur in hepatitis C virus-negative patients).

Note: Combined therapy (daily SC continuous deferoxamine 50 mg/kg/day + daily deferiprone 75 mg/kg/day) has been found to be safer and more rapid in successful reversal of cardiomyopathy in beta-thalassemia patients (Beatrix Wonke).

(Deferoxamine: Desferal 0.5 g vial injection, Deferiprone: Kelfer 250 mg, 500 mg cap).

ISONIAZID POISONING

Antidote: Pyridoxine

1.0 mg IV for each 1.0 mg of isoniazid ingested. Give 700 mg/kg; max 5g if amount of isoniazid ingested is unknown.

LEAD POISONING

Antidotes: Calcium Disodium Ethylenediaminetetraacetic Acid, British anti-Lewisite, 2,3-Dimercaptosuccinic Acid, and Penicillamine

- *For patients of lead poisoning with encephalopathy*: Ethylenediaminetetraacetic acid (EDTA) + BAL.
- *Lead poisoning with blood level more than 70 mg/dL but no encephalopathy*: EDTA + DMSA or BAL.
- *Lead poisoning with blood level between 45 mg/dL and 70 mg/dL*: DMSA or penicillamine.

Dosage and Duration of Therapy

- *Calcium disodium ethylenediaminetetraacetic acid*: 50 mg/kg/day as continuous 24-hour infusion or 1,000–1,500 mg/m^2/24 h IV (continuous or intermittent infusion) or IM divided q 6 h/12 h × 5 days.
- *British anti-Lewisite (Dimercaprol)*: 4 mg/kg/dose × 1 dose followed by 3–4 mg/kg/dose q 4 hours × 2–5 days.
- *2,3-dimercaptosuccinic acid (Succimer)*: 10 mg/kg/dose q 8 hours PO × 5 days, and then q 12 hours × 14 days.
- *D-penicillamine*: Initial 10 mg/kg/24 h × 2 weeks, increase slowly to 20–30 mg/kg/24 h divided q 12 hours PO × 10–20 weeks.

Note: Repeat chelation therapy if blood lead level rebounds to 45 mg/dL or greater but the interval must not be less than 3 days.

S/E of British anti-Lewisite: Injection site sterile abscess, vomiting, fever, hypertension, and nephrotoxicity.

S/E of ethylenediaminetetraacetic acid: Hypercalcemia, elevated blood urea nitrogen (BUN), acute zinc depletion, and nasal congestion; monitor urinary output strictly as chelated lead complex is nephrotoxic.

MERCURY POISONING

See under Arsenic and Mercury Poisoning.

METHANOL POISONING

Antidote: Fomepizole

(See under Ethylene Glycol and Methanol Poisoning).

METHEMOGLOBINEMIA

Antidote: Methylene Blue

Methylene blue antidote for drug-induced methemoglobinemia and cyanide toxicity:

1–2 mg/kg (0.1–0.2 mL/kg of 1% solution) IV slowly over 5–10 minutes, may repeat every 0.5–1 hour for severe cyanosis or methemoglobin more than 30%. Maximum 7 mg/kg.

CI: Renal insufficiency, glucose-6-phosphate dehydrogenase (G6PD) deficiency.

S/E: Vomiting, abdominal pain, bluish-green urine, and stools.

MORPHINE AND OTHER NARCOTICS OVERDOSE POISONING (PETHIDINE, PENTAZOCINE, AND OTHER OPIATES, e.g. HEROIN)

Antidote: Naloxone

Neonates and children:
- *Intravenous, IM, SC, endotracheal tube (ETT)*: 0.1 mg/kg/dose (maximum 2 mg/dose).
- May repeat every 2-3 minutes until desired response (maximum total dose 10 mg). Additional doses at 1-2 hours intervals PRN.

Adults: 0.4-2 mg/dose, may repeat every 2-3 minutes PRN.

Caution: May cause acute narcotic withdrawal symptoms (vomiting, sweating, tachycardia, tremulousness, and seizures in neonates addicted to opiates).

(Narcotan injection 20 µg/mL, 2 mL amp; 400 µg/mL 1 mL amp).

ORGANOPHOSPHATES POISONING (CHOLINESTERASE INHIBITOR INSECTICIDES)

Antidotes: Atropine/Pralidoxime

Atropine: 0.05 mg/kg IV every 5-10 minutes until full atropinization effect (when all secretions become dry); then every 1-4 hours; taper in the next 24 hours.

Pralidoxime (used with atropine for significant organophosphate poisoning): 20-50 mg/kg/dose IV (diluted to 50 mg/mL in normal saline); infuse over 15-30 minutes (maximum at the rate of 200 mg/min) or give 1M. May repeat after 1-2 hours if muscle weakness is not relieved and then q 10-12 hours as needed IV/IM.

(Pralidoxime available as Taurpam, Neopam, Meripam 500 mg in 20 mL vial/amp).

PHENOTHIAZINES AND METOCLOPRAMIDE TOXICITY (e.g. CHLORPROMAZINE, PROMETHAZINE, PROCHLORPERAZINE, TRIFLUOPERAZINE)-INDUCED EXTRAPYRAMIDAL REACTIONS

Antidote: Diphenhydramine

Initial: 1 mg/kg (maximum 50 mg) IV slowly over 2–5 minutes or IM, then 1 mg/kg/dose IM/PO q 6 hours for 48 hours (maximum dose 300 mg/24 h).

S/E: See under diphenhydramine.
(Benadryl 10 mg/mL vial).

Antidote 2: Benztropine (for Acute Dystonic Reaction)

- *Children > 3 years*: 0.02–0.05 mg/kg/dose PO/IM/IV 1–2 times/day.
- *Adults*: 1–4 mg/dose 1–2 times a day.

Note: For children < 3 years, use only for life-threatening emergencies.

PO: Administer with food to decrease GI upset.

Intramuscular/intravenous: Use IV only when oral or IM are not appropriate.

Onset of action: Oral: within 1 hour; parenteral: within 15 minutes.

Duration of action: 6–48 hours.

S/E: Tachycardia, orthostatic hypotension, gastrointestinal tract (GIT) upset, nervousness, and hallucinations.

SALICYLATES

Antidote: Sodium bicarbonate

Bolus: 1–2 mg/kg followed by a continuous infusion IV

Goal: Urine pH 7.5–8.0.

Follow potassium closely and repeat as necessary.

TRICYCLIC ANTIDEPRESSANTS

Antidote: Sodium bicarbonate.

Intravenous bolus 1–2 mEq/kg, repeat bolus doses as needed to keep QRS less than 110 msec.

Follow potassium level.

WARFARIN, DICOUMAROL POISONING/ TOXICITY

Antidote: Vitamin K1 (Phytonadione)

Infants and children: 1–2 mg/dose q 4–8 hours SC/IV; if life-threatening bleeding: 5 mg/dose IV.

Adults: 2.5–10 mg/dose SC/IV; PO: 2.5–5 mg/dose.

May repeat in 6-8 hours SC/IV. If given orally, may repeat after 12–48 hours.

Note: Rate of IV administration maximum 1 mg/min. Watch for hypertension and anaphylaxis especially when given intravenously

For more information, see under "Vitamin K1" in the section Pediatric Drug Formulary.

(Injection Kenadion 1 mg/0.5 mL, 10 mg/1 mL).

Medications Whose Single Dose may be Fatal for a Toddler

32
CHAPTER

The medications whose single dose may be fatal for a toddler are described in Table 32.1.

Table 32.1: Medications whose single dose may be fatal for a toddler.		
Medications[1]	Minimal potential fatal dose (mg/kg)	Maximal dose unit available (mg)
Oral hypoglycemics		
Chlorpropamide	5	250
Glibenclamide	0.1	5
Glipizide	0.1	10
Antimalarials		
Chloroquine	20	500
Quinine	80	600
Theophylline	8.4	600
Calcium channel blockers		
Diltiazem	15	180
Nifedipine	15	20
Verapamil	15	240
Antiarrhythmics		
Disopyramide	15	100
Procainamide	70	250
Quinidine	15	200
Narcotics		
Codeine	7–14	15

Contd...

Contd...

Medications[1]	Minimal potential fatal dose (mg/kg)	Maximal dose unit available (mg)
Tricyclic antidepressants		
Amitriptyline	15	75
Imipramine	15	75
Antipsychotics		
Chlorpromazine	25	200
Loxapine	30–70	50
Thioridazine	15	100

[1]*Assumptions:* Toddler would weigh 10 kg; the lowest described or estimated fatal dose (adjusted for body weight) was used; the toddler is healthy, with normal drug metabolism.

Source: Adapted from Bar-Oz B, Levichek Z, Koren G. Medications that can be fatal for a toddler with one tablet or teaspoonful: a 2004 update. Paediatr Drugs. 2004;6(2):123-6.

Note: Strength of maximal unit available (mg) of different drugs updated as per their availability in India now.

Section 4

Drugs in Pediatrics

33 Pediatric Drug Formulary

ANTIBACTERIAL DRUGS

Amikacin Sulfate

Aminoglycoside antibiotic:
- *Neonates*:
  - *> 2,000 g*:
    - ≤7 *days*: 7.5–10 mg/kg/dose q 12 h intravenous/intramuscular (IV/IM)
    - *> 7 days*: 10 mg/kg/dose q 8 h IV/IM
  - *1,200–2,000 g*:
    - ≤7 *days*: 7.5 mg/kg/dose q 12–18 h IV/IM
    - *> 7 days*: 7.5 mg/kg/dose q 8–12 h IV/IM
- *Children*: 15–22.5 mg/kg/day div q 8–12 h IV/IM
- *Adults*: 15 mg/kg/day div q 8–12 h IV/IM (maximum 1.5 g/day)

Caution: Adjust dose in patients with renal dysfunction. Loop diuretics (furosemide and bumetanide) enhance aminoglycoside-induced ototoxicity and nephrotoxicity. Central nervous system (CNS) penetration is poor beyond early infancy.

Side effects (S/E): Nephrotoxicity, ototoxicity, eosinophilia, and bone marrow suppression

(Inj Amicin, Amikef, Amitax, Mikacin, and Ivimicin 100 mg, 250 mg, and 500 mg 2 mL vial)

Amoxicillin

Aminopenicillin:

- *Infants > 3 months and children*: 25–50 mg/kg/day div q 8–12 h (maximum 1,500 mg/day) per oral (PO)
  - For treatment of acute otitis media (resistant *Streptococcus pneumoniae* infection)
  - 80–90 mg/kg/day div q 12 h PO
  - *For prophylaxis in recurrent otitis media*: 20 mg/kg/dose q HS
- *Adult*: 250–500 mg/dose q 8–12 h (maximum 3 g/day) PO

S/E: Rash and diarrhea

Caution: Increase dose interval in renal impairment cases
(Capsules: 250 mg and 500 mg; Novamox, Mox, Wymox, Lamoxy, and Blumox; DT: Novamox 125 mg and 250 mg; Wymox 250 mg; Lamoxy 250 mg, Blumox 125 mg, 250 mg, 500 mg; Tab: Novamox LB 250 mg and 500 mg; Mox 125 mg, 250 mg, and 500 mg; Wymox 125 mg and Lamoxy 125 mg; Syr: Novamox 125 mg and 250 mg/5 mL; Mox 125 mg and 250 mg/5 mL; Wymox, Lamoxy, and Blumox 125 mg/5 mL; Drops: Novamox, 100 mg/mL; Inj: Mox and Hipen; 250 mg and 500 mg)

Amoxicillin-clavulanic Acid

Aminopenicillin with Beta-lactamase Inhibitor

Dose based on amoxicillin component:

- *Oral*:
  - *Neonates and infants < 3 months*: 30 mg/kg/day q 12 h PO
  - *Children > 3 months*: 20–40 mg/kg/day q 8–12 h PO
  - *Children with otitis media (second-line drug)*: 80–90 mg/kg/day div q 12 h
  - *Adults*: 250–500 mg/dose q TID PO or 875 mg/dose q 12 h

Note: The above total daily dose can be given in two divided doses in the BID dose preparations of this drug.

- *Intravenous:**
  - *Premature and FT < 7 days*: 25 mg/kg dose q 12 h IV
  - *FT > 7 days–3 months*: 25 mg/kg/dose q 8 h IV
  - *> 3 months–12 years*: 25 mg/kg dose q 8–6 h IV
  - *Children >12 years and adults*: 1.2 g/dose q 8–6 h IV

Caution: Increase dose interval in patients with renal dysfunction

S/E: Diarrhea and skin rash.

[Enhancin, Augmentin Duo, and Clavam; 375 (250 + 125 mg), 625 mg (500 +125), and 1,000 (875 + 125 mg) tab; Enhancin, Moxclav, and Clavam (i) BD syr 228.5 mg (200 + 28.5 mg)/5 mL and (ii) 156.25 mg (125 + 31.25 mg)/5 mL syr; Augmentin Duo syrup 228.5 mg (200 +28.5 mg)/5 mL; and Enhancin DS 228.5 mg tab Enhancin, Augmentin, and Clavam inj. 1.2 g (1,000 + 200 mg), 600 mg (500 + 100 mg) and 300 mg (250 + 50 mg) inj vial]

Ampicillin

Aminopenicillin:
- *Neonates:*
  - See under 'dosage of antimicrobial agents in neonates', Chapter 34.
- *Children:* Mild-to-moderate infections
  - *PO*: 50–100 mg/kg/day div q 6 h (maximum PO 2–3 g/day)
  - *IM/IV*: 100–200 mg/kg/day div q 6 h
  - *Enteric fever PO*: 200 mg/kg/day div q 6 h.
  - *Meningitis, severe infections:* IM/IV 200–400 mg/kg/day div q 6 h (maximum IM/IV 12 g/day)

S/E: Diarrhea, rash, drug fever, and oral candidiasis
[Capsules 250 mg and 500 mg; Roscillin, Biocillin, Ampilin, and Campicillin].

*Note: IV preparation of the drug is not suitable for IM use. It should be used immediately after reconstitution and given IV slowly over 3–4 minutes. For administration as IV infusion, refer to drug literature

(DT: Roscillin DT 125 mg and Ampilin DT 250 mg; Syr Roscillin and Biocillin 125 mg/mL, 250 mg/5 mL; Syr Ampilin and Campicillin 125 mg/5 mL; Drops Biocillin, Roscillin, and Aristocillin 100 mg/mL; Inj Roscillin, Biocillin, Ampilin, and Aristocillin 250 mg, 500 mg vials).

Ampicillin-sulbactam

Aminopenicillin with Beta-lactamase inhibitor:
- *Children*: 100–200 mg/kg/day div q 6 h IM/IV
  - *Meningitis*: 200–400 mg/kg/day div q 6 h IV (maximum total dose 8 g/day of ampicillin)
- *Adults*: 1–2 g/dose q 6–8 h (maximum total dose 12 g/day) IM/IV.

Note: Dose based on ampicillin component

Caution: Increase dose interval in renal failure

S/E: Diarrhea, skin rash, drug fever, and injection site pain or thrombophlebitis

[Saltum 375 mg tab (ampicillin 220 mg + sulbactam 147 mg); kid tab 250 mg (ampicillin 146.6 mg + sulbactam 98 mg), inj 1.5 g vial (ampicillin 1 g + sulbactam 500 mg); and Sulbacin 375 mg tab, 1.5 g and 0.75 g vials].

Azithromycin

Macrolide antibiotic:
- *Children > 6 months*: 10 mg/kg/dose (maximum 500 mg) q OD PO × 3 days or 10 mg/kg/day (maximum 500 mg) q OD PO × 1 day; and then 5 mg/kg/day (maximum 250 mg) q OD PO × 4 days
  - *For streptococcal pharyngitis/tonsillitis:* 12 mg/kg/day div q OD × 5 days (maximum 500 mg/day)
  - *Typhoid fever:* 20 mg/kg/day (maximum 500 mg/day) div q OD × 7–14 days.
  - *Pertussis prophylaxis*:
  - *< 6 months*: 10 mg/kg/day q OD × 5 days PO

- *> 6 months*: 10 mg/kg/day (maximum 500 mg) q OD × 1 day PO, then 5 mg/kg/day q OD × 4 days PO.

Precaution: The drug should be taken on empty stomach at least 1 h before or 2 h after meals.

S/E: Gastrointestinal (GI) discomfort, elevated liver enzymes, and cholestatic jaundice.

(Azee—100 mg DT, 250 mg, 500 mg, and 1 g tab, Azithral Aziwok—100 mg KT, 250 mg, and 500 mg tab; Azee, Aziwok, and Zithrocin susp—200 mg/5 mL; and Azithral susp—100 mg/5 mL, 200 mg/5 mL).

Aztreonam

Monobactam antibiotic inhibitor:
- *Neonates > 2000 g*:
  - ≤7 *days*: 30 mg/dose q 8 h IM/IV
  - *> 7 days*: 30 mg/dose q 6 h IM/IV (*For more details see Table 34.1, Chapter 34*)
- *Children*: 90–120 mg/kg/day div q 6–8 h IM/IV

S/E: Diarrhea, rash, pancytopenia, eosinophilia, hypotension, and seizures

(Treonam inj 0.5 g, 1 g vials, Azenam, Aztres, and Trezam inj 0.5 g, 1 g, and 2 g vials)

Carbenicillin

Carboxypenicillin
- *Neonate > 2000 g*:
  - ≤7 *days*: 300 mg/kg/day div q 6 h IM/IV
  - *< 7 days*: 300–400 mg/kg/day div q 6 h IM/IV
- *Children IM/IV*: 400–600 mg/kg/day div q 4–6 h

Contraindications (CI): Hypersensitivity to penicillin

S/E: Phlebitis at IV injection site, platelet dysfunction, raised liver function tests (LFT), hypokalemia, and GI tract (GIT) disturbance.

(Carbelin inj 1 g and 5 g vial)

Cefaclor

Second-generation cephalosporin:
- *Children*: 20–40 mg/kg/day div q 8–12 h PO (maximum dose 2 g/day)
- *Adults*: 250–500 mg/dose q 6–8 h (maximum dose 4 g/day)

CI: Hypersensitivity to cephalosporins, cautious use in patients with penicillin allergy, and renal dysfunction

S/E: Vomiting, diarrhea, skin rash, eosinophilia, and serum sickness reaction

(Keflor, Distaclor DT 125, 250 mg tab; 125 mg/5 mL, 187.5 mg/5 mL susp, Keflor, Distaclor, Halocef 50 mg/mL drops; Keflor, Distaclor 250 mg cap; Keflor MR 375 mg, 750 mg tab; and Distaclor CD 375 mg tab and 500 mg cap)

Cefadroxil

First-generation cephalosporin:
- *Children:* PO—30 mg/kg/day div q 12 h (maximum 2 g/day)
- *Adults*: 1–2 g/day div q OD/BID (maximum 4 g/day)

Caution: Increase dose interval in renal impairment

S/E: As with cephalexin

(Droxyl, Cefadur, Cefoxid, and Kefloxin—125 mg, 250 mg DT and 500 mg tab, and Droxyl 250 mg/5 mL, Cefadrox, Cefadur, Kefloxin, and Kidrox—125 mg, 250 mg/5 mL susp; Cefoxid 125 mg/5 mL susp; and Cefadur, Kidrox 100 mg/mL drops)

Cefazolin

First-generation cephalosporin:
- *Neonates < 7 days*: 20 mg/dose q 12 h IM/IV
  > 7 days: 20 mg/dose q 8 h IM/IV

- *Children*: 50–100 mg/kg/day div q 8 h IM/IV (maximum dose 6 g/day)
- *Adults*: 2–6 g/day div q 6–8 h IM/IV (maximum dose 12 g/day)

Caution: Penicillin allergy. Also use cautiously with increase in dose interval in renal dysfunction.

S/E: Transient elevation of liver enzymes, phlebitis, leukopenia, and thrombocytopenia

(Cefazolin, Reflin inj 250 mg, 500 mg, 1 g vial)

Cefdinir

Third-generation cephalosporin:
- *Children 6 months to 12 years*: 14 mg/kg/day div q 12–24 h PO (maximum 600 mg/day)
- *> 12 years and adults*: 600 mg/day div q 12–24 h PO

Caution: Not recommended for infants below 6 months; reduce dose up to 7 mg/kg OD in patients with renal insufficiency (creatinine clearance < 30 mL/min)

S/E: Diarrhea, rash, vomiting, abdominal pain, and headache
(Adcef, Cefdiel, and Cefdinir 300 mg cap, syr 125 mg/5 mL)

Cefepime Hydrochloride

Fourth-generation cephalosporin:
- *Children > 2 months*: 100 mg/kg/day div q 12 h IM/IV (by infusion over 30 min)
  - *Serious infections and febrile neutropenic patients*: 150 mg/kg/day div q 8 h IV/IM
    Maximum dose: 6 g/24 h
- *Adults*: 2–4 g/day div q 12 h IV/IM (maximum 6 g/day)

Caution: Adjust dose (increase in dose interval and dose reduction) in renal impairment cases.

S/E: Vomiting, diarrhea, rash, thrombophlebitis, and headache

(Ceficad, Forpar, Ivipime 500 mg, 1 g inj vial)

Cefixime

Third-generation cephalosporin:
- *Children*: 8 mg/kg/day div q OD-BID PO (maximum 400 mg/day)
  - *Enteric fever*: 20 mg/kg/day div q 12 h PO
- *Adults*: 400 mg/day div q OD-BID PO

Caution: Use cautiously and reduce dosage in renal dysfunction patients

S/E: Nausea, abdominal pain, diarrhea, headache, and rash

(Zifi, Biotax, Topcef 100 mg, 200 mg DT tab, Zifi; Topcef, Xim, Taxim-O susp 50 mg/5 mL; Cefspan 100 mg/5 mL)

Cefoperazone

Third-generation cephalosporin:
- *Neonates*: 100 mg/kg/day div q 12 h IM/IV
- *Children*: 100–200 mg/kg/day div q 8–12 h IM/IV
- *Adults*: 2–4 g/day div q 8–12 h IM/IV (maximum 12 g/day)

Caution: Use cautiously in hepatic failure, biliary obstruction, penicillin allergy patients

Note: Not recommended for meningeal infection due to poor cerebrospinal fluid (CSF) penetration

(Myticef, Magnamycin 250 mg, 500 mg, 1 g, 2 g vial, Cefomycin 1 g, 2 g vial)

Cefoperazone-sulbactam

Third-generation cephalosporin with beta-lactamase inhibitor:
- *Children*: IV/IM 40–80 mg/kg/day (i.e. 20–40 mg/kg/day of cefoperazone) div q 6–12 h
  - *Maximum*: 160 mg/kg/day (i.e. 80 mg/kg/day of cefoperazone)
- *Adults*: 2–4 g/day (i.e. 1–2 g/day of cefoperazone) div q 12 h IV/IM

Note: Follow manufacturer's instructions regarding preparation of injection carefully. The use of this drug has not been extensively studied in premature infants and neonates

S/E: Diarrhea, vomiting, rash, eosinophilia, drug fever, and reversible neutropenia

(Sulbacef, Saltumex, Magnex 1 g, 2 g vial; 1 g vial contains 500 mg each of cefoperazone sodium and sulbactam sodium)

Cefotaxime

Third-generation cephalosporin:
- *Neonates*: > 2000 g:
  - < 7 *days*: 50 mg/dose q 12 h IV/IM
  - > 7 *days*: 50 mg/dose q 8 h IV/IM
  - < 2000 g: *see* "Dosage of antimicrobial agents in neonates" (Chapter 34).
- *Children*: 100–200 mg/kg/day div q 6–8 h IV/IM
  - *Meningitis*: 200 mg/kg/day div q 6 h IV (maximum 12 g/day)
- *Adults*: 1–2 g/dose q 8–12 h IM/IV (maximum 12 g/day)

Caution: Reduce dose in renal dysfunction patients

S/E: Rash, eosinophilia, neutropenia, elevated blood urea nitrogen (BUN), and liver enzymes.

(Taxim, Biotax 125 mg, 250 mg, 500 mg, 1 g vial; Omnatax, Claforan 250 mg, 500 mg, 1 g vial)

Cefotetan Disodium

Second-generation cephalosporin:
- *Children*: 40–80 mg/kg/day div q 12 h IM/IV
- *Adults*: 2–4 g/day div q 12 h IM/IV (maximum 6 g/day)

Caution: Increase dose interval in renal impairment patients

S/E: As with other cephalosporins

Cefoxitin Sodium

Second-generation cephalosporin:
- *Children*: 80–160 mg/kg/day div q 6–8 h IM/IV (maximum 12 g/day)
- *Adults*: 4–8 g/day div q 6–8 h IM/IV

Caution: Poor CSF penetration; reduce dose in renal failure

S/E: Similar to other cephalosporins

Cefpirome

Fourth-generation cephalosporin:
- *Children*: 100 mg/kg/day div q 12 h IV only
- *Adults*: 2–4 g/day div q 12 h IV only

Give prepared solution slowly IV over 3–5 min; or by infusion (1 g in 100 mL normal saline, Ringer's, 5% or 10% dextrose solution) over 20–30 minutes. Do not administer in sodium bicarbonate solution.

CI: Known allergy to cephalosporins

Caution: Previous hypersensitivity to beta-lactam antibiotic. Discontinue breast feeding if mother is receiving cefpirome. Adjust dose in renally impaired patients.

S/E: Overdosage may cause encephalopathy, may reverse following peritoneal dialysis and hemodialysis

(Forgen Inj 250 mg, 500 mg, 1 g vial; Bacirom inj 250 mg, 1 g vial; Tafron, Ceforth inj 1 g vial)

Cefpodoxime Proxetil

Third-generation cephalosporin:
- *Children > 2 months*: 10 mg/kg/day div q 12 h PO (maximum dose up to 12 years—400 mg/day)
- *Adults*: 200–800 mg/day div q 12 h PO

Caution: Poor CNS penetration; increase dose interval in renal failure

S/E: Diarrhea, nausea, vomiting, abdominal pain, and rarely hypersensitivity reactions

(Cepocor, Cepodem, Monocef O 100 mg, 200 mg tab, susp 50 mg/5 mL, 100 mg/5 mL)

Cefprozil

Second-generation cephalosporin:
- *Children*: 30 mg/kg/day div q TID/BID PO (maximum dose 1 g/day)

- *Adults*: 500 mg–1 g/day div q BID PO (maximum dose 1.5 g/day)

S/E: Rash, eosinophilia, headache, insomnia, diarrhea, vomiting, elevated liver enzymes, BUN, and serum creatinine (Refzil-0 tab 250 mg, 500 mg; susp 125 mg, 250 mg/5 mL).

Ceftaroline

Ceftaroline Fosamil

Fifth-generation cephalosporin:
- *Children < 6 months*: 24 mg/kg/day div q 8 h IV
  - *Weight < 33 kg*: 36 mg/kg/day div q 8 h IV
  - *Weight > 33 kg*: 400 mg/dose q 8 h IV
- *Adults*: 600 mg/dose q 12 h IV

Note: Safety and effectiveness in pediatric patients not yet established (Teflaro 600 mg or 400 mg ceftaroline powder in 20 mL vials)

Ceftazidime

Third-generation cephalosporin:
- *Neonates*:
  - *< 2,000 g < 7 days*: 100 mg/kg/day div q 12 h IV/IM
  - *< 2,000 g > 7 days*: 150 mg/kg/day div q 12 h IV/IM
  - *> 2,000 g 7 days or less*: 150 mg/kg/day div q 8 h IV/IM
  - *> 2000 g > 7 days*: 150 mg/kg/day div q 8 h IV/IM
- *Infants and children*: 100–150 mg/kg/day div q 8 h IV/IM
  - *Meningitis*: 150 mg/kg/day div q 8 h IV/IM
- *Adults*: 2–6 g/day div q 8–12 h IV/IM (maximum 6 g/day)

Special features: Good antipseudomonas activity and CSF penetration

Caution: Increase dose interval in renal failure (Fortum, Tazid 250 mg, 500 mg, 1 g vial)

(Inj C-zid, Fortum-ES, Tazid, Tizime 250 mg, 500 mg, 1 g)

Ceftibuten

Third-generation cephalosporin:
- *Children*: 9 mg/kg/day q OD PO (maximum dose 400 mg/day)
- *Adults*: 200–400 mg/day q OD PO

Note: Better give the drug on empty stomach, reduce dose in renal failure

(Procadex 400 mg cap, susp 90 mg/5 mL)

Ceftizoxime

Third-generation cephalosporin:
- *Infants > 1 month and children*: 150–200 mg/kg/day div q 6–8 h IV/IM (maximum dose—12 g/day)
- *Adults*: 1–2 g/dose q 6–8 h IV/IM (maximum dose 12 g/day)

Note: Good CNS penetration; increase dose interval in renal failure

S/E: As with other cephalosporins

(Ceftizox, 250 mg, 1 g vial; Eldcef 1 g vial)

Ceftriaxone Sodium

Third-generation cephalosporin:
- *Neonates*:
  - *2,000 g or less:* 50 mg/kg/day div q 24 h IV/IM
  - *> 2,000 g:* 7 days or less 50 mg/kg/day div q 24 h IV/IM
  - *> 2,000 g*: > 7 days—75 mg/kg/day div q 24 h IV/IM
- *Children*: 50–75 mg/kg/day div q 12–24 h IV/IM
  - *Meningitis*: 100 mg/kg/day div q 12–24 h IV/IM; maximum dose 4 g/24 h
- *Adults*: 1–4 g/24 h div q 12–24 h IV/IM; maximum dose 4 g/24 h

Note: Not recommended for use in neonates with hyperbilirubinemia; use cautiously in neonates, children with liver, gallbladder or pancreatic disease, penicillin allergy, or renal impairment.

S/E: Reversible gallbladder pseudolithiasis (emesis, right upper quadrant pain), rash, eosinophilia, GI intolerance, and leukopenia

(Becef, Cefaxone, Monocef, Oframax, Traxol 125 mg, 250 mg, 500 mg, 1 g vial)

Cefuroxime

Second-generation cephalosporin:
- *Cefuroxime sodium IV/IM:*
  - *Neonates*: 50–100 mg/kg/day div q 12 h IV/IM
  - *Infants and children*: 75–150 mg/kg/day div q 8 h IV/IM (maximum 6 g/day)
  - *Adults*: 750–1500 mg/dose q 8 h IV/IM (maximum 9 g/day)

Note: Use not recommended for meningitis due to poor efficacy. Administer IV slowly over 3–5 minutes at a maximum concentration of 100 mg/mL.

- *Cefuroxime axetil PO:*
  - *Children*: Suspension—20–30 mg/kg/day div q 12 h PO (maximum dose 500 mg/day; in otitis media 1 g/day)
    - *Tablets*: 125–250 mg/dose q 12 h

    Note: Cefuroxime axetil film coated tablets and suspension are not bioequivalent. Do not substitute on a mg/mg basis. Administer suspension with food
  - *Adolescents and adults*: PO 250–500 mg/dose q BID (tablets)

Caution: Penicillin allergy, increase dose interval in severe renal impairment

(Cefuroxime axetil tab—Zocef, Ceftum 125 mg, 250 mg 500 mg tab; susp Cefoxim, Widcef, Ceftum 125 mg/5 mL) (Cefuroxime sodium inj—Inj Zocef, Supacef 250 mg, 750 mg, 1.5 g vial)

Cephalexin

First-generation cephalosporin:
- *Children*: 25–100 mg/kg/day div q 6 h PO
- *Adults*: 1–4 g/day div q 6 h PO

For prophylaxis against urinary tract infection:
- Children: 10 mg/kg single dose HS

Note: Better administer on empty stomach; increase dose interval in renal failure; and some cross reactivity with penicillins

(Sporidex, Ceff, Sepexin, Phexin 250 mg, 500 mg cap, Kid tab 125 mg, DT 250 mg, Sporidex, Ceff syrup 125 mg/5 mL, 250 mg/5 mL, drops 100 mg/mL; Sepexin syrup 125 mg/5 mL; Phexin syrup 250 mg/5 mL, drops 100 mg/mL)

Chloramphenicol

Broad spectrum:
- *Neonates*:
  - *2000 g or less*: 25 mg/kg/day div q 24 h IV/PO
  - *> 2000 g*: 7 days or less 25 mg/kg/day div q 24 h IV/PO
  - *> 2000 g*: > 7 days—50 mg/kg/day div q 12 h IV/PO
- *Children*: 50–75 mg/kg/day div q 6 h IV/PO
  - *Meningitis*: 75–100 mg/kg/day div q 6 h IV (maximum dose 4 g/day)
- *Adults*: 50–100 mg/kg/day/ div q 6 h PO/IV (maximum dose 4 g/day)

Precaution: Risk of gray baby syndrome with too high dose in neonate; follow hematologic status; (risk of bone marrow suppression, and aplastic anemia)

(Chloromycetin, Paraxin, Enteromycetin 250 mg, 500 mg cap, susp 125 mg/5 mL, Paraxin inj 1 g vial)

Ciprofloxacin

Fluoroquinolone:
- *Neonates*: 20 mg/kg/day div q 12 h IV/PO
- *Children*:
  - *PO*: 20–30 mg/kg/day div q 12 h (maximum dose; oral 1.5 g, per day)
  - *IV*: 10–20 mg/kg/day div q 8–12 h; maximum dose: 800 mg/day

- *Adults*:
  - *PO*: 250–750 mg/dose q 12 h
  - *IV*: 200–400 mg/dose q 12 h

Note: Administer IV over 1 h at drug concentration of 1–2 mg/mL. Do not administer antacids with oral ciprofloxacin.

Caution: Use with caution in children < 18 years old (as with other quinolones) and in patients with seizure disorders; reduce dose in renal failure

S/E: Confusion, dizziness, skin rash, headache, epigastric distress, and rarely seizures

(Cifran, Ciplox, Ciprobid, Ciprolet 100 mg, 250 mg, 500 mg, 750 mg tab, inf 20 mg/10 mL (50 mL, 100 mL, 200 mL inf); Cifran OD, Ciplox OD, C-OD 500 mg, 1 g tab; Ciprolar susp 125 mg/5 mL; and Neocip susp 125 mg/5 mL)

Clarithromycin

Macrolide antibiotic:
- *Children*: 15 mg/kg/day div q 12 h PO
- *Adults*: 250–500 mg/dose q 12 h PO.

S/E: GI upset, abdominal cramps, and dyspepsia

(Crixan 250 mg, 500 mg tab, DT 125 mg, D. syr 125 mg/5 mL; Claribid 250 mg, 500 mg tab, D. syr 125 mg/5 mL; Clarie DT 125 mg, tab 250 mg)

Clindamycin

Lincosamide antibiotic:
- *IV/IM Neonates > 2000 g*:
  - *≤7 days*: 5 mg/kg/dose q 8 h IV/IM
  - *> 7 days*: 5 mg/kg/dose q 6 h IV/IM
    (For doses in neonates <2,000 g, *see* Chapter 34 "Dosage of Antimicrobial Agents in Neonates")
- *Children*:
  - *IV/IM*: 25–40 mg/kg/day div q 6–8 h
  - *PO*: 10–30 mg/kg/day div q 6–8 h

- *Adults*:
  - *IV/IM*: 1.2–1.8 g/day div q 12 h/6 h, (maximum 4.8 g/day)
  - *PO*: 150–450 mg/dose q TID/QID (maximum 1.8 g/day)

Caution: Administer slow IV over 30-60 min (infusion rate maximum 30 mg/min); rapid administration may cause hypotension and shock

S/E: Diarrhea, nausea, rash, pseudomembranous colitis, and bone marrow suppression

[Dalacin C 150 mg, 300 mg cap, inj 150 mg/mL (2 mL, 4 mL inj); Dalasearch 150 mg cap]

Cloxacillin

Penicillinase-resistant penicillin:
- *Children*: 50–100 mg/kg/day div q 6 h PO/IV
- *Adults*: 250–500 mg/dose q 6 h (maximum 4 g/day) PO/IV

Note: Give oral preparation 1 h before or 2 h after food

S/E: Nausea, rash, eosinophilia, and diarrhea

(Klox, Clopen, Bioclox 250 mg, 500 mg cap; Klox, Clopen syr 125 mg/5 mL; Klox, Bioclox inj 250 mg, 500 mg vials)

Colistin

(*Colistimethate sodium*: Polymyxin E)

For treatment of multidrug resistant Gram-negative organisms including *Pseudomonas aeruginosa* and *Klebsiella pneumoniae*
- *Children*: 2.5–5 mg/kg/day div q 6–12 hourly IV/IM
- *Adults*: 300 mg/day div q 6–12 hourly IV/IM

Caution: Neurotoxic, adjust dose for renal insufficiency

Precaution: Should not be administered concomitantly with polymyxins or aminoglycosides, its dose should be reduced in cases of renal dysfunction

S/E: Neurotoxicity (headaches paresthesia, ataxia), nephrotoxicity, respiratory insufficiency, and muscle weakness

(Injection xylistin, colinem, koolistin, 1, 2 and 3 million IU per vial).

Note: Colistin   1 mg = 13,333 units

2.5 mg = 33333 units

150 mg = 2 million units

300 mg = 4 million units

Cotrimoxazole

Trimethoprim-sulfamethoxazole

Dosage based on trimethoprim component:
- *Mild-to-moderate infections treatment:* 5–8 mg trimethoprim/kg/day div q BID PO
- *Pneumocystis carinii treatment:* 15–20 mg trimethoprim/kg/day div q 6 h PO
- *For prophylaxis in urinary tract infection (UTI):* 2–3 mg trimethoprim/kg/day OD PO or IV
- *For Typhoid fever:* 10 mg/kg/day div q 12 h
- *For prophylaxis against Pneumocystis carinii:* 10 mg trimethoprim/kg/day div q BID daily for 3 days in a week (maximum 320 mg/day)

Precaution: Not recommended for infants < 2 months

CI: Patients with glucose-6-phosphate dehydrogenase (G6PD) deficiency (can cause severe hemolysis); porphyria

S/E: Skin reactions (rash and Stevens-Johnson syndrome), blood dyscrasias, and renal or hepatic damage
[Bactrim, Septran, Ciplin, and Oriprim; Tab—trimethoprim 80 mg + sulfamethoxazole 400 mg; DS tab—trimethoprim 160 mg + sulfamethoxazole 800 mg; Susp—trimethoprim 40 mg + sulfamethoxazole 200 mg/5 mL; Bactrim, Septran Pediatric tab – trimethoprim 20 mg + sulfamethoxazole 100 mg; Inj Ciplin: (trimethoprim 160 mg + sulfamethoxazole 800 mg/3 mL) for IM use; Inj Oriprim IV (Trimethoprim 80 mg + sulfamethoxazole 400 mg/500 mL) for IV use]

Daptomycin

- *Children*: Dose not established yet
- *Adults*: 4 mg/kg/day OD IV

S/E: Rash, renal failure, anemia, headache, myopathy, and hypotension

(Cubicin 350 mg inj)

Demeclocycline

Tetracycline group antibiotic
- *Children*: 8–12 mg/kg/day div q 6–12 h PO
- *Adults*: 150 mg/dose q 6–8 h PO or 300 mg/dose q 12 h PO

Caution: Avoid in children below 8 years of age due to risk of permanent tooth staining.

S/E: Nausea, vomiting, diarrhea, and rarely diabetes insipidus
(Ledermycin 150 mg and 300 mg tab)

Doxycycline

Tetracycline derivative antibiotic:
- *Children > 8 years*: 2–5 mg/kg/day div q 12–24 h PO (maximum dose 200 mg/day)
- *Adults*: 100–200 mg/day

Precaution: Not recommended for children below 8 years (may cause tooth enamel hypoplasia and permanent staining)

S/E: Photosensitivity, GI upset, hemolytic anemia, and raised intracranial pressure (ICP)

(Doxy-1 mg, 100 mg, and 200 mg cap; Minicycline 100 mg cap, syr 25 mg/5 mL, 50 mg/5 mL)

Erythromycin

Macrolide antibiotic:
- *Neonates > 2000 g*:
  - ≤7 *days*: 20 mg/kg/day div q 12 h PO
  - *> 7 days*: 30 mg/kg/day div q 8 h PO

- *Neonates ≤2000 g and others: See* "Dosage of Antimicrobial Agents in Newborn," Chapter 34
- *Children*: 30–50 mg/kg/day div q 6–8 h (maximum dose 2 g/day) oral
  IV: 5 mg/kg/dose as infusion over 8 hr with normal saline or Ringer lactate or as intermittent bolus over 20–60 minutes every 6–8 h
   - *Pertussis and chlamydial pneumonia:* 40–50 mg/kg/day div q 6 h × (maximum 2 g/day) PO × 14 days
   - *Diphtheria:* 40–50 mg/kg/div q QID PO (maximum 2 g/day) × 14 days
   - *Rheumatic fever prophylaxis:* 500 mg/day div q 12 h PO

CI: Simultaneous use with terfenadine, astemizole, cisapride (may cause serious cardiac arrhythmias)

S/E: Nausea, vomiting, abdominal pain, and cholestatic jaundice (with use of estolate salt)

(Erythrocin 100 mg, 250 mg, 500 mg tab, Althrocin 100 mg tab, 125 mg KT, 250 mg, 500 mg tab, 250 mg DT; Eltocin 125 mg DT, 250 mg, 500 mg tab; Althrocin, Erythrocin susp 125 mg/ 5 mL; Althrocin, Erythrocin drops 100 mg/mL; Inj Erythromycin 1 g vial)

Furazolidone

Nitrofuran compound
Giardiasis:
- *Children*: 6 mg/kg/day div q QID PO × 7–10 days
- *Adults*: 100 mg/dose q QID PO × 7–10 days

S/E: Nausea, vomiting, dizziness, and headache

CI: Infants < 1 month, G6PD deficiency

(Furoxone 100 mg tab, susp 25 mg/5 mL)

Gentamicin

Aminoglycoside antibiotic:
- *Neonates*:
   - *> 2000 g*: ≤7 days—2.5 mg/kg/dose q 12 hourly IM/IV

- > 2000 g: > 7 days—2.5 mg/kg/dose q 8 hourly IM/IV
- ≤2000 g and others: *See* 'Antimicrobial Agents in Neonates', Chapter 34
- *Children*: 2.5 mg/kg/dose q 8-12 h IV/IM OR 5-7.5 mg/kg/day IM/IV div q OD
- *Adults*: 3-6 mg/kg/day div q 8 h or OD IV/IM

Caution: IV administration to be slow over 30-60 minutes; monitor renal function; increase dose interval in renal impairment patients

S/E: Ototoxicity and nephrotoxicity

(Genticyn, Garamycin 20 mg, 60 mg, 80 mg inj, Gentamicin, Laramycin 80 mg inj)

Imipenem-cilastatin

Broad spectrum antibiotic

- *Neonates*:
    - *> 2000 g; ≤7 days*: 20 mg/kg/dose q 12 h IV/ IM
    - *> 2000 g; > 7 days*: 20 mg/kg/dose q 8 h IV/ IM (for neonates ≤2,000 g *see* "Dosage of antibiotics in neonates", Chapter 34)
- *Children*: 60-100 mg/kg/day div q 6 h IV/IM (maximum 4 g/day)
- *Adults*: 2-4 g/day div q 6-8 h IV/IM (maximum dose 4 g/day)

Caution: Administer drug IV slowly over 30-60 minutes

S/E: Skin rash, seizures, hypotension, blood dyscrasias, and elevated LFT

(Inj Primaxin 500 mg, 1000 mg, 1500 mg containing imipenem 250 mg, 500 mg and 750 mg, respectively)

Kanamycin

Aminoglycoside; second-line antituberculosis drug:
- *Neonates*: *see* under section "Dosage of antimicrobial agents in neonates"

- *Children*: 15 mg/kg/day div q 8–12 h IM/IV (maximum 1 g/day)

S/E: Auditory, vestibular, and renal toxicity

Precaution and monitoring: When given IV, administer over 30–60 minutes, regularly monitor serum creatinine, auditory, and vestibular functions.

(Inj Kancin, Kanamac 500 mg, 1 g vial)

Levofloxacin

Antibiotic fluoroquinolone group:
- *Children*: 10 mg/kg/day div q 24 h PO/IV infusion (maximum 500 mg/day)
- *Adults*: 500–750 mg/dose q 24 h PO/IV

Precaution: Administer slow IV infusion over 60–90 minutes. Rapid infusion/bolus may cause hypotension

CI: Hypersensitivity, epilepsy; cautious use in patients with renal impairment, and children below 18 years.

(Levoflox, Loxof, Fynal, Glevo 250 mg, 500 mg, 750 mg tab, infn 500 mg/100 mL)

Lincomycin

Lincosamide antibiotic:
- *Children > 1 month*: PO: 30–60 mg/kg/day div q 6–8 h
  IM/IV: 10–20 mg/kg/day div q 12–24 h
- *Adults*: Oral 250–500 mg/dose q 6–8 h, IM/IV 600 mg/dose q 12–24 h

Precaution: Give IV lincomycin (300 mg/mL preparation) by slow infusion over 60 minutes. Rapid IV administration may cause hypotension and cardiac arrest.

Monitoring: LFT, renal function, and blood counts during prolonged therapy

S/E: Diarrhea, pseudomembranous colitis, stomatitis, serum sickness, vertigo, esophagitis, and aplastic anemia

(Lynx, Shelinc 250 mg, 500 mg cap, inj 300 mg, 600 mg; Lynx syr 125 mg/5 mL)

Linezolid

Oxazolidinone antibiotic:
- *Neonates < 7 days*: 20 mg/kg/day div q 12 h IV/PO
- *Neonates ≥ 7 days, infants and children*: 30 mg/kg/day div q 8 h IV/PO
- *Adults*: 1,200 mg/day div q 12 h IV/PO

S/E: Headache, nausea, diarrhea, myelosuppression, and pseudomembranous colitis

Monitoring: Monitor complete blood count (CBC), platelet counts and hemoglobin (Hb) during linezolid therapy especially when it exceeds 2 weeks or when there is pre-existing thrombocytopenia or myelosuppression

Caution: Do not mix any other medication with linezolid infusion while it is administered over 30–120 minutes.

(Linospan, Lizolid 600 mg tab, 200 mg/100 mL inf, 600 mg/300 mL inf; Lizomed susp 100 mg/5 mL)

Meropenem

Broad spectrum carbapenem antibiotic:
- *Neonates*: see Chapter 14 "Dosage of Antimicrobial Agents in Neonates"
- *Children*: 60 mg/kg/day div q 8 h IV (maximum dose 3 g/day)
  - *Meningitis*: 120 mg/kg/day div q 8 h IV (maximum dose 6 g/day)
- *Children > 50 kg and adults*: 1.5–3 g/day div q 8 h IV
  - *Meningitis*: 6 g/day div q 8 h IV

Note: Give IV as bolus over 5 minutes or by IV infusion over 15–30 minutes

CI: Hypersensitivity to carbapenems or other beta-lactam antibiotics

S/E: Diarrhea, rash, vomiting, headache, thrombocytopenia, neutropenia, and oral thrush

(Inj Meronem, Merocrit, Merotrol 500 mg, 1 g vial)

Mezlocillin Sodium
(*Antibiotic Class: Penicillin-ureidopenicillin*)

- *Neonates*:
  - 7 days or less 150 mg/kg/day div q 12 h IV
  - *> 7 days*: 225 mg/kg/day div q 8 h IV
- *Children*: 200–300 mg/kg/day div q 4–6 h IV
  - *Cystic fibrosis*: 300–450 mg/kg/day div 4–6 h IV
- *Adults*: 2–4 g/dose q 4–6 h IV (maximum 12 g/24 h)

S/E: Interferes with platelet aggregation, LFT results elevated, nausea, diarrhea, and edema

(Inj Mezlin)

Minocycline

Tetracycline derivative:
- *Children > 8 years*: 4 mg/kg/day div q 12 h PO (maximum 200 mg/day)
- *Adults:* Initial 200 mg, then 100 mg dose q 12 h PO

Caution: Not for children below 8 years

CI: Hepatic and renal dysfunction

(Cynomycin 50 mg, 100 mg cap; Nimolin 50 mg, 100 mg tab)

Nafcillin Sodium

Penicillinase-resistant penicillin:
- *Neonates*: *See* dose in section on Dosage of antimicrobial Agents in Newborn
- *Children*: IV/IM—50–200 mg/kg/day div q 4–6 h (maximum dose 12 g/day)
  PO: 50–100 mg/kg/day div q 6 h
- *Adults*: 4–12 g/day div q 4–6 h IV/IM

Caution: Oral route of administration is not recommended, since its absorption is highly variable and erratic. IM injection is very painful and it should be administered deep IM into a large muscle (gluteus maximus) using a solution containing 250 mg/mL.

Extravasation (during IV administration) may cause tissue sloughing and necrosis.

Precaution: Reduce dose in patients with severe renal and hepatic impairment.

S/E: Neutropenia, eosinophilia, elevated serum glutamic-oxaloacetic transaminase (SGOT), and skin rash

(*Nafcillin injection 1 g per vial*).

Nalidixic Acid

First-generation quinolone:
- *Children > 3 months*: 50–55 mg/kg/day PO div q 6 h PO
  - *Prophylaxis of UTI*: 30 mg/kg/day div q 12 h
- *Adults*: 1 g/dose q 6 h PO

CI: Infants below 3 months; porphyria, epilepsy, and G6PD deficiency.

S/E: Epigastric distress, pseudotumor cerebri, blood dyscrasias, skin rash, diplopia, vertigo.

(*Gramoneg, Enterodix 500 mg tab, susp 300 mg/5 mL; Ulix-P 150 mg, 250 mg tab*).

Neomycin

Aminoglycoside antibiotic:
- *Neonates*: 50 mg/kg/day div q 6 h
- *Children*: 50–100 mg/kg/day div q 6–8 h PO
  (*maximum dose:* 12 g/24 h, in hepatic coma cases)
- *Adults:* 500–2000 mg/dose q 6–8 h PO

Monitor: For nephrotoxicity and ototoxicity

(*Neomycin sulfate cap 350 mg*)

Netilmicin

Aminoglycoside antibiotic:
- *Neonate > 2000 g*:
    - ≤*7 days*: 2.5 mg/dose q 12 h IV
    - *> 7 days*: 2.5 mg/dose q 8 h IV
- *Neonate ≤2000 g*: see under Chapter 34 (Dosage of Antimicrobial Agents in Neonates)
- *Infants and children*: 2.5 mg/dose q 8 h IV or 5–7.5 mg/kg/day q OD IV
- *Adults:* 4–6 mg/kg/day; life-threatening infections: 7.5 mg/kg/day

Caution: Reduce dose and increase dose interval in renal impairment

S/E: Ototoxicity (tinnitus, nausea, and vertigo); nephrotoxicity

(Netromycin 10, 25, 50, 200, and 300 mg inj)

Nitrofurantoin

Urinary antiseptic:
- *Children > 1 month*: 5–7 mg/kg/day div q 6 h PO (maximum dose 400 mg/day)
    - *Urinary tract infection prophylaxis*: 1–2.5 mg/kg/day q HS PO (maximum dose 100 mg/day)
- *Adults*: 50–100 mg/dose q 6 h

CI: Infants below 1 month, G6PD deficiency, and severe renal impairment.

S/E: Dizziness, vomiting, rash, cholestatic jaundice, and hemolytic anemia.

(Furadantin 50 mg, 100 mg tab, susp 25 mg/5 mL).

Norfloxacin

Antibiotic; quinolone group:
- *Children*: 10–15 mg/kg/day div q 12 h PO (maximum 800 mg/day)
- *Adults*: 400 mg/dose q BID PO

CI: Hypersensitivity

S/E: Nausea, abdominal cramps, diarrhea, insomnia, and skin rash

(Norflox, Norbid, Norilet 100 mg DT, 200 mg, 400 mg tab; Flox 400 mg tab, susp 100 mg/5 mL); Bacigyl 400 mg tab; 100 mg/5 mL)

Ofloxacin

Quinolone antibiotic:
- *Children:* PO 15 mg/kg/day div q 12 h
  IV 5–10 mg/kg/day div q 12 h
- *Adults*: 400–800 mg/kg/day div q 12 h PO/IV

CI: Epilepsy, hypersensitivity to quinolones

S/E: Nausea, abdominal cramps, diarrhea, insomnia, skin rash, arthralgia, and neutropenia

(Zo 100, 200, 400 mg tab, Zanocin 100 mg, 200 mg, 400 mg, 800 mg tab, Tarivid, Supaxin, 200 mg, 400 mg tab, Oflomac 100, 200, 300, 400 mg tab, Tarivid infn 200 mg, 400 mg/100 mL Supaxin infn 200 mg/100 mL; Oflox, Zenflox 100 mg, 200 mg, 400 mg tab, susp 50 mg/5 mL; Zenflox Forte susp 100 mg/5 mL; Clofcin 50 mg/5 mL)

Oxacillin

Antistaphylococcal penicillin (beta-lactam antibiotic):
- *Neonates*
  - Postnatal age 7 days or less
    - *Weight 1,200–2,000 g*: 50 mg/kg/24 h div q 12 h IV
    - *Weight > 2000 g*: 75 mg/kg/24 h div q 8 h IV
  - *Postnatal* age > 7 days
    - *Weight < 1,200 g*: 50 mg/kg/24 h div q 12 h IV
    - *Weight 1,200–2,000 g*: 75 mg/kg/24 h div q 8 h IV
    - *Weight > 2000 g*: 1,000 mg/kg/24 h div 6 h IV
- *Infants*: 100–200 mg/kg/24 h div q 4–6 h IV

- *Children:* 50–100 mg/kg/24 h div q 4–6 h IV
- *Adults* 2–12 g/24 h div q 4–6 h IV (maximum 12 g)

S/E: Rash, GIT disturbance, hepatotoxicity, leukopenia, and thrombocytopenia

(Bactocill 1 g and 2 g vials—diluted with sterile water/0.9% sodium chloride to make solution 100 mg/mL)

Oxytetracycline

Group I tetracycline:

Children > 8 years: PO 25–50 mg/kg/day div q 6 h, IM 15–25 mg/kg/day div q 8–12 h

S/E: Same as with tetracycline

[Oxytetracycline 500 mg cap, inj 50 mg/mL (20 mL); Terramycin 250 mg, 500 mg cap, inj 50 mg/mL (10 mL)]

Pefloxacin

Quinolone group antibiotic:
- *Children*: 12 mg/kg/day div q 12 h PO
- *Adults*: 400 mg/dose q 12 h PO
  Adults IV: 400 mg/dose (by slow IV infusion) q 12 h

S/E: Nausea, skin rash, arthralgia, myalgia, insomnia, and thrombocytopenia

Special precautions: Avoid exposure to ultraviolet light during treatment due to risk of photosensitivity reactions.

(Pelox 200 mg, 400 mg tab, Pebact, Peflobid 400 mg tab, Pelox, Peflobid infn 400 mg/100 mL)

Penicillin G Aqueous

- *Neonates*:
  - > 2,000 g: 7 days or less 25,000–50,000 U/kg/dose q 8 h IV/IM (75,000–150,000 U/kg/day)
  - > 2,000 g: > 7 days—25,000–50,000 U/kg/dose q 6 h IV/IM (100,000–200,000 U/kg/day)

Neonatal meningitis:
- *> 2000 g: < 7 days*—300,000–400,000 U/kg/day div q 8 h IV
- *> 2000 g: ≥ 7 days*—400,000 U/kg/day div q 6 h IV
- *For neonates 2000 g or less see* Chapter 34 (Dosage of Antimicrobial Agents in Neonates)
- *Infants and children*: IM/IV 100,000 to 2,50,000 U/kg/day div q 4–6 h (maximum 400,000 U/kg/day)
- *Adults:* 2–24 million units/day div q 4–6 h IV or IM

CI: Hypersensitivity to penicillin

Precaution: Perform intradermal test of sensitivity before injecting penicillin

(Benzyl penicillin inj 5, 10 lac vial)

Penicillin G Benzathine

- *Treatment of asymptomatic congenital syphilis.*
  - *Neonate*: IM—50,000 U/kg single dose
- *Treatment of group A Streptococcal infection:*
  - *Children < 27 kg*: 600,000 U/dose IM single dose
    ≥ 27 kg: 1.2 million U/dose IM single dose
- *For Rheumatic fever prophylaxis (secondary):*
  - *Children < 27 kg:* 600,000 units IM every 3 weeks
  - *Children 27 kg or more*: 1.2 million units IM every 3 weeks

Caution: Do not administer this drug IV; may cause death due to cardiac arrest

S/E: Same as for penicillin G

(Penidure LA 6, LA 12, LA 24 containing penicillin benzathine G 0.6 million, 1.2 million, 2.4 million units per vial, respectively)

Penicillin G Procaine

- *Neonates*: 50,000 U/kg/dose q 24 h IM × 10 days (congenital syphilis cases)
- *Children*: 25,000–50,000 U/kg/day div q OD IM (maximum 4.8 million U/dose)

Caution: Not to be given intravenously

S/E: Similar to penicillin G

(Procaine penicillin inj 400,000 IU/vial)

Penicillin V Potassium

- *Systemic infection:*
  - *Children*: 25–50 mg/kg/day div q 6–8 h PO
- *Acute group A streptococcal pharyngitis:*
  - *Children*: 250–500 mg/dose q BID-TID × 10 days
  - *Adolescents and adults*: 500 mg/dose q BID-TID × 10 days
- *Rheumatic fever prophylaxis:*
  - *< 5 years*: 125 mg/dose BID PO
  - *≥ 5 years*: 250 mg/dose BID PO

Caution: Increase dose interval to q 8 h in severe renal impairment

S/E: Rash, eosinophilia, and allergy

(Kaypen 125 mg, 250 mg tab; Penivoral 65 mg, 130 mg tab; Crystapen 125 mg tab; susp Kaypen, Crystapen 125 mg/5 mL)

Piperacillin Sodium

Extended spectrum penicillin

- *Neonate*:
  - *≤7 days*: 50 mg/kg/dose q 8 h IM/IV
  - *> 7 days*: 50 mg/kg/dose q 6 h IM/IV
- *Children*: 200–300 mg/kg/day div q 4–6 h
- *Adults*: 2–4 g/dose q 4–6 h (maximum 24 g/day)

Precautions: IM injection painful; IV to be infused slowly over 30 minutes in concentration of 40 mg/mL; arrange minimum interval of 2 hours from any aminoglycoside infusion to avoid lowering of aminoglycoside serum level; increase dose interval if renal impairment; may give false positive Direct Coombs test and elevated alanine aminotransferase (ALT), aspartate aminotransferase (AST).

S/E: Eosinophilia, hemolytic anemia, neutropenia, and seizures

[Inj Piperacillin 2 g, 4 g (vials); Inj Piperapen 1 g, 2 g (vials)]

Piperacillin-tazobactam

Piperacillin with beta-lactamase inhibitor
Doses based on piperacillin content:
- *Infants < 6 months*: 150–300 mg/kg/day div q 6–8 h IV
- *Infants > 6 months and children*: 300–400 mg/kg/day div q 6–8 h (maximum 18 g piperacillin component/day) IV
- *Adults*: 12 g/day div q 6 h IV

Note: IV administration of drug to be done over 30 minutes at a maximum concentration of 200 mg/mL (piperacillin component)

Caution: Reduce dose in renal impairment

S/E: As with piperacillin

(Inj Tazar, Tazact, Zosyn 4.5 g vial contains piperacillin 4 g + tazobactam 500 mg)

Roxithromycin

Semisynthetic macrolide antibiotic:
- *Children*: 5–7.5 mg/kg/day div q 12 h PO
- *Adults*: 150 mg/dose q BID PO
  Maximum duration of treatment: 10 days

Caution: Use cautiously in hepatic insufficiency

S/E: Vomiting, epigastric pain, diarrhea, and rash

(Roxid, Roxee, Biorox, Roxisara, Roxeptin 50 mg, 150 mg tab, susp 50 mg/5 mL; Roxid, Biorox drops 25 mg/mL)

Sparfloxacin

Quinolone group antibiotic:
- *Children*: 4 mg/kg/day div q OD PO
- *Adults*: 200 mg/dose q OD PO

S/E: GI upset, skin allergy, insomnia, hallucinations, and convulsions

(Spardac 100 mg DT, 200 mg tab, Rexpar, Sparbact, Sparx 100 mg, 200 mg tab)

Streptomycin Sulfate

Aminoglycoside; antituberculosis drug
For treatment of tuberculosis: *See* section on "Antituberculosis drugs".

Sulfadiazine

- *Rheumatic fever prophylaxis:*
  - ≤30 kg: 500 mg OD PO;
  - > 30 kg: 1 g OD PO
- *Congenital toxoplasmosis:*
  - *Infants*: 100 mg/kg/day div q BID PO × 12 months
- *Toxoplasmosis:*
  - *Children*: 100–200 mg/kg/day div q QID PO

Note: Pyrimethamine and folinic acid are given along with sulfadiazine in the treatment of toxoplasmosis.

CI: Hypersensitivity to sulfonamides and porphyria

S/E: Rash, Stevens-Johnson syndrome, hepatitis, hemolysis in patients with G6PD deficiency, and leukopenia

(Sulfadiazine 500 mg tab)

Sulfamethoxazole-trimethoprim

See cotrimoxazole

Tetracycline

Children > 8 years: 25–50 mg/kg/day div q 6 h PO

CI: *Children < 8 years*. May cause retarded bone growth and permanent tooth discoloration

S/E: GI upset, stomatitis, rash, fever, and hepatotoxicity

(Hostacycline, Resteclin 250 mg, 500 mg cap; Achromycin inj IV 250, 500 mg; inj IM 100 mg)

Ticarcillin Disodium

Extended spectrum penicillin:
- *Neonates*:
  - > 2,000 g: ≤7 days—75 mg/dose q 8 h IV/IM
  - > 2,000 g: > 7 days—75 mg/dose q 6 h IV/IM
  - ≤ 2,000 g: *See* Chapter 34 (Dosage of Antimicrobial Agents in Neonates)
- *Infants and children*: 200–300 mg/kg/day div q 4–6 h IV/IM
- *Adults*: 2–4 g/dose q 4–6 h (maximum 24 g/day) IV

S/E: Bleeding diathesis (decreased platelet aggregation), elevated LFT, allergy, hypernatremia, and hypokalemia

(Inj Ticar 1 g, 3 g, 5 g/vial)

Ticarcillin-clavulanate

Penicillin + β-lactamase inhibitor
Dosage based on ticarcillin component:
- *Term neonates and infants < 3 months*: 200–300 mg/kg/day div q 6–8 h IV
- *Infants > 3 months and children*: 200–300 mg/kg/day div q 4–6 h IV
- *Adults*: 3 g/dose q 4–6 h (maximum 18–24 g/day) IV

Note: Administer by IV infusion over 30 minutes, preferred concentration less than or equal to 50 mg/mL. Must give a gap of 30–60 minutes between it and aminoglycoside administration (if latter required)

S/E: Rash, eosinophilia, raised LFT, and reduced platelet aggregation

[Inj Timentin–(ticarcillin 300 mg + clavulanate 100 mg)]

Tobramycin

Aminoglycoside antibiotic:
- *Neonates*:
  - > 2,000 g: ≤ 7 days—2.5 mg/kg/dose q 12 h IV/IM
  - > 2,000 g: > 7 days—2.5 mg/kg/dose q 8 h IV/IM
  - ≤ 2,000 g: *See* Chapter 34 (Dosage of Antimicrobial Agents in Neonates)
- *Children*: 6–7.5 mg/kg/day div q 8 h IV/IM (maximum 300 mg/day)
- *Adults*: 3–6 mg/kg/day div q 8 h IV/IM

Caution: Increase dose interval in patients with renal dysfunction

S/E: Nephrotoxicity, ototoxicity (vestibular/cochlear), and allergy

(Tobacin, Tobraneg 20 mg, 60 mg, 80 mg vial)

Vancomycin

Glycopeptide antibiotic:
- *Neonates*:
  - > 2,000 g: ≤ 7 days—15 mg/kg/dose q 12 h IV
  - > 2,000 g: > 7 days—15 mg/kg/dose q 8 h IV
  - ≤ 2,000 g: *See* Chapter 34 (Dosage of Antimicrobial Agents in Neonates)
- *Children*:
  - *IV*: General infections—40 mg/kg/day div q 6 h
  - *IV*: Staphylococcal meningitis and osteomyelitis; penicillin resistant pneumococcal meningitis—60 mg/kg/day div q 6 h (maximum 1 g/dose)
  - *PO*: *Clostridium difficile* associated colitis—40–50 mg/kg/day (maximum 2 g/day) div q 6 h
- *Adults*:
  - *IV*: 0.5 g/dose q 6 h (maximum dose 4 g/day)
  - *PO*: *C. difficile* associated colitis—0.5–2 g/day div q 6 h

Precautions: Infuse IV over 60 minutes (or slower) rapid IV infusion causes flushing of face (red man syndrome), fever, chills, and phlebitis. Do not use oral preparation for systemic infection since it is not absorbed.

Special indications: Vancomycin IV use especially indicated for penicillin and third-generation cephalosporin resistant *S. pneumoniae* infections and methicillin resistant staphylococcal infections.

S/E: Phlebitis, red man syndrome, ototoxicity, nephrotoxicity, and neutropenia.

(Vancogen, Vancorim, Forstaf 500 mg vial, Vancocin-CP 150 mg tab, 500 mg vial inj)

ANTITUBERCULOSIS DRUGS–FIRST LINE

Isoniazid

Antituberculosis drug:
- *Daily dose regimen*: 10* mg/kg/day div q OD PO (maximum 300 mg/day)
- *Intermittent therapy*: 15** mg/kg/day thrice weekly (maximum 600 mg/dose)

*The dose to be rounded off to the next higher dose, never less

**10 mg/kg/day as recommended under Revised National Tuberculosis Program, Government of India

Caution: If clinical jaundice and hepatomegaly develop during treatment, stop the drug (along with rifampicin and pyrazinamide). Start streptomycin and ethambutol. When serum glutamic pyruvate transaminase (SGPT) returns to near normal (usually 2–4 weeks), restart isoniazid at 5 mg/kg. Continue streptomycin and ethambutol. If no deterioration, restart rifampicin after 1 week. If tolerated, stop streptomycin and ethambutol. (If the child was earlier on pyrazinamide, restart it after 1 week to complete its course).

CI: Hepatic damage

S/E: Hepatotoxicity, rash, and peripheral neuropathy (uncommon in children); rarely giddiness, optic neuritis, psychosis, convulsions, and hematologic abnormalities

Note: In the opinion of members of Indian Academy of Pediatrics (IAP) Working Group on Childhood Tuberculosis (1997) pyridoxine supplementation is not necessary in children taking INH

(Isonex, Isokin 100 mg, 300 mg tab; syr Isokin, Ipcazide, Siozide 100 mg/5 mL)

Rifampicin

Antimycobacterial drug:
- *For treatment of tuberculosis:*
    - *Dose (daily regimen)*: 10 mg/kg/day div q OD PO (maximum 600 mg/day)
    - *Dose (thrice-weekly regimen):* 15* mg/kg/day div q OD PO, maximum 600 mg/day (three times/week)
    (*Dose as recommended under Revised National Tuberculosis Program, Government of India)
- *For treatment of leprosy*: 10 mg/kg/day div q OD PO (maximum 600 mg/day)
- *For prophylaxis in contacts of N. meningitidis meningitis*: 20 mg/kg/day (maximum 600 mg/day), div q 12 h PO × 4 days;
    - *Infants < 6 months*: 10 mg/kg/day div q 12 h PO × 4 days
- *For prophylaxis of H. influenzae contacts:*
    - 20 mg/kg/day div q OD PO (maximum 600 mg/day) × 4 days

Note: The drug should be administered on empty stomach. It causes orange-red discoloration of sweat, saliva, tears, and urine.

S/E: Hepatotoxicity, GI upset, rash, pruritus, flu like syndrome, leukopenia, and thrombocytopenia

Caution: Watch for evidence of hepatotoxicity. If noted, stop the drug and follow steps as advised under "isoniazid"

(R-cin, Rimactane, Rimpin, Ticin 150 mg, 300 mg, 450 mg cap/tab; syr 100 mg/5 mL)

Pyrazinamide

Antituberculosis drug:
- *Dose* (daily regimen): 30 mg/kg/day div q OD PO
- *Dose* (thrice-weekly regimen): 30–35 mg/kg/day div q OD (three times/week)

CI: Hepatic damage

Caution: Cautious use in renal failure with reduction of dosage. Watch for evidence of jaundice or hepatic dysfunction. Stop the drug if these develop and take further steps as advised under "isoniazid"

S/E: Hepatotoxicity, GI upset, rash, arthralgia, hyperuricemia, cutaneous hypersensitivity, and photosensitization

(PZA-Ciba 250, 500, 750, 1000 mg tab, susp 250 mg/5 mL; Pyzina 300, 500, 750, 1000 mg tab.; P-Zide 500, 750, 1000 mg tab)

Streptomycin Sulfate

Aminoglycoside; antituberculosis drug
For treatment of tuberculosis:
- *Dose (daily regimen)*: 15* mg/kg/day div q OD IM (maximum 1 g/day)
- *Dose (thrice-weekly)*: 30** mg/kg/day div q OD IM (maximum 1 g/day)

*Dose as per Consensus Statement Recommendations of IAP 1997

**Dose as recommended under Revised National Tuberculosis Program, Government of India

Caution and precautions:
- *Use with caution in patients with renal impairment, increase dose interval and monitor renal function (for details, see section on "Drugs in renal impairment")*
- *Stop the drug if patient develops tinnitus, loss of hearing, dizziness or loss of balance, and review regarding its further use or alternative drug administration.*

S/E: Tinnitus, ataxia, vertigo, loss of hearing, and renal impairment

(Inj Streptomycin 1 g vial, inj Ambistryn-S 0.75 g, 1 g vial)

Ethambutol

Antituberculosis drug

Children > 6 years:
- *Dose (daily regimen)*: 15–20 mg/kg/day div q OD PO
- *Dose (intermittent, thrice-weekly regimen)*: 30 mg/kg/day once in a day PO

Caution: Better avoid in renal failure. If used, reduce dose and monitor drug concentration and renal function.

S/E: Optic neuritis, arthralgia, hepatitis, cutaneous hypersensitivity, and peripheral neuropathy

(Combutol, Mycobutol, Themibutol 200 mg, 400 mg, 600 mg, 800 mg, 1,000 mg tab)

Antitubercular drug combinations—some trade preparations:
- *Combinations of rifampicin 450 mg + INH 300 mg* (Rcinex 450, Rimactzid, Ticinex, Binex, Montinex Forte)
  - *Rifampicin 100 mg + INH 50 mg* (Rcinex 50 DT, Rimactazid Disped, Ticinex kid, Montinex kid)
- *(i) Combination of rifampicin 225 mg + INH 150 mg + pyrazinamide 750 mg* (Rcinex Z, Tricox 1500, Monotrip Forte)
  - *Combination of rifampicin 450 mg + INH 300 mg + pyrazinamide 2 tab 750 mg* (Rimactazid + Z, Anticox-Z, Ter-3)
  - Combination of rifampicin 100 mg + INH 50 mg + pyrazinamide 300 mg (Monotrip kid, RHZ kid)

ANTITUBERCULOSIS DRUGS—SECOND LINE

Capreomycin

Second-line antituberculosis drug:

Children: 15 mg/kg/day IM (maximum 1 g/day)

Precaution: Perform audiogram at baseline and at least every other month and conduct periodic examinations for vestibular function while patient is receiving therapy.

S/E: VIII cranial nerve damage (hearing loss before vestibular dysfunction), renal toxicity

(Inj Kapocin 0.5 g, 0.75 g, 1 g vial)

Cycloserine

Second-line drug in multidrug-resistant (MDR) tuberculosis:

Children: 10–20 mg/kg/day div q 12 h PO (maximum 1 g/day)

Precaution: Give pyridoxine supplement especially when cycloserine is given along with INH

Monitoring: Regular assessment of mental status

CI: Epilepsy and renal failure

S/E: Depression, psychosis, seizures, and peripheral neuropathy

(Cyclorine, Coxerin, and Myser 250 mg cap)

Ethionamide

Second-line antituberculosis drug in MDR cases:

Children: 15–20 mg/kg/day div q 8–24 h PO (maximum 1 g/day)

S/E: Vomiting, anorexia, abdominal pain, hepatotoxicity, arthralgia, and photosensitivity

(Ethide, Ethomid, and Myobid 250 mg tab)

Kanamycin

Aminoglycoside; second line antituberculosis drug:

Children: 15 mg/kg/day div q 8–12 h IM/IV (maximum 1 g/day)

S/E: Auditory, vestibular, and renal toxicity

Precaution and monitoring: When given IV, administer over 30 minutes. Regularly monitor serum creatinine, auditory, and vestibular functions

(Inj Kancin, Kanamac 500 mg, 1 g vial)

PAS (Para-aminosalicylic Acid)

Second-line antituberculosis drug:

Children: 150 mg/kg/day div q 8 h PO (after food)—maximum dose 10–12 g/day

S/E: Vomiting, diarrhea, hypersensitivity reactions, and rarely hepatitis

(Q-PAS powder 100 g jar)

ANTILEPROSY DRUGS

Clofazimine

Leprosy, multibacillary (in combination with rifampicin and dapsone):
- *Children*:
  - 1 mg/kg/day div q OD PO (maximum 50 mg/day)
  - Or 4–6 mg/kg/day PO once a month (maximum dose 300 mg)

S/E: Cutaneous hyperpigmentation, ichthyosis, xerosis, and enteritis

(Clofazine, Hansepran 50 mg, 100 mg cap)

Dapsone

Children: 1 mg/kg/day oral once daily × 36 months, maximum dose 100 mg/day

Caution: Risk of hemolytic anemia in G6PD deficiency cases, dermatitis, hepatitis and methemoglobinemia, and rarely life-threatening granulocytopenia

(Dapsone 25 mg, 50. mg, 100 mg tab)

Rifampicin

Antimycobacterial drug:

For treatment of leprosy: 10–20 mg/kg/day div q OD PO (maximum 600 mg/day)

Note: The drug should be administered on empty stomach. It causes orange–red discoloration of sweat, saliva, tears, and urine.

S/E: Hepatotoxicity, GI upset, rash, pruritus, flu like syndrome, leukopenia, and thrombocytopenia

Caution: Watch for evidence of hepatotoxicity. If noted, stop the drug and follow steps as advised under "isoniazid".

(R-cin, Rimactane, Rimpin, Ticin 150 mg, 300 mg, 450 mg cap/tab; syr 100 mg/5 mL)

ANTIMALARIAL DRUGS

Artemether

Indications:
- *Chloroquine resistant Plasmodium falciparum malaria (without complications)*
- *Severe malaria with complications*
  - *Uncomplicated malaria*:
    - 4 mg/kg OD PO × 3 days (plus mefloquine base 25 mg/kg in 2 divided doses on third day PO)
  - *Complicated malaria*:
    - *Initial*: 3.2 mg/kg IM (day 1); followed by 1.6 mg/kg IM OD × 6 days (total 7 days)

(Inj Larither, Paluther 80 mg/mL 1 mL amp; Larither 40 mg cap)

Artesunate

i. *For treatment of severe malaria with complications due to Plasmodium (all species) infection (mostly P. falciparum)*:

- *Children*: *Initial*: 2.4 mg/kg/dose (maximum 120 mg) IV/IM, then 1.2 mg/kg/dose (maximum 60 mg) IM/IV at 12 and 24 h, then 1.2 mg/kg/dose (maximum 60 mg) IM/IV OD for 6 days or earlier when patient can be shifted to oral artesunate + plus sulfadoxine – pyrimethamine therapy. For details, given in Chapter 7.

ii. *For uncomplicated chloroquine resistant P. falciparum malaria*
    Artesunate 4 mg/kg PO × 3 days plus sulfadoxine pyrimethamine single dose PO on day 1 (sulfadoxine 5 mg/kg + pyrimethamine 1.25 mg/kg)

(Falcigo, Falcynate 50 mg tab, inj 60 mg vial)

Chloroquine

Antimalarial and antiprotozoal drug:

- Malaria: Treatment *(All chloroquine sensitive plasmodium species)*
    - *Uncomplicated cases*:
        ◦ *Oral*: Initial—10 mg of chloroquine base/kg (maximum dose 600 mg); followed by 5 mg/kg 6 hours later on first day, and then 5 mg/kg/day OD for next 2 days (at 24 h and 48 h). Total dose 25 mg/kg
- *Malaria*: Prophylaxis
    - *Chloroquine sensitive areas*: 5 mg/kg/dose PO once a week (maximum dose 300 mg/dose)
- *Amoebic liver abscess*: *As a follow-up therapy after initial treatment with metronidazole, tinidazole or dehydroemetine*: 10 mg base/kg (maximum 300 mg base)/day div q BID-TID × 2–3 weeks

S/E: Hypotension, headache, vomiting, rash, and tinnitus

[Lariago, Resochin, Emquin, Nivaquine 250 mg tab (150 mg base), 500 mg tab (300 mg base), susp 50 mg base/5 mL, inj 40 mg base/mL]

Mefloquine

Chloroquine Resistant Plasmodium falciparum Malaria (Uncomplicated Cases)

Prophylaxis:

Single dose once a week; dose as given below

< 5 kg—5 mg/kg; 5–9 kg—31.25 mg (1/8 of 250 mg tab); 10–19 kg—62.5 mg (1/4 tab); 20–30 kg—125 mg (1/2 tab); 31–45 kg—187.5 mg (3/4 tab); > 45 kg—250 mg (1 tab)

Start 1–2 weeks prior to departure and continue for 4 weeks after last exposure

Caution: Concomitant administration of quinine (exacerbates side effects)

CI: Known hypersensitivity, H/O epilepsy, severe psychiatric disorder, and cardiac conduction abnormalities

S/E: Vertigo, nausea, GI upset, visual disturbances, headache, insomnia, rarely seizures, and psychosis

(Meflotas, Mefloquine, Falcital 250 mg tab – 228 mg base per tablet)

Primaquine

- *Plasmodium vivax and ovale malaria—for prevention of relapse*: 0.25 mg/kg/day (of base) div q OD PO × 14 days
- *Treatment of P. falciparum malaria (uncomplicated):*
  As adjunct to artesunate and sulfadoxine-pyrimethamine combination therapy.
  For details see under Drug Therapy in Malaria, Chapter 7

Caution: May cause hemolytic anemia in G6PD deficiency cases. In cases of borderline G6PD deficiency, may give primaquine 0.6–0.8 mg/kg once a week × 6 weeks

CI: Infants below 1 year, pregnancy

S/E: Occasionally, neutropenia, GI disturbance, and methemoglobinemia

(PMQ-INGA 2.5 mg, 7.5 mg tab; Malirid 7.5 mg, 15 mg tab)

Proguanil + Atovaquone

For chemoprophylaxis against malaria in chloroquine resistant areas

Please *see* in Chapter 7 on Malaria.

Quinine Dihydrochloride

Severe and Complicated Malaria Treatment

All Chloroquine sensitive plasmodium species and chloroquine resistant P. falciparum infection:

- *IV*: Loading dose—20 mg/kg (by infusion given in a concentration of 1 mg/mL of 5% dextrose saline) over 4 h; then
  - 10 mg/kg/dose IV (by infusion over 2 h) every 8 h calculated from beginning of previous infusion. Shift to oral quinine sulfate as soon as possible to complete a course of 7 days (parenteral + oral)
- *Alternative*: IM quinine (if facilities for IV administration not available)

  Loading dose: 20 mg/kg (available quinine solution to be diluted in normal saline to 60–100 mg salt per mL), then divided into two parts and injected on either side in the anterolateral thigh by a 1.5 inch needle (not in buttock).

  Subsequently 10 mg/kg every 8 h (after dilution as explained) (Note—undiluted quinine preparation (300 mg/mL) is strongly irritant). Patient should be switched to oral quinine as soon as possible
- *Quinine sulfate oral follow up:*
  - *PO*: 10 mg/kg/dose (maximum 600 mg/dose) q TID. Total duration of therapy (parenteral + oral) 7 days (tetracycline, doxycycline or clindamycin as described later under quinine sulfate).
  - *Follow-up Primaquine:* 0.75 mg/kg single dose (maximum 45 mg) to eradicate gametocytes so as to prevent transmission of infection

CI: Severe quinine allergy, cardiac disorders, and G6PD deficiency; coagulopathy is a relative contraindication to IM quinine.

Precautions:
- *Avoid loading dose if the patient has received quinine or mefloquine or halofantrine in the past 12 hr (both mefloquine and halofantrine produce additive toxicity)*
- *Reduce follow-up oral quinine dose to 5–7 mg/salt/kg, if parenteral quinine is required for > 48 h or patient develops acute renal failure.*

Caution: Lethal hypotension may develop if injected rapidly intravenously.

Monitoring: Frequent blood glucose monitoring must be done during parenteral quinine administration for early detection and proper management of hypoglycemia

S/E: Tinnitus, deafness, headache, nausea, and visual disturbances (termed as "cinchonism")

(Inj Cinkona, Rez-Q, Quininga 300 mg/2 mL amp)

Quinine Sulfate

Uncomplicated chloroquine resistant P. falciparum malaria:

30 mg/kg/day div q TID PO × 7 days (maximum 650 mg/dose and total 2 g/day)

Note: Oral quinine sulfate is used in combination with a second another antimalarial drug, either
- *With tetracycline*: 40 mg/kg/day div q 8 h × 3 days; maximum 250 mg/dose (not recommended for children below 8 years of age) or
- *With doxycycline*: 2 mg/kg/day × 7 days (not recommended for children below 8 years of age) or
- *With clindamycin*: 20–40 mg/kg/day div q 8 h × 3 days

S/E: Tinnitus, blurred vision, headache, nausea, pruritus, giddiness

(Cinkona, Quininga 100 mg, 300 mg tab; Rez-Q 100 mg, 300 mg, 600 mg tab)

Sulfadoxine–pyrimethamine

Chloroquine resistant P. falciparum malaria (uncomplicated) treatment:

Children: Please *see* under ACT-SP treatment in Chapter 7 (Malaria Treatment)

Caution: *Not recommended for prophylaxis;*

CI: Infants < 2 months of age, H/O sulfonamide or pyrimethamine intolerance, pregnancy at term, and severe hepatic dysfunction

(Reziz, Pyralfin tab contain pyrimethamine 25 mg, sulfadoxine 500 mg, Forte tab: pyrimethamine 37.5 mg, sulfadoxine 750 mg, susp: pyrimethamine 12.5 mg and sulfadoxine 250 mg per 5 mL; Malocide, Croydoxin-FM tab pyrimethamine 25 mg and sulfadoxine 500 mg)

ANTIHELMINTHICS

Albendazole

- *Round worm, pin worm, and hook worm*
  - *Children 1–2 years: 200 mg PO single dose*
  - *> 2 years children and adults*: 400 mg/dose PO single dose
  - Repeat one dose after 2 weeks for pinworm and roundworm infections.
  - *Whipworm and cutaneous larva migrans*: Above dose × 5 days
  - *Visceral larva migrans:* 400 mg BD × 5 days PO
- *Hydatid cyst (not amenable to PAIR or surgery)*
  - 15 mg/kg/day div q BD PO (maximum 800 mg/day) × 28 days

May need to repeat a total of three cycles with 15 days drug free intervals for eradication of cysts

- *Neurocysticercosis*: 15 mg/kg/day div q BID PO × 7 days (maximum 800 mg/day)

Note: Administer prednisone 2 mg/kg/day once daily × 2-3 days before and then during albendazole therapy to prevent cerebral edema and worsening of symptoms.

- *Trichuriasis*: 400 mg PO × 3 days for all ages
- *Strongyloidiasis*: 400 mg BD PO × 7 days as an alternative to Ivermectin
- *Trichinellosis*: 400 mg BD PO × 8-10 days
- *Trichinosis*: 400 mg/dose q BID PO ×8-14 days + steroids for CNS or severe symptoms
- *Giardiasis: 10 mg/kg/day (maximum 400 mg/day) × 5 days*

CI: Ocular and spinal cysticercosis

(Zentel, Noworm, Wormin-A, Vermital, Combantrin-A 400 mg tab, susp 200 mg/5 mL)

Diethylcarbamazine

- *Tropical pulmonary eosinophilia:*
  - 6 mg/kg/day div q TID PO × 10-20 days
- *Visceral larva migrans*
  - 10 mg/kg/day div q 8 h PO × 7 days
- *Lymphatic filariasis (asymptomatic microfilaremic patients)*
  - *Day 1:* 1 mg/kg/day × single dose PO, p.c.
  - *Day 2:* 3 mg/kg/day div q TID PO
  - *Day 3:* 3-6 mg/kg/day div q TID PO
  - *Day 4 to 14:* 6 mg/kg/day div q TID PO
- *Löffler pneumonia 15 mg/kg/day single oral dose:* 4 days

S/E: Headache, malaise, arthralgia, nausea, and rarely acute psychotic reaction; during treatment of filariasis: nodules along lymphatics, lymphadenitis, transient hydrocele, or lymphedema

(Banocide, Hetrazan 50 mg, 100 mg tab, 120 mg/5 mL susp, Banocide susp 50 mg/5 mL)

Ivermectin

- *Scabies, pediculosis, ascariasis, cutaneous larva migrans, strongyloidiasis × 2 days, onchocerciasis*

Children age 6 years or more: 0.2 mg/kg PO × single dose to be taken on empty stomach; contraindicated in children below 5 years

S/E: Pruritus, fever, rash, nausea, vomiting, and giddiness.

(Iverin, Ivermectol 3 mg, 6 mg, 12 mg tab)

Mebendazole

- *Ascariasis, hookworm, whipworm (trichuris):*
  Children and adults: 100 mg/dose q BID PO × 3 days; repeat in 3-4 weeks if not cured
- *Pinworms*: 100 mg/dose q BID PO × 1 day; repeat in 2 weeks (to kill the ova that have developed later)
- *Trichinellosis:* 200-400 mg/dose q TID × 3 days, then 400-500 mg/dose q TID × 10 days PO
- *Visceral larva migrans*: 100-200 mg/dose q BID PO × 5 days + corticosteroids to limit inflammatory responses

(Mebex, Wormin, Eben 100 mg tab, susp 100 mg/5 mL)

Niclosamide

- *Taenia saginata and T. solium (beef and pork tapeworm) infection, Diphyllobothrium latum, and Hymenolepis nana:*
  Children: 1 g empty stomach followed by another dose after 1 hour. Give a brisk purgative 2 hours after last dose. For *H. nana* dose (Dwarf tapeworm; single dose as above, followed by half the dose for next 6 days. Use half of this dose in children < 6 years

Note: The tablet should be chewed thoroughly and not swallowed as a whole

S/E: Headache, rash, dizziness, nausea, and abdominal pain

(Niclosan 500 mg tab)

Piperazine Citrate

- *Roundworm: 50-75 mg/kg/day q OD PO × 2 days (maximum 3.5 g/day)*
- *Pinworm*: 65 mg/kg/day q OD PO × 7 days (maximum 2.5 g/day). May repeat q 1 week PRN

CI: Renal or hepatic impairment and seizures

Note: Piperazine citrate is drug of choice for ascariasis complicated by intestinal or biliary obstruction. Second-line drug for ordinary ascariasis and pinworm infection

(Piperazine citrate 500 mg tab, susp 750 mg/5 mL)

Praziquantel

- *Taenia saginata and T. solium:* 10–20 mg/kg single dose PO in morning
- *Hymenolepis nana:* 25 mg/kg single dose PO in morning
- *Schistosomiasis:* 20 mg/kg/dose q TID × 1 day
- *Neurocysticercosis:* 50 mg/kg/day div q TID × 15 days

Precaution: Give corticosteroids for 3 days before and during drug therapy for neurocysticercosis to prevent worsening of symptoms (headache, seizures, intracranial hypertension) as the patient responds to the dying parasite with increased inflammation. Some authorities recommend a higher dose of praziquantel 100 mg/kg/day divided in three doses when given along with corticosteroids. The tablets should be taken with food and not chewed (bitter taste)

CI: Ocular cysticercosis and spinal cysticercosis

S/E: Drowsiness, dizziness, diarrhea, headache, and malaise

(Distocide 600 mg tab; Cysticide 500 mg tab)

Pyrantel Pamoate

- *Roundworm and pinworm:* 11 mg/kg/dose once PO; repeat same dose once after 2 weeks in pinworm infestation
- *Hookworm:* 11 mg/kg/dose OD PO × 3 days

S/E: Vomiting, headache, rash, and transient AST elevation

(Nemocid, pyranthel 250 mg tab, susp 250 mg/5 mL)

Thiabendazole

- *Dose*: 50 mg/kg/day div q BID (maximum 3 g/day)
  - *Strongyloidiasis:* × 2 days;
  - *Intestinal nematodes:* × 2 days

- *Cutaneous larva migrans:* × 2–5 days
- *Visceral larva migrans:* × 5–7 days
- *Trichinosis:* × 2–4 days

S/E: Rash, vomiting, vertigo, and leukopenia

(Mintezol 500 mg tab, susp 500 mg/5 mL)

ANTIPROTOZOAL OR ANTIPARASITIC DRUGS

Amphotericin B

See under "Antifungal Drugs".

Chloroquine

See under "Antimalarial Drugs".

Dehydroemetine Hydrochloride

Amebicidal Drug

- *Fulminant invasive amebiasis of intestines or liver:*

Children: 1 mg/kg/day IM × 7–10 days

Caution: Never give IV. Patient must be hospitalized, watch for cardiotoxicity. Stop if tachycardia, T-wave depression, arrhythmia, or proteinuria.

(Dehydroemetine, Tilmetin inj 30 mg, 60 mg; dehydroemetine 10 mg tab)

Diloxanide Furoate

Intestinal amebiasis (intraluminal):
- *Children > 2 years*: 20 mg/kg/day div q 8 h PO × 10 days
- *Adults*: 500 mg/dose q TID PO

Caution: Not effective in hepatic amebiasis

S/E: Nausea, flatulence, and skin rash

(Furamide 500 mg tab)

Furazolidone

Giardiasis:
- *Children*: 6 mg/kg/day div q QID PO × 7–10 days
- *Adults*: 100 mg/dose q QID PO × 7–10 days

S/E: Nausea, vomiting, dizziness, and headache

CI: Infants < 1 month, primaquine sensitivity

(Furoxone 100 mg tab, susp 25 mg/5 mL)

Metronidazole

- *Amebiasis (amoebic colitis, liver abscess, and metastatic amebiasis):*
  - *Children*: 30–50 mg/kg/day div q TID PO × 7–10 days
  - *Adults*: 600–800 mg/dose q TID PO × 7–10 days
- *Giardiasis:*
  - 15 mg/kg/day div q TID PO (maximum 750 mg/day) × 5–7 days
  - *Adults*: 200 mg/dose q TID PO × 5–7 days
- *Trichomoniasis:* 15 mg/kg/day div q TID PO ×7 days
- *Anaerobic infection:*
  - *Neonates*:
    - \> 2,000 g ≤ 7 days:
      7.5 mg/kg/dose q 12 h PO/IV
    - \> 7 days: 7.5 mg/kg/dose q 8 h PO/IV
    - ≤ 2,000 g: *see* Chapter 34 (Dosage of Antimicrobial Agents in Neonates)
  - *Children and Adults*: 30 mg/kg/day div q 6 h PO/IV
- *Pseudomembranous colitis (C. difficile infection)*
  - *Children*: 30 mg/kg/day div q 6 h PO × 7–10 days
  - *Adults*: 800 mg/dose q TID PO

Precaution: Give IV infusion slowly over 30–60 minutes

Caution: Severe liver or renal disease; reduce dose, and monitor regularly

S/E: Nausea, headache, metallic taste, paresthesia, transient leukopenia, and rarely seizures

(Flagyl, Metrogyl, Aristogyl 200 mg, 400 mg tab; Flagyl, Metrogyl susp 200 mg/5 mL; Aristogyl susp 100 mg/5 mL; Metrogyl, Metronidazole IV (Core, Albert) 500 mg /100 mL inf)

Miltefosine

- *Visceral leishmaniasis:* 2.5 mg/kg day div q BID/OD PO after meals ×28 days

S/E: Vomiting, diarrhea, transient elevation of liver enzymes, blood urea, and serum creatinine

(Impavido 10 mg, 50 mg capsules)

Nitazoxanide

- *Giardiasis; cryptosporidiosis; E. histolytica and C. difficile infection; and ascariasis*
  - *Children*:
  - *12–47 months*: 100 mg/dose q 12 h PO × 3 days
  - *4–11 years*: 200 mg/dose q 12 h PO × 3 days
  - *Adults*: 500 mg/dose q 12 h PO × 3 days

Note: The drug should preferably be taken with food for better absorption.

Caution: Use with caution in patients with hepatic, biliary, and renal disease

S/E: Abdominal pain, diarrhea, vomiting, and headache

(Nitarid, Nitcol, Nitacure, Nizonide: DT 200 mg, 500 mg tab, susp 100 mg/5 mL)

Paromomycin

- *Giardiasis:* 25–30 mg/kg/day div q TID (maximum 1.5 g /day) PO × 5–10 days
- *Intraluminal intestinal amebiasis:* 25–35 mg/kg/day div q TID (maximum 1.5 g /day) PO × 7 days
- *Visceral leishmaniasis:* 11 mg/kg/day div q OD IM × 21 days
- *Cryptosporidiosis:* 25–35 mg/kg/day PO × 7 days

S/E: Myalgia, vertigo, GI upset, skin eruptions, and hematuria

(Humatin 250 mg cap)

Pentamidine Isothionate

Leishmaniasis (cases unresponsive or intolerant of antimony):
- *Localized cutaneous leishmaniasis*: 2-3 mg/kg/dose IM alternate days × 4-7 doses
- *Visceral leishmaniasis*: 3-4 mg/kg/dose IM on alternate days × 15 doses
- *Pneumocystis carinii*: Treatment—4 mg/kg/day IM/IV OD × 14 days
- *Prophylaxis*: 4 mg/kg/dose IM/IV every 2-4 weeks

Precaution: IV administration to be done slowly in dextrose solution over 1 h, IM injection should be deep IM.

Caution: Hypotension and renal damage

(Inj pentacarinate, pentam 300 mg vial)

Pyrimethamine

Congenital Toxoplasmosis

- *Pyrimethamine*:
    - *Load*: 2 mg/kg/day div q 12 h PO × 2 days
    - *Maintenance*: 1 mg/kg/day div q OD PO × 2-6 months, then 1 mg/kg/day for 3 alternate days in a week × till completion of total 12 months of treatment PLUS

    + *Sulfadiazine*: *Loading dose*: 100 mg/kg/day, then 100 mg/kg/day div q BD PO × 12 months PLUS

    + *Leucovorin (folinic acid)*: 5-10 mg per day × 3 days in a week

Acquired Toxoplasmosis

- *Pyrimethamine*:
    Children:
    - *Loading dose*: 2 mg/kg/day div q BD PO (maximum 100 mg/day) × 2 days

- *Maintenance dose*: 1 mg/kg/day div q BD PO (maximum 25 mg/day) × 4–6 weeks

Note: Must administer folinic acid (calcium leucovorin) concomitantly since pyrimethamine inhibits folic acid synthesis resulting in bone marrow depression.

Doses of sulfadiazine and calcium leucovorin (given along with pyrimethamine)
+ *Sulfadiazine*: Loading dose—75 mg/kg/day, then 50 mg/kg/day
+ *Calcium leucovorin*: 5–20 mg/kg/day × 3 days in a week or daily

S/E: Bone marrow depression, seizures, glossitis, rash, and photosensitivity

(Daraprim tab 25 mg)

Sodium Stibogluconate

- *Localized cutaneous and diffuse cutaneous leishmaniasis*: 20 mg/kg/day IV/IM × 20 days
- *Mucosal leishmaniasis and visceral leishmaniasis:* 20 mg/kg/day IV/IM × 28 days

S/E: Arthralgia, myalgia, nausea, elevated hepatic transaminases, nonspecific T-wave flattening or inversion, reduced white blood cell (WBC), Hb, and platelets

(Pentavalent antimony inj 100 mg/mL)

Spiramycin

- *For treatment of pregnant women with T. gondii infection to prevent congenital toxoplasmosis in the fetus:*

Dose: 1 g/dose (3 MIU/dose) q 8 h PO (without food) —during first trimester

S/E: Paresthesias, rash, vomiting, and diarrhea

Note: Pyrimethamine and sulfadiazine are given during remainder of pregnancy

(Rovamycin tab 1.5 million IU; Forte tab 3 MIU; susp 0.375 MIU/5 mL)

Tinidazole

- *Giardiasis and trichomoniasis*:
  - *Children*: 50 mg/kg single dose once (maximum 2 g) PO
  - *Adults*: 2 g single dose once
- *Amebiasis; mild-to-moderate intestinal disease* (colitis):
  - *Children*: 50 mg/kg/dose (maximum 2 g) q OD PO × 3 days
  - *Adults*: 2 g/dose q OD PO × 3 days
- *Severe intestinal amebiasis and amoebic liver abscess*: 50 mg/kg/dose (maximum 2 g) q OD PO × 5 days

S/E: Metallic taste, nausea, vomiting, and rash

(Tini 300 mg, 500 mg, 1 g tab, Tiniba, 300 mg, 500 mg, 1 g tab; Tini susp 75 mg/5 mL, 150 mg/5 mL; Fasigyn 500 mg, 1 g tab; Tiniba, Tinipidi 800 mg/400 mL inf)

ANTIVIRAL DRUGS

Acyclovir

- Herpes Simplex
  - *Neonates herpes simplex virus (HSV) infection; HSV encephalitis and HSV infection in immunocompromised children (all ages)*:
    - 30 mg/kg/day div q 8 h IV × 14–21 days (may increase dose to 45 mg/kg/day to 60 mg/kg/day in term infants)
  - *Mucocutaneous HSV infection (including genital)*:
    - *For initial infection:*
      - *Older adolescents and adults*: 200 mg/dose q 5 times a day PO × 7–10 days
      - *Younger children*: 10–20 mg/kg/dose q QID PO (maximum 200 mg/dose) × 7–10 days
  - *For recurrence in older adolescents and adults*: Same dose per day as for initial infection in older adolescents and adults × 5 days
  - *For daily suppressive therapy in older adolescents and adults*: 400 mg/dose q BID/TID PO

Chapter 33: Pediatric Drug Formulary

- Herpes Zoster
  - *Children*: 20 mg/kg/dose × 5 times a day (maximum 800 mg/dose) PO × 7 days
  - *Immunocompromised children*: 10 mg/kg/dose q 8 h IV × 7–10 days
- Varicella

Guidelines regarding use of acyclovir in varicella:

A. *Neonates:* Acyclovir IV 10 mg/kg/dose q TID
   - For skin or eye involvement × 14 days
   - For disseminated or CNS disease × 21 days
B. *Infants (0–1 year):* Acyclovir PO 20 mg/kg/dose q QID × 7–10 days
C. *Healthy child 1–13 years: uncomplicated varicella:*
   - Routine use of acyclovir not recommended (marginal benefit of drug use, low risk of disease complications)
D. *Indications for acyclovir therapy:*
   i. *Children 1 year or more: In following special situations*
      - With chronic cutaneous or pulmonary disease: PO
      - Having corticosteroids therapy (short-term or intermittent oral corticosteroids or aerosolized corticosteroids): PO
      - Receiving long-term salicylates therapy: PO
      - IV acyclovir therapy is recommended in children with evidence of disseminated varicella infection (e.g. pneumonia, encephalitis, thrombocytopenia, and severe hepatitis): IV
      - May employ acyclovir in second cases in household contacts: PO
   ii. *Adolescents (>13 yr):*
      Acyclovir PO 20 mg/kg/dose × QID × 7–10 days
      - *Timing of therapy*:
        For optimum results treatment should begin as soon as possible, preferably within 24 hours of onset of the exanthem. The benefit is dubious if it is delayed beyond 72 hours
      - *Dose:*
        * *Children 1 year or more: PO 20 mg/kg/dose × 4 times a day × 5 days (maximum 800 mg/dose)*

- « *IV (in severe disseminated disease and immunocompromised children): 30 mg/kg/day div Q 8 h × 7–10 days*
- « *For IV administration, dilute the drug to final concentration of 5 mg/mL and infuse over 1–3 hours. Reduce dose in renal impairment*

S/E: Nephrotoxicity, bone marrow suppression, GI irritation, fever, and rash

(Zovirax, Ocuvir 200, 400, 800 mg tab, susp 400 mg/5 mL; Acivir DT 200 mg, 400 mg, 800 mg; Zovirax, Zoylex, 250 mg/inj 1 mL amp.; Acivir, Virex 5% cream)

Amantadine Hydrochloride

- *For prophylaxis and treatment of influenza A:*

Note: Its value now doubtful due to present high levels of resistance to it among influenza A ($H_3 N_2$) and (HINI) viruses.

1–9 years or < 40 kg: 5 mg/kg/day div q 12 h (maximum 150 mg/day) PO

> 9 years or > 40 kg: 200 mg/kg/day div q 12 h PO

Caution: Reduce dose in renal impairment

S/E: Drowsiness, dizziness, hypotension, and urinary retention

(Amantrel, Neaman 100 mg cap, 50 mg/5 mL)

Foscarnet

- *Cytomegalovirus (CMV) retinitis:*
  - *Initial*: IV 180 mg/kg/day div q 8 h × 14–21 days
  - *Maintenance*: IV 90–120 mg/kg/day q once daily
- *Herpes simplex resistant to acyclovir:*
  - *IV*: 120 mg/kg/day div q 8 h × up to 3 weeks or until lesions heal
  - *Recommended dilution for IV infusion 12 mg/mL*: infusion rate 60 mg/kg/h

Precaution: Reduce dose in renal insufficiency

S/E: Hypertension, seizures, bronchospasm, and nephrotoxicity

(Inj Foscavir 500 mg, 1 g vials)

Ganciclovir

- *Treatment of CMV infection in pediatric acquired immunodeficiency syndrome (AIDS) cases:*
  - 12 mg/kg/24 h div q 12 h IV × 6 weeks; then

Maintenance: 5 mg/kg/day div q OD IV

Note: Treatment schedules for CMV infection are still under assessment and evolution

S/E: Neutropenia, thrombocytopenia, liver dysfunction, reduced spermatogenesis, renal abnormalities, and retinal detachment

(Inj Cytovene 500 mg per vial)

Interferon Alpha–2b

- *Treatment of chronic active hepatitis B:*
  - *Children 2-18 years*: 3-10 million units/m^2 3 times weekly s/c × 24 weeks
- *Treatment of chronic active hepatitis C:*
  - *Children 3-18 years:* 3-10 million units/m^2 three times weekly s/c (in combination with oral ribavirin—*see* under "ribavirin" for its dosage)

Caution: Closely monitor in cases of mild and moderate hepatic and renal impairment. Avoid if severe hepatic impairment or renal clearance < 10 mL/min/1.73 m^2

S/E: Anorexia, nausea, lethargy, occular, depression, myelosuppression, hypotension, hypertension, nephrotoxicity, and hepatotoxicity

(Shanferon, Viraferon 3 million IV, 5 million IU inj vial)

Isoprinosine—Antiviral Agent

- *For subacute sclerossing panencephalitis and viral encephalitis:*

Dose: Initial and during peak stage of disease—100 mg/kg OD Subsequently—50 mg/kg OD as maintenance

S/E: Dizziness, mild stomach pain, itching (Inosiplex tab 500 mg)

Oseltamivir

- *For treatment and prophylaxis of influenza A and B:*
  - *Treatment:* (treatment should begin within 2 days of onset of symptoms):
    - *Infant < 1 year*: 3 mg/kg/dose q BID × 5 days
    - *Children 1 year–12 years*:
    - *≤ 15 kg:* 30 mg/kg/dose q BID × 5 days
    - *> 15–23 kg*: 45 mg/dose q BID × 5 days
    - *> 23–40 kg*: 60 mg/dose q BID × 5 days
    - *> 40 kg*: 75 mg/dose q BID × 5 days
    - *Children > 12 years and adults*: 75 mg/dose q BID × 5 days
- *Prophylaxis of influenza*
  - *Adults*: 75 mg/dose q OD × 7 days (up to 6 week)

S/E: Nausea, vomiting, diarrhea, dizziness, headache, rash, and arrhythmia

Peginterferon

Pegylated Interferon Alpha–2b

Treatment of chronic hepatitis C
Children > 3 years and adults:
1–1.5 µg/kg SC PO once weekly
a. For genotypes 1 and 4: 48 weeks
b. For genotypes 2 and 3: 24 weeks.
This drug is given in combination with ribavirin in both cases

Precautions: The dose of drugs should be reduced by 25% in cases with moderates renal failure and by 50% in cases of severe renal failure

S/E: Flu-like symptoms, headache, bodyache, angioedema, urticaria, myelosuppression, seizures and arrhythmia

(Pegintron M.S. and D 50, 80, 120, 150, µg per 0.5 mL vial/redipen)

Ribavirin

- *For serious respiratory syncytial virus (RSV) bronchiolitis, RSV pneumonia (controversial value):*
  - *Aerosol*: 6 g ribavirin vial diluted in 30 mL sterile water (20 mg/mL) is administered as aerosol via a specialized small particle aerosol generator over 12–18 h OD × 3–7 days

  Caution: Do not give in patients with endotracheal tube
  - *Oral:* < 10 years—10 mg/kg/day maximum 150 mg/day
  - *> 10 years*: 10 mg/kg/day maximum 200 mg/day

S/E: Hypotension, worsening of respiratory distress, and cardiac arrest

(Ribavin, Virazide 100 mg, 200 mg cap, syr 50 mg/5 mL; Virazole aerosol 6 g)

Rimantadine

For prophylaxis of influenza A infection (all ages above 1 year) and treatment > 13 years:

- *Prophylaxis*:
  - *Children 1–9 years*: 5 mg/kg/day q OD (maximum dose 150 mg/day)
  - *Children > 10 years and adults*: 100 mg/dose q BID
- *Treatment*:
  - *Adolescents > 13 years and adults*: 100 mg/dose q BID

Note: During influenza epidemic, administer rimantadine for prophylaxis × 2–3 weeks after influenza vaccination (till development of postvaccination adequate protective antibodies)

Caution: Reduce dose to 1/2 in persons with severe liver or renal dysfunction

S/E: Drowsiness, confusion, urinary retention, (other anticholinergic effects), and hypotension

(Flumadine 100 mg tab. by Carico pharma)

Valganciclovir

Antiviral agent:
- *For prevention of CMV disease following transplantation:*
    - *Children*: 15–18 mg/kg/day PO × first 100 days post-transplant
    - *Adolescents and adults:* 900 mg/day PO × first 100 days post-transplant
- *CMV retinitis:*
    - *Adolescents and adults*: Induction—900 mg q BID × 21 days PO, then maintenance—PO 900 mg OD

S/E: Fever, headache, seizure, blood dyscrasia, renal function decreased, and peripheral neuropathy

(*Valcept, valgan 450 mg tab*)

Zanamivir

- *Treatment of influenza A and B:*
  Children 7 years and above and adolescents:
    - 2 inhalations (10 mg) q 12 h × 5 days
    - May administer two doses on first day (minimum interval >2 h)
- For prevention (household exposure)
    - Start within 36 hours of exposure
    - 10 mg single dose × 10 days

Caution: May cause bronchospasm in children with hyperreactive airway disease

S/E: Nausea, sinusitis, diarrhea, cough, and dizziness

(*Relenza rotadisk: Blister for oral inhalation: 5 mg; Rotadisk with diskhaler*)

ANTIRETROVIRAL—HIV DRUGS

Abacavir

Nucleoside/Nucleotide Reverse Transcriptase Inhibitor
- *For treatment of human immunodeficiency virus (HIV) infection:*
    - Children 3 months to 13 years:

- ▫ 8 mg/kg/dose q BID (maximum dose 300 mg BID)
- \> *30 kg*: 300 mg BID
- *Adolescents > 16 years and adults:* 600 mg/dose q OD

S/E: Nausea, vomiting, headache, diarrhea, and rash

(*Abavir, abammune, virol, ABC tab 300 mg, susp 20 mg/mL*)

Didanosine

- *Neonates and infants < 3 months*: 100 mg/m^2/day div q 12 h PO
- *Children < 13 years*: 180–300 mg/m^2/day div q 12 h PO
- *Adolescents and adults < 60 kg:*
  - 125 mg/dose q 12 h PO (tablets);
  - *Adults > 60 kg:* 200 mg BD PO

S/E: Headache, GIT upset, peripheral neuropathy, rash, and CNS depression

(*Dinex 100 mg chew tab, 250 mg, 400 mg cap, oral susp 10 mg/mL*)

Efavirenz (EFV)

Non-nucleoside reverse transcriptase inhibitor:
- *Anti-HIV-1 infection:*
  - *Children*:
    - ▫ ≥ *3 years, 10–15 kg*: 200 mg/dose q OD HS PO
    - ▫ *15 to < 20 kg*: 250 mg/dose q OD HS;
    - ▫ *20 to < 25 kg*: 300 mg/dose q HS
    - ▫ *25 to < 32.5 kg*: 350 mg/dose q OD HS
    - ▫ *32.5 to < 40 kg*: 400 mg/dose q HS
    - ▫ *> 40 kg*: 600 mg/dose q OD HS

Note: If using an oral suspension, use a 30% higher dose

Precaution: Do not give with fatty food which raises absorption by 50%.

S/E: Depression, psychiatric disturbance, and rash if combined with nelfinavir (NFV)

(*Efavir 200 mg, 600 mg cap; Sustiva cap 50 mg, 100 mg, 200 mg, Eferven 200 mg, 600 mg tab; suspension 30 mg/mL*)

Indinavir

Protease inhibitor and antiretroviral HIV drug:
- *Children*: 500 mg/m^2/dose (maximum 800 mg/dose) q 8 h PO
- *Adolescents and adults*: 800 mg/dose q 8 h PO

Caution: Patients with mild-to-moderate hepatic impairment (reduce dose by 25%)

S/E: Headache, nausea, hyperbilirubinemia, nephrolithiasis, and hyperglycemia.

Precaution: Liable to have serious interaction with several drugs (check literature carefully)

(Indivan 400, Indivir 400 mg cap)

Lamivudine

Antiviral drug for HIV infection:
- *Neonates*: 4 mg/kg/day div q 12 h PO
- *Children*: 8 mg/kg/day div q 12 h PO (maximum 300 mg/day)

S/E: Headache, fatigue, GI intolerance, rash, pancreatitis, and peripheral neuropathy

(Lamivir 100 mg, 150 mg tab, Lamidac, Lamivir-HBV 100 mg tab)

Lopinavir + Ritonavir (LPVr)

Non nucleoside reverse transcriptase inhibitors:
- *For treatment of HIV infections:*
  - *14 days to 18 years*: 300 mg/m^2 lopinavir (LPV) + 75 mg/m^2 RTV BID PO
  - *Adolescent (>18 years) and adult*:
    - 400 mg LPV + 100 mg ritonavir (RTV) BID or
    - 800 mg LPV + 200 mg RTV Q OD PO

S/E: Diarrhea, headache, nausea, vomiting, hepatitis, and pancreatitis

(Ritocom, ritomax-L cap contain lopinavir 133.3 mg and RTV 33.3 mg)

Nelfinavir (NFV)

Protease inhibitor drug for HIV infection:
- < 2 years: Not recommended
- > 2–13 years: 110–130 mg/kg/day div q 12 h PO
- > 13 years and adults: 750 mg/dose q 8 h or 1,250 mg/dose q 12 h PO

S/E: Headache, dizziness, diarrhea, hypertension, anemia, leukopenia, and hepatitis

(Nelvir 250 mg tab)

Nevirapine

Non-nucleoside reverse transcriptase inhibitor (anti-retroviral-HIV drug):
- *Prophylaxis for infant (with no antepartum treatment of mother*
  - 1st dose: 2 mg/kg birth to 48 h;
  - 2nd dose: 2 mg/kg 48 h after first dose,
  - 3rd dose: 2 mg/kg 96 h after 2nd dose
- *Treatment:*
  - *Age < 8 years*: 200 mg/m^2 OD × 14 days; then same dose BID (maximum 200 mg per dose)
  - *> 8 years*: 120–150 mg/m^2 OD × 14 days, then BID
  - *Adolescents and adults*: 200 mg/dose q OD × 14 days; then if tolerated 400 mg/day div q 12 h PO

Caution: Patients with liver or renal dysfunction

S/E: Skin rash, Stevens-Johnson syndrome, GI discomfort, headache, and diarrhea

(Nevipan, Neve, Nevimune 200 mg tab, 100 mg/5 mL susp)

Stavudine

Antiretroviral Drug for HIV infection:

- *Neonates (0–13 days) 0.5 mg/kg/dose*
- *Neonates 14 days to children < 30 kg*: 1 mg/kg/dose q 12 h PO
- *Children and adults 30–60 kg*: 30 mg/dose q 12 h PO
  - *> 60 kg*: 40 mg/dose q 12 h PO

S/E: Headache, GI intolerance, rash, peripheral neuropathy, and pancreatitis

(Stavir 30 mg, Stag 30 mg, 40 mg cap)

Tenofovir

For treatment of HIV infection:
- *Children > 2–12 years:*
  - *Dose*: 8 mg/kg per dose q OD
- Children > 12 years and 35 kg, and adult
  - *Dose*: 300 mg/dose q OD

S/E: Nausea, vomiting, and diarrhea

(Ricovir, teevir, and tenatide tabs—100 mg, 150 mg, 200 mg, and 300 mg)

Zalcitabine

Nucleoside reverse transcriptase inhibitor:
- *Children*: 0.01 mg/kg/dose q TID PO
- *Adolescents*: 0.75 mg/dose q TID PO
- *Adults*: 1 mg/dose q BID PO

Precaution: Reduce dose in renal disease—cautious use in patients with liver disease and pancreatitis.

S/E: Headache, malaise, GIT disturbance, and peripheral neuropathy

(Hivid 0.375, 0.75 mg caps.)

Zidovudine

Antiretroviral-HIV drug:
A. *Prophylaxis*: 0–6 weeks—premature infants; gestational age < 35 weeks: 1.5 mg/kg IV q12; hr;

For gestational age >35 weeks: 3 mg/kg/dose IV q12 hr or 4 mg/kg/dose PO q12 hr

B. *Treatment:*
   - *6 weeks–18 year:*
     - *4 to < 9 kg*: 12 mg/kg/dose twice daily PO
     - *9 to < 30 kg*: 9 mg/kg/dose twice daily PO
   - *> 30 kg (adolescent and adult):*
     - 300 mg twice daily PO or
     - 200 mg thrice daily

S/E: Headache, seizure, bone marrow suppression, rash, cholestatic hepatitis, and diarrhea

(Zoylex DT 200 mg, 400 mg, tab 800 mg, vial 250 mg per 10 ml, Zydowin tab 100 mg, 300 mg, Zidovir 100 mg, 300 mg tab, oral solution 50 mg/5 mL)

ANTIFUNGAL DRUGS

Amphotericin B Deoxycholate (Conventional)

- *Severe and serious systemic fungal infections:*
  - *Initial*: In infants < 10 kg give a test dose of 0.1 mg (diluted in 1 mL 5% dextrose) and in children > 10 kg, give test dose of 1 mg (diluted in 10 mL 5% dextrose solution) by slow-infusion over 30 minutes. If tolerated, follow-up by remaining initial dose of 0.25–0.5 mg/kg by IV infusion over 4–6 h. Increase as tolerated by 0.25–0.5 mg/kg/day
  - *Maintenance dose*: 0.5–1 mg/kg/day q OD by infusion over 6–8 h
- *Leishmaniasis Visceral:*
  - *Initial*: Give as explained above (under fungal infections)
  - *Maintenance*: 1 mg/kg on alternate days by infusion over 4 h × 15 injections over 30 days period

S/E: Fever, rigors, hypotension, hypertension, anemia, thrombocytopenia, hypokalemia, hepatic dysfunction, renal failure, and anaphylactoid reaction.

Monitoring: Monitor hematologic, electrolyte, renal, and hepatic status regularly. Consult manufacturer's information sheet for more details prior to administration of this drug

(Fungizone, Amfocan, Mycol Inj 50 mg vial)

Amphotericin B Lipid Complex

- *Serious and life-threatening fungal infections:*
    - *Infants ≥ 1 month, children and adults*:
      Dose: 3–5 mg/kg/day div q OD by IV infusion
- *Leishmaniasis visceral:*
  Dose: 2 mg/kg/day div q OD by IV infusion ×5 days

Note: Check drug literature of the product proposed to be used for dose and mode of administration and follow instructions carefully

Monitoring and S/E: As with amphotericin B conventional drug (given earlier)

[Ampholip 10 mg, 50 mg, 100 mg; AmBisome® (Liposome Amphotericin B); Amphocil® (Amphotericin B cholesterol dispersion)]

Anidulafungin

- *Antifungal agent (broad spectrum) for candida infections:*
    - *Children*:
        ▫ Loading dose 1.5 mg/kg/day IV
        ▫ *Maintenance dose:* 0.75 mg/kg/day IV

Note: Few clinical studies of its use in pediatric patients
- *Adults*:
    - Loading dose 100–200 mg IV;
    - *Maintenance dose*: 50–100 mg/day IV

The drug to be reconstituted with companion diluent provided with the injection vial and administered in IV infusion as per given instructions.

S/E: Eye pain, visual disturbance, nausea, vomiting, and abdominal pain
(Eraxis 50 mg vial)

Caspofungin

- *Invasive candidiasis and aspergillosis:*
  - *Children:* 70 mg/m² IV loading dose, followed by 50 mg/m² daily OD IV
  - *Adults:* 50–150 mg/day

Cautious use in hepatic impairment and in children below 3 years

S/E: Rash, fever, diarrhea, vomiting, hypotension, thrombophlebitis

(*Casfung, Casporan, Cancidas 50 mg, 70 mg vials*)

Clotrimazole

- *Topical antifungal agent for oral and vaginal candidiasis and ringworm infections*

For local application or use

(*Candid, Canesten, Surfaz lotion and gel 1% and 2%; Candid, Lotril and Surfaz 100 mg vaginal pessaries*)

Fluconazole

Antifungal agent
- *Oropharyngeal or esophageal candidiasis:*
  - *Neonate > 14 days, infants and children*:
    - *Day 1:* 6 mg/kg (maximum 200 mg) PO/IV q OD; then 3 mg/kg/day (maximum 100 mg) PO/IV div q OD × 14–21 days
- *Systemic candidiasis:*
  - 6–12 mg/kg/day q 24 h PO/IV × 28 days
- *Cryptococcal meningitis:*
  - *Acute:* 12 mg/kg/day (maximum 400 mg/day) div q OD first day, then 6–12 mg/kg/day div q OD PO/IV × 10–12 weeks after CSF culture becomes negative
  - *Relapse:* 6 mg/kg/day q OD PO/IV

Note: Neonates < 14 days—dose same as for older children in all above conditions but administered q 24–72 h

Precaution: Reduce dose if renal impairment, monitor renal function test (RFT) and LFT

S/E: GI upset, elevated LFT, and rash

(Flumed, Fungal, Zocon 50 mg, 150 mg, 200 mg tab; Fluzide 50 mg DT, Forcan 100 mg DT; Syscan, Forcan 200 mg/100 mL IV infusion)

Flucytosine

Antifungal agent
- *Candida and Cryptococcus sepsis treatment*:
  - *Neonates*: 50–100 mg/kg/day div q 6 h
  - *Children and adults:* 100–150 mg/kg/day div q 6–8 h

Note: Use of this drug is recommended in combination with amphotericin-B, especially in cases with CNS, kidney, and disseminated disease. Resistance to this drug develops rapidly if used singly.

Monitoring: Renal function, CBC, LFT, and platelets

S/E: Serious bone marrow depression, increased BUN, hepatotoxicity, and CNS disturbance

[Ancoban 500 mg tab; inj 10 mg/mL (250 mL bottle)]

Griseofulvin

Children > 2 years: Microsize or micronized formulation 10–20 mg/kg/day div q 12–24 h PO (maximum dose 1 g/24 h)

CI: Hepatic dysfunction, porphyria, and monilial infection

Monitoring: Hematologic, hepatic, and renal functions

S/E: Headache, nausea, diarrhea, rash, and leukopenia

(Fungivin 125 mg, 250 mg, 375 mg tab; Dermonorm 250 mg, 500 mg tab)

Itraconazole

- *> 12 years children*: 3–5 mg/kg/day div q OD-BD PO (maximum 10 mg/kg/day)

- *Adults*: 200–400 mg/day div q BD PO

CI: Concomitant use with terfenadine, astemizole, cisapride, and quinidine

Caution: Cautious use in hepatic impairment cases

S/E: Nausea, headache, dizziness, rash, hepatitis, and hypertension

(Canditral, Itaspor 100 mg cap)

Ketoconazole

Antifungal agent:
- *Children > 2 years*:
  - *Esophageal candidiasis:* 3–6 mg/kg/day div q OD
  - *Disseminated coccidioidomycosis (outside CNS):* 3–15 mg/kg/day div q OD/BID
- *Adults:* 200–400 mg OD/BD after meals

Monitoring: LFTs to be closely monitored

S/E: Vomiting, rash, fever, pruritus, and headache

(Fungicide, Nizral, Ketozole 200 mg tab)

Miconazole

Antifungal agent:

2% cream lotion, gel, powder for local application

(Daktarin, decanazole, zole 2% cream/gel, zole 2% lotion and powder)

Nystatin

Antifungal

- *Oral candidiasis:*
  - *Neonate*: 100,000 units to each side of mouth × QID
  - *Infant*: 200,000 units to each side of mouth × QID
  - *Children and adults*: 400,000–600,000 units to each side of mouth × QID

Note: One nystatin tablet (500,000) units dissolved in 5 mL glycerine provides 100,000 units per mL

(Mycostatin 500,000 U tab)

Terbinafine

- *Children < 20 kg*: 62.5 mg/day div q OD
- *Children 20–40 kg*: 125 mg/day div q OD
- *Children > 40 kg and adults*: 250 mg/day div q OD

Duration of treatment: For fingernails infection 6 weeks; toenails infection 12 weeks; tinea 2 weeks

Precaution: Avoid below 2 years age

S/E: Nausea, diarrhea, skin irritation, and leukopenia

(Sebifin 250 mg, Exifine 125 mg, 250 mg tab)

Voriconazole

- *Invasive aspergillosis, candidemia, and fluconazole resistant serious candida infections in non-neutropenic patients:*
  - *Children 2–11 years*: 9 mg/kg/dose IV/PO q BID loading for 2 doses followed by
    8 mg/kg/dose IV/PO q BID maintenance
  - *Children ≥ 12 years and adults:*
    - 6 mg/kg/dose IV/PO q 12 h for 2 doses followed by 4 mg/kg/dose IV/PO q 12 h

Note: Dose in children in higher than in adults on pharmacokinetic basis. Oral medication should be taken on empty stomach.

S/E: Transient visual disturbances, hepatotoxicity, fever, rash, nausea, and vomiting

(Fungior, Voritek, Vorage 50 mg, 200 mg tabs; inj 200 mg vial)

CVS DRUGS FOR SHOCK AND CHF

Adrenaline

See under "Epinephrine".

Amrinone

Adrenergic agonist:
- *Neonates*:
  - *Initial*—0.75 mg/kg bolus (over 2–3 minutes), then
  - *Maintenance*: 3–5 µg/kg/min continuous infusion
- *Infants and children*:
  - *Initial*: 0.75 mg/kg bolus (over 2–3 minutes), then
  - *Maintenance*: 5–10 µg/kg/min continuous infusion (maximum dose 10 mg/kg/24 h)

Monitor: For arrhythmia, hypotension, thrombocytopenia, and hepatotoxicity

(Inj Amicor, Cardiotone 100 mg/20 mL)

Digoxin

Cardiac inotrope and antiarrhythmic:
- *Congestive heart failure (CHF) and supraventricular tachyarrhythmia*
  - For dosage please, see Table 33.1

Monitoring: Watch heart rate, electrocardiography (ECG) for cardiac arrhythmia, and serum digoxin level in refractory CHF, and renal dysfunction cases

Table 33.1: Oral total digitalizing and maintenance dose of digoxin.

Oral total digitalizing dose	Oral maintenance dose
• *Premature* 0.02 mg/kg/day	1/4 of TDD
• *F.T.* 0.03 mg/kg/day	1/4 of TDD
• *Infant or child < 10 years*: 0.03–0.04 mg/kg/day	1/4 of TDD, maximum 0.2–0.5 mg/day
• *> 10 years and adult* 0.01–0.015 mg/kg/day or 0.5–1 mg/day	1/4 of TDD, maximum 0.2–0.5 mg/day

Note: IV doses are about 75% of oral doses. For rapid digitalization—1/2 of total digitalizing dose is given stat, followed by one-fourth dose each 8 h later and then 16 h later. The maintenance dose is started 12 h after full digitalization.

CI: Ventricular arrhythmia, atrioventricular (AV) block, and constrictive pericarditis

S/E: Nausea, vomiting, bradycardia, arrhythmias, vertigo, diplopia, photophobia, and yellow or green vision

[Lanoxin, Cardioxin 0.25 mg tab; Digoxin Pediatric syr 0.05 mg/mL; Digoxin, Cardioxin inj 0.25 mg/mL (2 mL amp)]

Dobutamine

Beta-adrenergic agonist:

- *Hypotension, low cardiac output CHF:*
  IV: infusion 5–20 µg/kg/min (maximum 40 µg/kg/min), start at lower end, titrate upwards as per patient's response. Do not mix with sodium bicarbonate
  CI: Idiopathic hypertrophic subaortic stenosis (IHSS), atrial fibrillation, and atrial flutter
  Caution: Watch for tachyarrhythmias, angina, and ectopics

Note: See formula for dose calculation under "Dopamine".

[Dobucin, Doburan, Dobustat 50 mg/mL (5 mL amp); Dobutrex 250 mg inj vial]

Dopamine

Sympathomimetic agent:

- *Low dose infusion*: 2–5 µg/kg/min—improves renal blood flow
- *Intermediate dose*: 5–15 µg/kg/min—increases cardiac contractility and cardiac output, induces rise in blood pressure (BP)
- *High dose*: More than 20 µg/kg/min—may cause reduced renal blood flow

CI: Tachyarrhythmia, hypovolemia, and pheochromocytoma

S/E: Ectopics, hypertension, tachyarrhythmia, and vasoconstriction

Note: Start dopamine infusion at the rate of 5 µg/kg/min, titrate upwards slowly PRN till desired effect; maximum 20 µg/kg/min; Formula for dose calculation:

$$6 \times \frac{\text{infant's weight (kg)} \times \text{desired dose in μg/kg/min}}{\text{desired fluid rate (mL/h)}}$$

= mg dopamine per 100 mL solution

For example:

$$\frac{6 \times 5 \text{ (wt in kg)} \times 10 \text{ (desired dose rate/min)}}{30 \text{ mL/h (fluid rate desired)}}$$

= Add 10 mg dopamine per 100 mL fluid

(Inj Dopamine, Dopinga 5 mL amp contains 40 mg dopamine per mL)

Epinephrine

Adrenaline—sympathomimetic agent:

- *For cardiac arrest and severe bradycardia:*
  - *Neonates:*
    - *IV, intratracheal*: 0.1-0.3 mL/kg of 1 in 10,000 solution; may repeat 2-3 times every 3-5 minutes *(Caution: Use 1—1,000 solution only after diluting it 10 times)*
  - *Infants and children:*
    - *Initial*: IV 0.1 mL/kg of 1 in 10,000 solution (maximum 10 mL/dose)
    - *If no response*: 0.1 mL/kg of 1 in 1,000 solution IV, repeat q 3-5 minutes PRN; if still not effective, give 0.2 mL/kg (of 1 in 1,000 solution) IV.
    - *If IV route not feasible, the second and subsequent doses can be given through endotracheal tube*: 0.1 mL/kg of 1 in 1,000 solution diluted in 3-5 mL of saline
- *For bronchospasm:*
  - *Infants and children*: SC 0.01 mL/kg of 1 in 1,000 solution; maximum single dose 0.3 mL; may repeat every 20 minutes for 3 doses
- *For anaphylaxis*: 0.01 mL/kg of 1 in 1,000 solution (maximum 0.3 mL/dose) intramuscular injection, repeat

every 15–20 minutes, if required. (IM injection achieves higher and quicker effective plasma concentration).

If anaphylactic reaction is secondary to a Hymenoptera sting, dilute 1/2 of the dose of epinephrine in 2 mL normal saline and infiltrate S/C at the site of sting to slow absorption and give the rest IM.

In case of persistent hypotension, under careful cardiac monitoring give slow IV infusion at an initial infusion rate of 0.1 µg/kg/min (gradually raised up to 1 µg/kg/min, if required) to sustain a systolic BP of 80 (+ 2 × age in years) mm Hg under close cardiac monitoring.

S/E: Tachycardia, hypertension, arrhythmia, restlessness, vomiting, and tremor

(Adrenaline tartrate (P and B Labs) inj 1 mL amp)

Isoproterenol

Beta-adrenergic agonist:

- *For low cardiac output CHF and shock (selected cases)*:
  IV infusion: 0.10–0.5 µg/kg/min; titrated against continuous determination of BP and heart rate in an ICU; dose may be raised up to 1.5 µg/kg/min.

CI: Significant tachycardia and aortic stenosis

S/E: Atrial and ventricular premature beats and cardiac arrhythmias

(Inj Isuprel 0.2 mg/mL 5 mL amp; Inj Isoprin 4 mg/2 mL amp)

Milrinone—Inotrope

Children:
- *Initial loading dose*: 50 µg/kg IV bolus over 10 minutes
- *Subsequently IV infusion*: 0.25–1 µg/kg/min

S/E: Hypotension, dysrhythmia, hypokalemia, and vomiting

CI: Severe aortic and pulmonary stenosis

(Amicor, Cardiotone 100 mg per 20 mL amp)

Norepinephrine

Adrenergic agonist
Hypotension:

Children: Initial—0.05–1 µg/kg/min; increase slowly as needed. Maximum dose 2 µg/kg/min

Precaution: Avoid extravasation as it may cause severe tissue necrosis

S/E: Hypertension, cardiac arrhythmia, headache, renal ischemia, and oliguria

(Adrenor 4 mg/2 mL amp)

Phenylephrine Hydrochloride

Alpha-adrenergic receptor antagonist:
- *Hypotension or shock:*
  - *Children*: By continuous infusion 0.5–2 µg/kg/min according to BP response

S/E: Sudden hypertension, increase in O_2 consumption, angina, arrhythmias, and restlessness

Vasopressin

- *Catecholamine refractory vasodilatory shock*

0.3 to 2 mu/kg/in IV infusion

For details *see* chapter on "Management of shock (For other indications, *see* under Drugs section on Hormones)"

(Inj pitressin, vasopin 20 units/mL)

ANTIHYPERTENSIVE DRUGS (TABLES 33.2 TO 33.9)

Table 33.2: Class I—angiotensin–converting enzyme inhibitors.

Drug	Starting dose	Maximum dose
Benazepril	0.02 mg/kg/day q OD (maximum 10 mg/day)	0.6 mg/kg/day (maximum 40 mg/day)
Captopril	0.3–0.5 mg/kg/dose q BID/TID	6 mg/kg/day
Enalapril	0.08 mg/kg/day q OD	0.6 mg/kg/day (40 mg/day)
Fosinopril	0.1 mg/kg/day up to 10 mg day q OD	0.6 mg/kg/day (40 mg/day)
Lisinopril	0.07 mg/kg/day up to 5 mg/day q OD	0.6 mg/kg/day (40 mg/day)
Quinapril	5–10 mg/day q OD	80 mg/day

Table 33.3: Class II—angiotensin receptor blockers.

Candesartan	*1–6 years:* 0.2 mg/kg/day q OD	Maximum 16 mg q OD
	> 6–17 years <50 kg: 4–8 mg q OD	Maximum 32 mg q OD
Losartan	0.75 mg/kg/day up to 50 mg/day q OD	Maximum 100 mg/day
Olmesartan	*20 to < 35 kg:* 10 mg; ≥35 kg 20 mg q OD;	Maximum 20 mg/40 mg q OD
Valsartan	*< 6 years:* 5–10 mg/day q OD	Maximum 80 mg OD
	6–17 years: 1.3 mg/kg/day up to 40 mg OD	Maximum 160 mg OD

Table 33.4: Class III—α and β-adrenergic antagonists.

Drug	Starting dose	Maximum dose
Labetalol	2–3 mg/kg/day div q BID	10–12 mg/kg/day; 12 g/day
Carvedilol	0.1 mg/kg/dose up to 15 mg q BID	0.5 mg/kg/dose; 25 mg BID

Table 33.5: Class IV—β-adrenergic antagonists.

Drug	Starting dose	Maximum dose
Atenolol	0.5–1 mg/kg/day div q OD/BID	2 mg/kg/day; 100 mg/day
Bisoprolol	0.04 mg/kg/day (2.5 mg/day q OD)	6.25–10 mg/day
Metoprolol	1–2 mg/kg/day div q BID	6 mg/kg/day (200 mg/day)
Propanolol	1 mg/kg/day div q BID/TID	16 mg/kg/day (640 mg/day)

Table 33.6: Class IV—calcium channel blockers.

Amlodipine	0.06 mg/kg/day q OD	0.3 mg/kg/day (10 mg/day)
Felodipine	2.5 mg/day q OD	10 mg/day
Isradipine	0.05–0.15 mg/kg/dose q TID/QID	0.8 mg/kg/day (20 mg/day)
Nifedipine extended release	0.25–0.5 mg/kg/dose q OD/BID	3 mg/kg/day (120 mg per day)

Table 33.7: Class V—central £-agonists.

Clonidine	5–10 µg/kg/day div q BID/TID	25 µg/kg/day (0.9 mg/day)

Table 33.8: Class VI—vasodilators.

Hydralazine	0.25 mg/kg/dose q TID/QID	7.5 mg/kg/day (200 mg/day)
Minoxidil	0.1–0.2 mg/kg/day div q BID/TID	1 mg/kg/day (50 mg/day)

Table 33.9: Class VII—central α-agonist.

Clonidine	5–10 µg/kg/day div q BID/TID	25 µg/kg/day (0.9 mg/day)

AMLODIPINE

Calcium channel blocker:

Children: 0.06 mg/kg/day OD PO; maximum 0.3 mg/kg/day, up to 10 mg/day

Precautions: Impaired liver or renal function

S/E: Peripheral edema, hypotension, headache, dizziness, rash, pruritus, and abdominal pain

(Amcard, Amdepin, Amlogard 2.5 mg, 5 mg, 10 mg, tablets)

Atenolol

Beta-1 adrenergic blocker:

Children: 0.5–1 mg/kg/day q OD PO (maximum 2 mg/kg/day or 100 mg/day)

Caution: Reduce dose in renal impairment. Do not discontinue abruptly, taper over 1–2 weeks, may cause rebound hypertension.

S/E: Bradycardia, wheezing, and hypotension

(Betacard, Catenol, Tenolol 25 mg, 50 mg, 100 mg tab; Tenolol 12.5 mg tab)

Bisoprolol

β-adrenergic antagonist (beta-blocker):
Hypertension:

Children: Starting dose 0.04 mg/kg/day up to 2.5 mg/day q OD PO; maximum dose 10 mg/day

S/E: Dizziness, headache, cold fingers, or toes

(Concor, Corbis 2.5 mg, 5 mg, 10 mg tab)

Captopril

Angiotensin converting enzyme inhibitor; antihypertensive and afterload reducing agent:
- *Hypertension and CHF:*
  - *Neonates:* Initial—0.05–0.1 mg/kg/dose q 8–24 h PO
  - *Infants:* Initial—0.15–0.3 mg/kg/dose q 8–24 h PO
  - *Children:* Initial—0.3–0.5 mg/kg/dose q 8–24 h PO
  - *Adolescents and adults:* Initial—12.5–25 mg/dose q 8–12 h PO

Subsequently, after commencing with initial doses as indicated above, titrate dose upwards weekly as required till minimum effective dose is reached.

Maximum dose:
Neonates: 2 mg/kg/day
Children: 6 mg/kg/day
Adolescents and adults: 450 mg/day

Caution: Reduce dose in renal impairment patients

S/E: Oliguria, hyperkalemia, proteinuria, neutropenia, and rash

(Captopril 12.5 mg, 25 mg tab; Aceten 25 mg tab)

Candesartan

Angiotensin receptor blocker:
- *Hypertension:*
  Children:
  i. *1–6 years*: 0.2 mg/kg/day q OD PO (maximum 0.4 mg/kg/day
  ii. *> 6–17 years*: < 50 kg—4–8 mg q OD PO (maximum 16 mg per day)
  iii. *> 6–17 years*: Over 50 kg: 8–16 mg q OD PO (maximum 32 mg per day)
  iv. *Adults*: 4 mg q OD; maximum 32 mg q OD

(Candesar 4 mg, 10 mg tab, Candelong 4 mg, 8 mg, 16 mg tab)

Carvedilol

Beta-receptor blocker vasodilator:
- *Hypertension and CHF:*

  Initial: 0.08 mg/kg/day div q 12 h PO; gradual increase PRN, maximum 0.5 mg/kg/div IV q 12 h (25 mg BD)

  S/E: Bradycardia, AV block, arrhythmia, worsening of asthma or CHF, and excessive hypotension

  (Carloc, Carvil, Caslot, Oricar 3.125 mg, 6.25 mg, 12.5 mg, 25 mg tab)

Clonidine

Alpha-2 adrenergic agonist:

Initial: 5–10 µg/kg/day div q 6 h PO; titrate upwards weekly PRN, maximum dose 0.9 mg/day

Caution: Abrupt discontinuation of the drug can cause severe rebound hypertension and tachycardia. Taper gradually over 10–14 days

S/E: Sedation, constipation, and withdrawal rebound hypertension

(Arkamin, Catapres 0.1 mg tab)

Enalapril Maleate or Enalaprilat

Angiotensin converting enzyme inhibitor:
- *Enalapril*
  - *Hypertension and CHF:*
    - *Infants and children*: Initial—0.1 mg/kg/day div q OD/BID PO; may increase slowly over 2 weeks up to 0.6 mg/kg/day (maximum—40 mg in 24 h)
    - *Adolescents and adults*: 2.5–5 mg/day div q OD/BID PO, titrate to maximum 40 mg/day
- *Enalaprilat*
  - *Hypertensive emergency:*
    - *Children*: 5–10 µg/kg/dose (say, 0.005–0.01 mg/kg/dose)
      Up to 1.25 mg per dose IV bolus

Caution: Reduce dose in renal impairment

S/E: Hypotension, syncope, hyperkalemia, hypoglycemia, cough, and renal failure

(Enalapril, Envas, Enace, Enpril 2.5 mg, 5 mg, 10 mg tab; inj Envas 1.25 mg/1 mL amp)

Esmolol

Beta-blocker:
- *Initial*: 100–500 µg/kg IV over 1 minute

- *Maintenance*: 25–100 µg/kg/min infusion, titrate slowly upwards every 10 minutes PRN (maximum 500 µg/kg/min)

CI: CHF and heart block

(Esocard inj 100 mg/mL)

Hydralazine

Vasodilator:
- *Chronic hypertension:*
  - *Infants and children*: *Initial*: 0.75–1 mg/kg/day q 6–12 h PO (maximum 25 mg/dose). Later increase dose slowly PRN over 4 weeks to a maximum of 5–7.5 mg/kg/day or 200 mg/day. Reduce dose in renal failure
- *Hypertensive emergency*: 0.2–0.6 mg/kg/dose IV/IM q 4–6 h PRN

S/E: Tachycardia, nausea, flushing, salt retention, and lupus like syndrome

(Nepresol 25 mg tab, Apresoline 25 mg tab; inj Apresoline 20 mg per mL ampoule)

Isradipine

Calcium channel blocker:
- *Hypertension:*
  Children: Starting dose 0.05–0.15 mg/kg/dose q TID/QID Maximum dose 0.8 mg/kg/day up to 20 mg per day

S/E: Dizziness, headache, vomiting, swelling hands and feet, chest pain (Dynacirc, Prescal 2.5 mg, 5 mg cap)

Labetalol

Alpha-1 and β-nonselective adrenergic blocker:
- *Chronic hypertension:*
  - *Initial*: 2–3 mg/kg/day div q BID PO; may increase gradually (maximum 10–12 mg/kg/day up to 1.2 g/day)
- *Hypertensive emergency:*

- *Initial*: 0.2–1 mg/kg/dose IV bolus (maximum 20 mg/dose) and then continuous IV infusion 0.4–1 mg/kg/h (maximum 3 mg/kg/h)

CI: Asthma, cardiogenic shock, pulmonary edema, heart block, and diabetes mellitus

S/E: Orthostatic hypotension, CHF, AV conduction disturbance, and urinary retention

(Normadate 50 mg, 100 mg, 200 mg cap, Lobert 100 mg tab, inj 5 mg/mL–4 mL, 20 mL)

Lisinopril

Antihypertensive agent
Angiotensin-converting enzyme inhibitor:
- *Children > 6 years*: 0.07 mg/kg q OD (maximum 5 mg per day)
- *Adults*: 10–40 mg/day q OD

Precaution: Use with caution and modify dose in renal impairment, especially renal artery stenosis, severe CHF, concurrent directive therapy

S/E: Orthostatic hypotension, dizziness, rash, and angioedema

(Lisoral, listril, linvas, cipril 2.5 mg, 5 mg, 10 mg tabs;

Lisonil 2.5 mg, 5 mg, 10 mg, 20 mg tab)

Losartan

Angiotensin II receptor blocker
Antihypertensive:
Children: 0.75 mg/kg/day up to 50 mg/day (starting dose); maximum 1.4 mg/kg/day (100 mg per day)

S/E: Postural hypotension, headache, dizziness, diarrhea and renal dysfunction

(Losar, Covance, Lara, Tozaar 25 mg, 50 mg tablets)

Metoprolol

Beta-blocker
- *Hypertension:*
  - *Children*:
    - *1 month–12 years*: Initially 1 mg/kg/dose q BID; increase if necessary to maximum 6 mg/kg/day div q BID/QID PO
    - *Children > 12–18 years*: Initially 50–100 mg/day; increase PRN to 200 mg/day div q OD/BID, maximum 400 mg/day
- *For cyanotic spell* 0.1 mg/kg IV over 1–2 minutes, repeat SOS q 5–10 minutes
- *Arrhythmias:*
  - *Children*: 12–18 years—50 mg/dose q BID/TID PO; maximum 300 mg/day

CI: Uncontrolled CHF, marked bradycardia, hypotension, and sick sinus syndrome

(Betaloc, Cardibeta, Tololol-XR 12.5 mg; Metolor, Metar, Metapro 25 mg, 50 mg tab; inj Betalock, Metolar 1.0 mg/mL in 5 mL ampoule)

Minoxidil

Arterial vasodilator:
- *Hypertension*:
  - *Initial*: 0.2 mg/kg/day div q 12 h PO (maximum 5 mg/day to begin with). Increase dose by 0.1 mg/kg/day at 3 days interval PRN
  - *Usual maintenance dose*: 0.2–1 mg/kg/day divided q OD/BD PO (maximum 50 mg/day)

CI: Pheochromocytoma

S/E: Hypertrichosis, fluid retention, bone marrow depression, and CHF

(Loniten tab 2.5 mg, 5 mg, 10 mg)

Nifedipine

Calcium channel blocker:
- *For chronic hypertension*: Extended release nifedipine
  - *Initial*: 0.25–0.5 mg/kg/day div q OD/BID;
  - *Later*: Can ↑ dose gradually; maximum 3 mg/kg/day (120 mg/day)
- *For hypertensive emergency*; immediate release nifedipine 0.25–0.5 mg/kg/dose; maximum dose 10 mg/dose; may repeat q 4–6 h, if needed

S/E: Facial flushing, tachycardia, acute hypotension, and dizziness

(Nifelat, Calcigard, Depin 5 mg, 10 mg cap; Nifedine 5 mg, 10 mg tab; Extended release – Calblac Retard ER tab 10 mg, 20 mg; Depin Retard SR tab 20 mg, Cardipin Retard ER 20 mg tab)

Olmesartan

Angiotensin receptor blocker
- *Hypertension*:
  Children:
  - *20 to < 35 kg*: 10 mg q OD PO (maximum 20 mg q OD)
  - *≥ 35 kg*: 20 mg q OD PO (maximum 40 mg q OD)

(Olmezest, Olmy 20 mg tab; Olmat 20 mg, 40 mg tab)

Phentolamine Mesylate

Alpha-1 adrenergic blocker
- *Pheochromocytoma diagnosis*:
  0.05–0.1 mg/kg/dose; maximum dose 5 mg IM/IV
- *Preoperative management of hypertensive crisis during pheochromocytoma surgery*
  0.05–0.1 mg/kg/dose; maximum dose 5 mg IM/IV 1–2 h prior to surgery; repeat q 1–4 h PRN

S/E: Hypotension and arrhythmias

(Fentanor 10 mg/mL, 1 mL inj)

Propranolol

Nonselective beta-adrenergic blocker:
- *Hypertension:*
  - *Initial*: 0.5–1 mg/kg/day div q 6–12 h PO; titrate upwards every 3–5 days PRN. Usual dose required 1–5 mg/kg/day (maximum 16 mg/kg/day)
- *Tetralogy of Fallot—cyanotic spells:*
  - *Acute stage*: IV 0.1–0.2 mg/kg/dose; slow IV bolus. May repeat in 15 minutes once.
  - *For reduction in frequency and severity of cyanotic spells:* PO 0.5–1 mg/kg/dose q 6 h
- *Arrhythmias [SVT, premature ventricular complexes (PVCs), long QT syndrome (LQTS)]:*
  - *Initial*: PO 0.5–1 mg/kg/day div q 6–8 h; increase dose every 3–7 days PRN
  - *Usual maintenance dose*: 2–4 mg/kg/day div q 6–8 h PO
- *For life-threatening arrhythmia:*
  - *IV*: 0.01–0.1 mg/kg/dose infused over 10–15 minutes; repeat at 6–8 h intervals PRN
  - *Maximum dose*: Infants 1 mg/dose; children 3 mg/dose
- *Migraine: prophylaxis:*
  - *Children 2–12 years:* 0.6–2 mg/kg/day div q 8–12 h PO; maximum 4 mg/kg/day; usual dose 10–20 mg/dose q BID/TID PO
  - *Children 12–18 years*: 20–40 mg/dose q BID/TID PO
  - *Maintenance*: 80–160 mg/day PO
- *Thyrotoxicosis (as supplement therapy):*
  - *Neonates*: 2 mg/kg/day div q 6–12 h PO (to control tachycardia and CHF)
  - *Children*: 0.5–2 mg/kg/day div q 8 h PO

CI: Heart failure, heart block, asthma, and cautious use in hepatic or renal disease

S/E: Bronchospasm, hypotension, bradycardia, hypoglycemia, heart block, CHF, and depression

(Inderal 10 mg, 40 mg, 80 mg tab, Ciplar 10 mg, 40 mg tab; Ciplar cap LA 40 mg, 80 mg; LOL-SR 40 mg, 80 mg tab; Propranolol-Samarth 1 mg/mL-1 mL amp)

Valsartan

Angiotensin receptor blocker:

- *Hypertension*:

    Children below 6 years: 5–10 mg/day; maximum 80 mg/day PO

    Children 6–17 years: 1.3 mg/kg/day up to 40 mg/day; maximum 2.7 mg/kg/day up to 160 mg/day PO

    Adults: 40 mg q BID; maximum 160 mg BID PO

    (Valzaar, Starval 80 mg, 160 mg cap; Diovan 40 mg, 80 mg, 160 mg tab)

DRUGS FOR CARDIAC ARRHYTHMIAS

Adenosine

Antiarrhythmic agent:

- *Paroxysmal SVT:*

    Initial: 50–300 µg/kg/dose IV push (increase by 50–100 µg/kg as needed) (maximum 12 mg/dose)

    CI: Second and third degree AV block, and sick sinus syndrome

    Monitor: ECG, BP, and respiration

    Caution: May precipitate bronchoconstriction

    S/E: Dyspepsia, flushing, and transient chest pain

    (Inj Adenocor, Adenoject, Tachyban 3 mg/mL 2 mL amp)

Amiodarone

Antiarrhythmic agent:

- *Supraventricular tachycardia, junctional ectopic tachycardia, and ventricular tachycardia:*

- *Oral*: 10 mg/kg/24 div q OD/BID × 4–14 days; reduce to 5 mg/kg/day for several weeks; if no recurrence reduce to 2.5 mg/kg/day
- *IV*: Loading dose—5 mg/kg over 1 h; then continuous infusion @ 2–10 mg/kg/24 h; maximum 15 mg/kg/day

CI: Second and third degree heart block, severe sinus node dysfunction

Caution: Maximum concentration of continuous IV infusion 2 mg/mL; dilute drug only with 5% dextrose solution

(Cordarone, Duron 100 mg, 200 mg tab; inj 150 mg per 3 mL amp)

Digoxin

Cardiac inotrope and antiarrhythmic:
- CHF, supraventricular tachyarrhythmia, atrial tachycardia, atrial fibrillation.

Dosage: Table 33.10.

Note: IV doses are about 75% of oral doses. For rapid digitalization—one-half of total digitalizing dose is given stat, followed by one-fourth dose each 8 h later and then 16 h later. The maintenance dose is started 12 h after full digitalization.

Table 33.10: Congestive heart failure and supraventricular tachyarrhythmia.		
Age	Oral total digitalizing dose	Oral maintenance dose
Premature	0.02 mg/kg/day	1/4 of TDD
FT	0.03 mg/kg/day	1/4 of TDD
Infant or child < 10 years	0.03–0.04 mg/kg/day	1/4 of TDD (maximum 0.2–0.5 mg/day)
>10 years and adult	0.01–0.15 mg/kg/day	1/4 of TDD (maximum 0.2–0.5 mg/day)

CI: Ventricular arrhythmia, AV block, and constrictive pericarditis

Monitoring: Watch heart rate, ECG for cardiac arrhythmia, serum digoxin level in refractory CHF, and renal dysfunction cases

S/E: Nausea, vomiting, bradycardia, arrhythmias, AV block, vertigo, diplopia, photophobia, and yellow or green vision

[Lanoxin, Cardioxin 0.25 mg tab; Digoxin Pediatric syr 0.05 mg/mL; Digoxin, Cardioxin inj 0.25 mg/mL (2 mL amp)]

Disopyramide

Antiarrhythmic agent

- *Supraventricular tachycardia, atrial fibrillation, and atrial flutter:*
    - < 2 years: 20–30 mg/kg/day div q 6 h PO or div q 12 hr (long acting forms)
    - 2–10 years: 9–24 mg/kg/day div q 6 h PO or div q 12 h (long acting forms)
    - 11–18 years: 5–13 mg/kg/day div q6 h PO or div q 12 h (long acting forms)
    - Maximum dose: 1.2 g/24 h

CI: Second or third degree heart block, CHF

Monitoring: Renal function, ECG, BP, and signs of CHF

(Norpace 100 mg, 150 mg cap; Regubeat 100 mg tab)

Flecainide Acetate

- *For resistant supraventricular tachycardic and life-threatening ventricular arrhythmia:*

Children: Initial 1–3 mg/kg/day div q TID PO; may increase up to 8 mg/kg/day div q TID PO

CI: Heart failure, abnormal left ventricular (LV) dysfunction, second degree or greater AV block, and bundle branch block

Precaution: Reduce dose in renal and hepatic dysfunction

S/E: Edema, bradycardia, heart block, CHF, headache, fatigue, rash, nausea, blurred vision, hepatic dysfunction, and tremor

(*Tambocor 100 mg tablets*)

Lidocaine

Antiarrhythmic agent and local anesthetic:
- *Ventricular premature contraction (VPC), ventricular tachycardia, and ventricular fibrillation:*

Loading dose: 1 mg/kg bolus slowly IV; can repeat in 5–10 min × 2 times followed by continuous IV infusion 20–50 µg kg/min (maximum dose 3 mg/kg)

CI: Heart block without a pacemaker

S/E: Convulsions, paresthesias, AV heart block, asystole, and respiratory arrest

(Inj Xylocard 2%; Gesicard 2% 50 mL vial, 1 mL: 21.33 mg of lidocaine)

Phenylephrine

See under cardiovascular system (CVS) drugs for shock and CHF.

Phenytoin

See under "Anticonvulsant drugs".

Procainamide

Antiarrhythmic agent class IA:
- *Supraventricular tachycardia, atrial fibrillation, atrial flutter, VPC, ventricular tachycardia:*
    - *Loading dose*: 3–6 mg/kg/dose IV over 5 minutes; repeat dose q 5–10 minutes PRN to a total of 10–15 mg/kg over 30–45 minutes

- *Maintenance dose*:
  - *IV*: 20–80 ug/kg/min by continuous IV infusion (maximum dose 2 g/day)
  - *PO*: 15–50 mg/kg/day q 4–6 h (maximum dose 4 g/day)

CI: Cardiogenic shock, myasthenia gravis, and sinus node dysfunction

Caution: Liver and renal dysfunction and CHF

S/E: Nausea, rash, fever, agranulocytosis, thrombocytopenia, systemic lupus erythematosus (SLE), hypotension, and AV block

[Pronestyl 250 mg tab, inj 100 mg/mL (10 mL)]

Propranolol (Nonselective Beta-adrenergic Blocker)

- *Arrhythmias (SVT, PVCs, and LQTS)*:
  - *Initial*: PO 0.5–1 mg/kg/day div q 6–8 h; increase dose every 3–7 days PRN
  - *Usual maintenance dose*: 2–4 mg/kg/day div q 6–8 h PO
  - *Maximum dose*: 60 mg/24 h
- *For life-threatening arrhythmia*:
  - *IV*: 0.1–0.15 mg/kg/dose infused over 5 minutes; repeat at 6–8 h intervals PRN
  - *Maximum dose*: IV—10 mg

Note: For information regarding use in other conditions, see Propranolol under Antihypertensive drugs

CI: Heart failure, heart block, asthma, and cautious use in hepatic or renal disease

S/E: Bronchospasm, hypotension, bradycardia, hypoglycemia, heart block, CHF, and depression

(Inderal 10 mg, 40 mg, 80 mg tab, Ciplar 10 mg, 40 mg tab; Ciplar cap LA 40 mg, 80 mg; LOL-SR 40 mg, 80 mg tab; Propanolol-Samarth 1 mg/mL–1 mL amp)

Propafenone

Antiarrhythmic:
- Supraventricular tachycardia, atrial tachycardia, atrial fibrillation, and ventricular tachycardia:
  - *Children*: 150–300 mg/m^2/day div q 8 h PO
  - *Adults*: 450 mg/day div q 8 h PO

Caution: May cause CHF, angina, worsen arrhythmia, GIT upset, dizziness and hypotension

(Rytmonorm 150 mg tab)

Quinidine Sulfate

Antiarrhythmic
- Supraventricular tachycardia, atrial fibrillation, atrial flutter, and VPC:
  - *Test dose*: 2 mg/kg/dose PO to exclude idiosyncratic reaction (QRS interval increase by 0.02 sec or more, stop drug use)
  - *Therapeutic dose*: 20–60 mg/kg/day div q 6 h PO; maximum dose 2.4 g/24 h

Caution: In atrial flutter, first give digoxin or verapamil or propranolol to prevent 1:1 conduction and fast ventricular rate.

S/E: GI upset, cinchonism, hypotension, AV node block, asystole, and blood dyscrasias

[Quinidine sulfate (GSK/200 mg tab; Natcardine (quinidine phenylethyl-barbiturate) 100 mg tab]

Verapamil

Calcium channel blocker:
- Supraventricular tachycardia
  Children > 1 year:
  - *IV loading dose*: 0.1–0.2 mg/kg (maximum 5 mg) over 2–3 minutes stat; repeat once after 20 minutes PRN (maximum second dose 10 mg)

Caution: Give under ECG monitoring. If myocardial depression, give IV calcium chloride for reversal.
- *Oral*: 2–7 mg/kg/day div q 8 h

CI: Ventricular tachycardia, severe CHF, atrial fibrillation with WPW, AV block, IV administration contraindicated in infants below 1 year

(Calaptin, Verap 40 mg, 80 mg tab; Verap 2.5 mg/mL inj-2 mL)

ANTICONVULSANT DRUGS

Adrenocorticotropic hormone
- *Infantile spasms:*
    - *Adrenocorticotropic hormone (ACTH) Gel*: 20 units/dose IM q OD × 2 weeks; if no response, increase dose to 30–40 units/dose IM q OD × additional 4 weeks

Note: Taper dose over several weeks; prednisolone 2 mg/kg/day has been found to be almost equally effective
- *Anti-inflammatory:*
    - *Adrenocorticotropic hormone aqueous*: 1.6 units/kg/day div q 6–8 h IM/SC
    - *Adrenocorticotropic hormone gel*: 0.8 units/kg/day div q 12–24 h IM

CI: Acute psychosis, CHF, peptic ulcer, and hypertension

S/E: As with other corticosteroids (see under prednisolone)

(Acton Prolongatum 60 IU/mL-0.5 mL amp, 5 mL vial; Inj conticotrophin, synacthen, acthar gel 40 units and 80 units per mL in 2 mL and 5 mL vials)

Carbamazepine

- *Partial and generalized tonic-clonic seizures; trigeminal neuralgia, diabetic neuropathy, bipolar disorders, benign childhood epilepsy with centrotemporal spikes (BCECT): Children*:
    - *Initial*: 10 mg/kg/day, div q TID; increase dose by 5 mg/kg/day at 1 week intervals PRN.
    - *Maintenance*: 10–30 mg/kg/day div q TID

Adults:
- *Initial*: 200 mg/dose q BID.
- *Maintenance*: 1200–1600 mg/day (usual)

Comments: Desired therapeutic serum level 3–12 µg/mL; check pretreatment CBC and LFT. Monitor blood counts and LFT closely for bone marrow and hepatic toxicity especially during the first four months.

S/E: Dizziness, diplopia, liver dysfunction, aplastic anemia, and leukopenia

(Mazetol 100 mg, 200 mg, 400 mg tab, SR tab 200 mg, 400 mg, syr 100 mg/5 mL; Tegretol 100 mg, 200 mg, 400 mg tab; CR tab 200 mg, 400 mg, syr 100 mg/5 mL; Zen 200 mg, 400 mg tab, CR tab 200 mg, 400 mg)

Clobazam

- *Lennox-Gastaut syndrome*:

All ages above 2 years: 10–20 mg/day div q BID/TID mg/kg/day div q BID/TID

Therapeutic level – 60–200 µg/L

S/E: Dizziness, ataxia, behavior problems, and weight gain

(Clozam, Frisium, Lobazam 5 mg, 10 mg, 20 mg tab)

Clonazepam

- *Absence, myoclonic, infantile spasms, partial, Lennox-Gestaut and akinetic seizures:*
  < 10 years or < 30 kg:
  - *Initial*: 0.01–0.03 mg/kg/24 h div q 8 h PO;
  - *Increment*: 0.25–0.5 mg/day (not per kg) every 3 days until seizures controlled or adverse effects appear.
  - *Maintenance dose*: 0.05–0.2 mg/kg/day div q BID/TID
  ≥ 10 years or ≥ 30 kg and adults:
  - *Initial*: 1.5 mg/day div q TID PO
  - *Increment*: 0.5–1 mg/day every 3 days (not per kg) PRN
  - *Maximum dose*: 20 mg/day
  - *Therapeutic level*: 25–85 µg/L

CI: Severe liver disease; watch for hematopoietic toxicity

S/E: Drowsiness, irritability, depression, and excessive salivation

(Clonotril, Epitril, Rivotril 0.25 mg, 2 mg tab)

Diazepam

- *Status epilepticus:*
  - *IV*: 0.1–0.3 mg/kg slow IV bolus (at the rate of 1 mg/min); maximum dose 10 mg. May repeat twice at 15–30 minutes interval as needed. Maximum total dose 0.75 mg/kg or 30 mg whichever is less over 8 h
  - *PR*: (when IV administration is not possible); prior to reaching hospital
    - 0.3–0.5 mg/kg (IV form of diazepam)
    - 0.2–0.5 mg/kg (diazepam rectal solution) depending upon age; 2–5 years—0.5 mg/kg; 6–11 years—0.3 mg/kg; ≥ 12 years—0.2 mg/kg
- *Prophylaxis of febrile seizures recurrence:*
  - *PO*: 0.3 mg/kg/dose q 8 h (1 mg/kg/24 h) at onset of febrile illness for duration of fever (usually 2–3 days)
  - *PR*: 0.5 mg/kg per dose as rectal suppository every 8 h
- *Sedation:*
  - *PO*: 0.2–0.3 mg/kg/dose q 6–8 h
  - *IM/IV*: 0.04–0.2 mg/kg/dose q 2–4 h (maximum dose 0.6 mg/kg in 8 h period)

Note: For rectal administration, IV diazepam preparation may be diluted in 3 mL of normal saline and placed in rectum by a syringe and a flexible tube. Ready-to-use rectal solution is also now available for use with a rectal applicator.

S/E: Hypotension, bradycardia, and respiratory depression

(Valium, Placidol, Anxol 2 mg, 5 mg, 10 mg tab; Calmpose 5 mg, 10 mg tab; Calmpose susp 2 mg/5 mL; Calmpose, Placidol, Anxol inj 10 mg/2 mL amp; Rec-DZ rectal application 2.5 mg/mL, 5 mg/mL; Direc-2 rectal application 2 mg/mL)

Ethosuximide

- *Absence seizures (first-line drug); and akinetic seizures (second-line drug):*
  Children >3 years: Initial: 15 mg/kg/day div q BID; increase 4–7 days PRN
  Maintenance: 20–30 mg/kg/day div. q BID/TID (maximum 1.5 g/day or 40 mg/kg/day)
  Therapeutic level 40–100 µg/mL; toxic level 150 µg/mL

Caution: Use cautiously in hepatic and renal disease. May increase tonic clonic seizures in mixed seizure patients

S/E: Abdominal discomfort, skin rash, leukopenia, and liver dysfunction

(Zarontin tab 250 mg; syrup 250 mg/5 mL)

Felbamate

Anticonvulsant (For Restricted Use Only)

- *Partial seizures (>14 years); Lennox-Gestaut syndrome (>2 years):*
  Children: 15–45 mg/kg/day div q BID PO
  Initial: 15 mg/kg/day; increase by 15 mg/kg/day at weekly intervals

Warning: Aplastic anemia and fatal hepatic failure have been reported following its use. Restrict use of this drug to cases of refractory epilepsies not amenable to other drugs.

Caution: Reduce initial and maintenance dose by 50% in patients with renal impairment.

S/E: Headache, dizziness, sleep disturbance, weight loss, GIT upset, pancytopenia, and aplastic anemia

(Felbatol by Med Pointe: 400, 600 mg tab; 600 mg/5 mL susp)

Fosphenytoin Sodium

- *Anticonvulsant (esp. for acute seizures):*

Each 1.5 mg fosphenytoin = 1 mg phenytoin

Note: The dose of this drug is calculated according to its equivalent in phenytoin (PE).

- *Children and adults*:

  Loading dose: 15–20 mg PE/kg IV

  Mode of administration: Dilute fosphenytoin pharmaceutical trade preparation with dextrose 5 % in water (D_5W) or NS to 1.5–25 mg PE/mL and then administer slowly at the rate of 3 mg PE equivalent/kg/min, not exceeding 150 mg PE equivalent per minute

  Maintenance dose (initial): 4–6 mg PE equivalent IM/IV

Note: Refer to phenytoin in this section for more information regarding usage, side effects, etc.

(Fosolin 2 mL, 10 mL inj, fosphen inj 2 mL ampoule contains 50 mg phenytoin equivalent per mL)

Gabapentin

- *Add on drug for refractory partial seizures*:

  Children > 3 years: 30–60 mg/kg/day div q TID

  Caution: Withdrawal of drug must be slow over at least one week

S/E: Dizziness, ataxia, headache, tremor, vomiting, nystagmus, and weight gain

(Gabapin, Gabantin, Neurontin 300 mg, 400 mg tab)

Lamotrigine

- *A broad spectrum adjunctive or monotherapy drug for all types of seizures including resistant complex partial, generalized tonic clonic, absence, myoclonic, clonic seizures, and Lennox-Gestaut*:
  - *If patient is not on valproate therapy*:
    - 2 mg/kg/day div q BID PO × 2 weeks, then 5 mg/kg/day div q BID PO × 2 weeks, then 10 mg/kg/day div q BID PO, if still uncontrolled

- Maximum dose 15 mg/kg/day but not exceeding 400 mg/day
- *If patient also on valproate:*
  - 0.1–0.2 mg/kg/day div q BID PO × 2 weeks, then
  - 0.2–0.5 mg/kg/day div q BID PO × 2 weeks, and then
  - 0.5–1 mg/kg/day div q BID PO, maximum 5 mg/kg/day or 150 mg/day

Caution: Initiate therapy with small dose and increase gradually at 2 week intervals. Serious risk of life-threatening Stevens-Johnson syndrome if rapid increase in dosage especially when combined with valproate.

Risk factors: Risk of life-threatening Stevens-Johnson syndrome, angioedema, toxic epidermal necrolysis especially in association with valproate

S/E: Nausea, headache, dizziness, blurred vision, diplopia, and rash

(Lametec, Lamitor 5 mg, 25 mg, 50 mg, 100 mg tab)

Levetiracetam

- *For partial and generalized tonic clonic seizures, myoclonic seizures, and BCECT:*
  - *Children* ≥4 years – <16 years*:
  - *Initial*: 20 mg/kg/day div q BID

*Note: Drug safety and efficacy not yet established in children below 4 years.

  - *Later*: May increase by 20 mg/kg/day every 2 weeks. Maximum 60 mg/kg/day div q BID
  - *Adolescents ≥ 16 years and adults*:
    - *Initial*: 500 mg/dose q BID;
    - *Later*: May increase every 2 weeks by 1,000 mg/day; maximum 3,000 mg/day

S/E: Somnolence, nervousness, asthenia, behavior disorder, aggression, GIT upset, accidental injury, and rarely psychosis

Caution: Taper dose slowly when discontinuing therapy. Abrupt withdrawal may enhance seizure frequency. Reduce dose in patients with renal dysfunction. Monitor Hb and WBC count.

(*Levroxa, levera, levecetam 250 mg, 500 mg, 750 mg tab, levroxa, levilex, kepra 100 mg/mL*)

Lorazepam

Benzodiazepine, anticonvulsant and anxiolytic:
- *Status epilepticus:*
  - *Neonates, infants and children:*
    - *IV*: 0.05–0.1 mg/kg/dose over 2–5 minutes. May repeat 0.05 mg/kg IV once in 10–15 minutes. Maximum dose 4 mg/dose
    - *PR*: 0.05–0.1 mg/kg, (if IV administration not feasible)
    - *Sublingual*: 0.05–1 mg/kg (home treatment of serial seizures to prevent progress to status epilepticus)
  - *Adults*:
    - *IV*: 4 mg/dose (not per kg) over 2–5 minutes. May repeat in 10–15 minutes.
    Total maximum dose in 12 h period: 8 mg
- *Anxiety or sedation*:
  - *Children*: 0.05 mg/kg/dose every 4–8 h PO/IV/IM; maximum dose 2 mg/dose
- *Adjunct to antiemetic therapy*:
  - *Children*: 0.04–0.08 mg/kg/dose IV (maximum single dose 4 mg); repeat q 6 h PRN

CI: Severe hypotension

S/E: Respiratory depression, sedation, depression, tachycardia, rash, and diplopia

(*Larpose, Calmese, Trapex 1 mg, 2 mg tab; Calmese, Trapex inj 2 mg/mL 2 mL amp*)

Midazolam

Benzodiazepine:
- *Status epilepticus:*
  - *Infants > 2 months and children*
    - *IV*: Loading dose—0.15 mg/kg followed by continuous infusion at the rate of 1 µg/kg/min;

titrate dose upward every 5 minutes until clinical seizure activity is controlled (usual infusion rate around 2.5 µg/kg/min), maximum 12 µg/kg/min
- *Buccal*: If IV access not available—0.3 mg/kg (maximum 5 mg), before reaching hospital
- *Neonatal seizures and febrile seizures:*
  - For details *see* in chapter 15
- *Sedation (preoperative sedation or conscious sedation for procedure):*
  - *IV*: 0.05–0.2 mg/kg load then continuous infusion at the rate of 1–2 µg/kg/min
  - *IM*: 0.1–0.15 mg/kg 30–60 minutes before surgery or procedure (maximum total dose—10 mg)
  - *Buccal, intranasal*: 0.15–0.3 mg/kg; may repeat in 5–15 minutes once
  - *Neonates*:
    - *Sedation*: Continous infusion 0.15–0.5 µg/kg/min

S/E: Respiratory depression, apnea, tonic/clonic movement, muscle tremor, sedation, paradoxical excitement, cardiac arrest, hypotension, and diplopia

(Fulsed, Sedeven, Shortal 5 mg/mL, 1 mL inj; 1 mg/mL, 5 mL, 10 mL inj)

Nitrazepam

- *Infantile spasms, myoclonic seizures, absence, and syndromes with multiple types of seizures:*

  Initial: 0.2 mg/kg/day div q TID PO; increase slowly to 1 mg/kg/day div q TID

S/E: Drowsiness, irritability, behavior abnormalities, and hallucinations

(Nitravet, Nitavan, 5 mg, 10 mg tab; Hypnotex 5 mg, 10 mg cap)

Oxcarbazepine

- *Partial seizures, BCECT:*
  Children > 3–17 years:

- *Initial*: 8–10 mg/kg/day div q BID PO (maximum 600 mg/day); increase slowly over 2 weeks
- *Usual maintenance dose*: 20–40 mg/kg/day div q BID PO (maximum 1800 mg/day)

Adults:
- *Initial*: 600 mg/day div q BID PO; increase slowly over 2 weeks;
- *Usual maintenance dose*: 1,200 mg/day div q BID PO (maximum 2,400 mg/day)

S/E: Headache, dizziness, somnolence, cognitive disturbance, rash, GIT upset, diplopia, hyponatremia, and rarely hypersensitivity reaction

(Oxcarb, Oxeptal, Oxetol 150 mg, 300 mg, 600 mg tab)

Paraldehyde

- *Status epilepticus in children:* Refer to chapter 15 for details
  - *IV* (paraldehyde 5% solution in D5W):
    Loading dose: 150–200 mg/kg IV slowly over 15–20 minutes followed by IV infusion at the rate of 20 mg/kg/h. Lower the IV drip rate as the seizures improve.
    Note: Prepare 5% solution of paraldehyde by adding 1.75 mL of paraldehyde (1 g/mL) to 5% dextrose solution to make a total volume of 35 mL. The paraldehyde solution must be administered only in a glass bottle as the drug is incompatible with and dissolves plastic. Shield the solution in the bottle with brown paper or aluminum foil to prevent paraldehyde from getting oxidized by exposure to light into highly toxic acetic acid.
  - *IM*: 0.15 mL/kg deep IM (as an alternative to IV administration). Use a glass (and not plastic) syringe.

Note: Always use a freshly opened paraldehyde bottle (for IV or IM use) since old outdated paraldehyde may have deteriorated to acetaldehyde and acetic acid.

- *Refractory neonatal seizures:* For dosage and mode of administration, see under on "Drug therapy in Epilepsy and Neonatal Seizures".

- *For agitation*:
  - *PR (diluted in equal amount of olive oil)*: 0.15 mL/kg/dose every 6–24 h PRN

Pentobarbital

Barbiturate; anticonvulsant; hypnotic; and general anesthetic:
Children:
- *Hypnotic*: 2–6 mg/kg/dose IM (maximum 100 mg/dose)
- *Conscious preoperative sedation*: Children > 18 months:
  - *Initial 2 mg/kg/IV*; may repeat 1–2 mg/kg q 5–10 minutes until adequate sedation (maximum total dose 6 mg/kg or 150–200 mg)
- *Pentobarbital coma:* Loading dose 10–15 mg/kg IV slowly over 1–2 h; maintenance infusion—initial 1 mg/kg/h; may increase to 2–3 mg/kg/h; maintain burst suppression on EEG

S/E: Drowsiness, CNS excitation or depression, respiratory depression, hypotension, and arrhythmia

(Nembutal sodium solution 20 mL and 50 mL multiple dose vials 50 mg/mL)

Phenobarbitone

Barbiturate:
- *Neonatal seizures and status epilepticus (neonates and children)*:
  - *IV*:
    - *Loading dose in neonate:* 15–20 kg IV slowly. May repeat 5 mg/kg q 15 minutes in neonate to a total maximum dose of 30 mg/kg
    - *Loading dose infants and children*: 5–10 mg/kg
- *Generalized tonic clonic, partial, and myoclonic seizures (maintenance dose)*
  - *Children below 5 years*: PO 3–5 mg/kg/day div q 12–24 h
  - *Children 5 years and above*: PO 2–3 mg/kg/day div q 12–24 h
- *Sedation:*
  - *Children*: PO/IM/IV: 2 mg/kg/dose; may repeat q TID PRN

- *Hyperbilirubinemia (neonatal)*
  - 3–8 mg/kg/day div q BID/TID PO

Precautions: IV phenobarbitone to be given slowly at the rate of not more than 1 mg/kg/min. Watch closely for hypotension and respiratory depression. Use cautiously in hepatic and renal disease.

CI: Acute intermittent porphyria and hyperkinetic children

S/E: Drowsiness, cognitive function impairment, paradoxical hyperactivity, rash, and hypotension

(Gardenal, Phenobarb 30 mg, 60 mg tab, Luminal 30 mg tab; Luminalettes 15 mg tab; Gardenal syr 20 mg/5 mL; Phenobarbitone sodium 200 mg/mL 1 mL inj)

Phenytoin

Anticonvulsant and antiarrhythmic:
- *Status epilepticus:*
  - *Loading dose IV*: 15–20 mg/kg (by slow infusion diluted in N. saline and not dextrose) at the rate of maximum 1 mg/kg/min. May repeat 10 mg/kg/IV after 1 hour. Maximum dose 1500 mg/24 h
- *Generalized tonic clonic and partial seizures*
  - *Maintenance*:
    - *Neonates*:
      - *< 6 months*: 8–10 mg/kg/day div q BID-TID PO/IV
    - *6 months–6 years*: 7.5–9 mg/kg/day div q BID-TID PO/IV
    - *7 years–16 years*: 6–8 mg/kg/day div q BID-TID PO/IV
    - *Adults*: 300–600 mg/day PO/IV div q BID-TID
- *Digoxin-induced arrhythmias*
  - *Loading doses IV*: 1.25 mg/kg and then every 5 minutes until desired effect (up to total dose of 15 mg/kg)
  - *Maintenance*:
    - *PO/IV*: 5–10 mg/kg/day div q 8–12 h (maximum 600 mg/day)

Precautions: Administer the drug IV diluted only with N. saline or 1/2 N. saline; do not give in glucose solution. Monitor closely for bradycardia, arrhythmia and hypotension

Therapeutic level: 10–20 µg/mL (free and bound), check after 7–10 days of regular dosing; desired timing of sampling: within 30 minutes prior to the next scheduled dose

S/E: Hirsutism, gum hypertrophy, ataxia, rash, Stevens-Johnson syndrome, nystagmus, coarsening facial features, liver damage, and blood dyscrasias

(Eptoin 50 mg, 100 mg tab, susp 125 mg/5 mL; Dilantin 25 mg, 100 mg cap, susp 125 mg/5 mL; Inj Dilantin, PE 50 mg/mL 2 mL amp)

Primidone

- *Generalized tonic clonic and partial seizures:*
    - *Children < 8 years*: 10–25 mg/kg/day div q BID-TID PO
    - *> 8 years and adults: Initial*: 125–250 mg/day PO; increase by 125–250 mg/day every 3–7 days

Usual dose: 750–1500 mg/day div q TID-QID PO maximum: 2 g/day

S/E: Personality changes, aggressive behavior, sedation, rash, and ataxia

(Mysoline 250 mg tab)

Propofol

- *Sedative and general anesthetic:*
    - *Sedation*: 1.5–3 mg/kg/dose IV over 1–2 minutes
- *Status epilepticus seizures unresponsive to other anticonvulsants:*
    - *Loading dose*: 1–2 mg/kg IV bolus followed by 1–2 mg/kg/h infusion (maximum 5 mg/kg/h). To be given for maximum period of 48 h

(Inj Propavan 1%, 10 mL, 20 mL vial; 2% 10 mL, 25 mL vial; Inj Propofol 2%)

Thiopental Sodium (Pentothal)

- *Cerebral edema*: 1.5–5 mg/kg/dose IV, repeat PRN
- *Status epilepticus:*
  - IV *loading dose*: 5 mg/kg and then 3–5 mg/kg/h infusion titrated to achieve a burst suppression EEG pattern. Start tapering after 24 h seizure period
- *Anesthesia induction*: 5–8 mg/kg IV
- *Sedation*: PR 5–10 mg/kg/dose; up to 30 mg/kg for deep sedation (maximum 1 g/dose)

(*Inj pentothal 250 mg, 500 mg, 1 g vials*)

Tiagabine

- *Adjunctive therapy for complex partial seizures:*
  - *Children*: Age above 12 years 0.5–2 mg/kg/day div q BID/QID PO
  - *Adolescents and adults*:
    - *Initial*: 4 mg/dose q OD; later increase by 4–8 mg every week until response (maximum 32 mg/day)

S/E: Dizziness, tiredness, drowsiness, depression, tremor

(*Gabitril 2 mg, 4 mg, 12 mg, 16 mg tab*)

Topiramate

- *Adjunctive therapy for refractory generalized tonic clonic, juvenile myoclonic epilepsy, complex partial seizures, infantile spasms and in Lennox–Gestaut syndrome:*

  1–9 mg/kg/day div q BID PO; slow titration

  S/E: Fatigue, cognitive depression, and glaucoma

  (*Topex, Topamac 25 mg, 100 mg tab*)

Valproic Acid (Sodium Valproate)

- *Broad spectrum for all types of seizures including generalized tonic clonic, absence, myoclonic, partial, and akinetic seizures:*
  - *Initial*: 10–15 mg/kg/day div q TID PO; increase weekly by 5–10 mg/kg/day until seizures controlled or side effects occur; maximum dose 60 mg/kg/day.

- *Usual maintenance dose*: 15–40 mg/kg/day div q TID PO. May need up to 100 mg/kg/day div q TID/QID, when child is receiving multiple anticonvulsants (e.g. phenytoin, carbamazepine)

CI: Hepatic disease

Caution: Fatal hepatic failure reported in few, especially in children below 2 years of age when under treatment with other anticonvulsants simultaneously

S/E: Drowsiness, tremor, hepatotoxicity, vomiting, weight gain, alopecia, thrombocytopenia, and rash

Serum therapeutic level: 50–100 µg/mL; toxic more than 150 µg/mL

(Valparin 200 mg, 500 mg tab, susp 200 mg/5 mL; Valtec 200 mg, 300 mg, 500 mg tab, susp. 200 mg/5 mL; Valparin chrono, Valtec CR 200 mg, 300 mg, 500 mg tab)

Vigabatrin

- *Infantile spasms (especially in children with tuberous sclerosis) and as adjunctive therapy for poorly controlled partial seizures:*
  - *Initial*: 30 mg/kg/day div q OD/BID
  - *Maintenance*: 50–150 mg/kg/day div q OD/BID

S/E: Bilateral visual field defects, CNS depression, behavior disturbance, and GIT intolerance

Monitoring: Do baseline eye examination and then every 6 months

(Sabril tab 500 mg)

Zonisamide

- *Anticonvulsant for treatment of partial epilepsy:*
  For children > 16 years: 4–8 mg/kg/day div q BID or QID

S/E: Fatigue, dizziness, anorexia, ataxia, and rarely hallucinations

(*Zonisep cap 25 mg, 50 mg, Zonegram tab 25 mg, 100 mg; Zorit, Zonimid 50 mg, 100 mg*)

BRONCHODILATORS AND DRUGS FOR ASTHMA

Adrenaline

See Epinephrine below

Aminophylline*

- *Apnea of prematurity, neonatal apnea:*
  - *Loading dose*: 6 mg/kg IV (infuse over 30 min)
  - *Maintenance dose*: 5-6 mg/kg/24 h div q 8 h IV/PO
- *Asthma (acute attack):*
  - *Loading dose*: 6 mg/kg IV (over 20 minutes)
  - *Maintenance dose*: IV
  - *Neonates*: 5 mg/kg/day
  - *Infants*:
    - *6 weeks–6 months*: 12 mg/kg/day (0.5 mg/kg/h)
    - *6 months–1 year*: 17 mg/kg/day (0.7 mg/kg/h)
    - *Note:* Infant is up to < 1 year
  - Children:
    - *1–9 years*: 24 mg/kg/day (1 mg/kg/h)
    - *9–12 years*: 21 mg/kg/day (0.9 mg/kg/h)
    - *> 12 years*: 16 mg/kg/day (0.6 mg/kg/h)

The above total doses per day may either be given by continuous IV infusion or administered IV div q 4-6 h

*Aminophylline is the ethylenediamine salt of theophylline. (100 mg of aminophylline = 80 mg theophylline)

Caution: Avoid initial loading dose or reduce it to 50% if patient has received theophylline within previous 24 h

S/E: Nausea, anorexia, nervousness, and tachycardia and at toxic levels—seizures, arrhythmia, and hypotension

Note: For oral use and dose see under theophylline [Aminophylline (Glaxo), inj 250 mg/2 mL; 10 mL ampoule; Aminophylline tab 100 mg]

Bambuterol Hydrochloride

Long acting beta-2 adrenergic agonist
- *Chronic bronchial asthma and nocturnal asthma:*
  - *Children*:
    - *2–5 years*: 5 mg single dose, shortly before bed time
    - *6–12 years*: 10 mg single dose, shortly before bed time
  - *Adults*: 10–20 mg single dose, shortly before bed time

(Bambudil, Betaday 10 mg, 20 mg tab, oral solution 1 mg/1 mL)

Beclomethasone Dipropionate

Corticosteroid (for oral inhalation)
- *Bronchial asthma:*
  - *5–12 years*: 150–400 µg/day div q TID/QID maximum 500 µg/day
  - *> 12 years and adults*: 400–800 µg/day div q BID/TID/QID; maximum 1,000 µg/day

Note: The number of inhalations to be adjusted according to drug content in each metered dose or Rotacap

S/E: Oropharyngeal candidiasis, dysphonia, suppression of hypothalamic-pituitary-adrenal axis following prolonged therapy at high doses

(Beclate inhaler 50 µg, 100 µg, 200 µg, 250 µg/puff, rotacap 100 µg, 200 µg, 400 µg/cap; Becoride inhaler 50 µg, 100 µg, 250 µg/puff)

Budesonide

Adrenal corticosteroid for oral inhalation, by nebulization and nasal spray:
- *Asthma*
  - *Oral inhaler*:
    - *Children 5 years or more*: Start at 1 inhalation (100 µg) BID and increase as needed. Maximum 800 µg/day

- *Adults*: Start at 1 inhalation (200 µg) BID and increase as needed. Maximum 1,600 µg/day
  - *Nebulization*
    - *Children*: Start at 0.5–1 mg q BID in acute exacerbation
      - Maintenance: 0.25 mg to 0.5 mg q BID
    - *Adults*: Start at 1–2 mg q BID in acute exacerbation
      - Maintenance: 0.5–1 mg q BID

S/E: Pharyngitis, cough, epistaxis, and nasal irritation. Rinsing mouth after each oral inhalation reduces chances of pharyngitis

- *Allergic Rhinitis*
  - *Children > 6 years and adults*:
    - *Initial*: 2 sprays 50 µg per spray, i.e. 100 µg in each nostril morning and at bed time or 4 sprays in each nostril morning. Maximum total dose 8 sprays/400 µg/day.
    - Reduce dose gradually to lowest effective dose

S/E: Oropharyngeal candidiasis, dysphonia, epistaxis, nasal irritation, and suppression of hypothalamic-pituitary-adrenal axis following prolonged therapy at high doses

Note: Rinsing mouth after each oral inhalation reduces incidence of pharyngitis.

(*Budecort inhaler 100 µg, 200 µg/dose; Rotacap 100, 200, 400 µg/cap; respules 0.25 mg, 0.5 mg, 1 mg/2 mL. Pulmicort inhaler 100 µg, 200 µg, 400 µg/puff; for nebulization 0.5 mg and 1 mg in 2 mL; Rhinocort nasal spray 50 µg per spray*)

Ciclesonide

- *Allergic rhinitis*
  - *Child 2–12 years*: 1–2 spray in each nostril once daily
  - *> 12 years*: 2 spray in each nostril once daily
- *Bronchial asthma*
  - *Child 12–18 years*: 160 ug single dose OD; reduce to 80 ug OD if control maintained

S/E: As with other inhaled corticosteroids

(*Ciclez inhaler 80 µg, 160 µg; Osonide inhaler 80 µg, 160 ug*)

Cromolyn (Sodium Cromoglycate)

Antiallergic agent: Mast cell stabilizer
- *For prevention of asthma:*
  Inhaler 5 mg/dose:
  - *Initial*: 2 puffs q QID;
  - *Maintenance*: 1 puff q QID

  Rotacaps 20 mg/dose:
  - *Initial*: 1 Rotacap q QID;
  - *Maintenance*: 1 cap q BID-TID

  Nebulization solution: (20 mg/2 mL): 20 mg q TID-QID

S/E: Hoarseness, coughing, and stinging sensation (more with Rotacap)

Note: Not indicated for relief of acute bronchospasm

(Cromal aerosol inhaler 5 mg/puff, Rotacap 20 mg/cap; respule 2 mg/2 mL: Ifiral Rotacap 20 mg/cap)

Epinephrine (Adrenaline)

Sympathomimetic agent:
- *For cardiac arrest and severe bradycardia:*
  - *Neonates*:
    - *IV and intratracheal*: 0.1–0.3 mL/kg of 1 in 10,000 solution; may repeat 2–3 times every 3–5 minutes

  Caution: Use 1: 1,000 solution only after diluting it 10 times
  - *Infants and children*:
    - *Initial*: IV 0.1 mL/kg of 1 in 10,000 solution (maximum 10 mL/dose). If no response: 0.1 mL/kg of 1 in 1,000 solution IV, repeat q 3–5 minutes PRN; if still not effective, give 0.2 mL/kg (of 1 in 1,000 solution) IV.

      If IV route not feasible, the second and subsequent doses can be given through endotracheal tube—0.1 mL/kg of 1 in 1,000 solution diluted in 3–5 mL of saline

- *For bronchospasm:*

Infants and children: SC 0.01 mL/kg of 1 in 1,000 solution; maximum single dose 0.5 mL; may repeat once after 15–30 minutes

- *Anaphylaxis*: 0.01 mL/kg of 1 in 1,000 solution (maximum 0.3 mL/dose) intramuscular injection, repeat twice every 15–20 minutes, if required. (IM injection achieves higher and quicker effective plasma concentration).

If anaphylactic reaction is secondary to a Hymenoptera sting, dilute one-half of the dose of epinephrine in 2 mL normal saline and infiltrate S/C at the site of sting to slow absorption and give the rest IM.

In case of persistent hypotension, under careful cardiac monitoring give slow IV infusion at an initial infusion rate of 0.1 µg/kg/min with gradual rise up to 1 µg/kg/min to sustain a systolic BP of 80 + (2 × age in years) mm Hg, under close cardiac monitoring

S/E: Tachycardia, hypertension, arrhythmia, restlessness, vomiting, and tremor

[Adrenaline tartrate (P&B Labs) inj 1 in 1,000 soln; (1 mg/mL); 1 mL amp]

Fluticasone Propionate

- Bronchial asthma
  By inhalation
  - *Children ≤ 12 years:*
    - *Low dose*: 100–200 µg/day div q BID
    - *Medium dose*: 200–500 µg/day div q BID
    - *High dose*: >500 µg/day div q BID
  - *Children > 12 years and adults:*
    - *Low dose*: 100–250 µg/day div q BID
    - *Medium dose*: >250–500 µg/day div q BID
    - *High dose*: >500 µg/day div q BID

(*Floease 50 µg, 125 µg/MDI, puff; Flutiflo 50 µg MDI; Ventiflo 50, 100, 200 mg 1 cap*)

Formoterol Fumarate

Long acting beta-2 agonist inhaler
- Bronchial asthma:

For inhalation; children > 5 years: 12 µg per inhalation (1 puff) BID;

Adults: 1–2 puff BID

Note: This drug is for long-term control of asthma. Not indicated for relief of acute bronchospasm

(Foratec inhaler 12 µg/dose, Rotacap 12 µg/cap)

Hydrocortisone Sodium Succinate

Corticosteroid:
- *Status asthmaticus*:
  - *Initial*: 4–8 mg/kg/dose (maximum 250 mg dose) followed by 8 mg/kg/day IV div q 6 hours
- *Anti-inflammatory*:
  - *PO*: 2.5–10 mg/kg/day div q 6–8 h
  - *IM/IV*: 1–5 mg/kg/day div q OD/BID
- *Acute adrenal insufficiency*:
  - *Load*: 1–2 mg/kg/dose IV bolus;
  - *Maintenance*:
    - *Infants and young children*: 25–150 mg/day div q 6–8 h
    - *Older children*: 150–250 mg/day div q 6–8 h
- *Anaphylaxis (as adjunct to other essential treatment)*
  - 5 mg/kg/dose q 6 h IV PRN
- *Shock*
  - *Children IV*:
    - *Initial*: 50 mg/kg, may repeat after 4 h and then 50–150 mg/kg/day div q 6 h/24 h for 48–72 h
  - *Adults*: 500 mg–2 g/dose q 2–6 h IV
- *Neonatal hypoglycemia (refractory to glucose infusion)*
  - *Neonates*: IV 5 mg/kg/day div q 8–12 h or 1–2 mg/kg/dose q 6 h

Note: Use only sodium succinate salt of hydrocortisone for IV/IM use. The acetate salt is meant for intra-articular, intra-synovial or intralesional injection only.

S/E: As with prednisone

[Inj Efcorlin, Hydrocortisone sodium succinate (Lyka, Samarth), (Hydrocortisone sodium succinate 134 mg equivalent to 100 mg hydrocortisone) vial]

Ipratropium Bromide

Anticholinergic bronchodilator:
- *Inhaler*:
  - *Below 12 years*: 1–2 puffs q TID/QID (20 µg/puff)
  - *> 12 years*: 2–3 puffs q QID (maximum 12 inhalation/24 h)
- *Rotahaler*:
  - *> 12 years and adults*: 1–2 Rotacaps TID/QID (40 µg/cap)
- *Nebulization*:
  - *< 12 years*: 125–250 µg/dose q TID-QID
  - *≥ 12 years*: 250–500 µg/dose q TID-QID

S/E: Dry mouth, blurred vision, urinary retention, and headache

(Ipravent inhaler 20 µg/puff, Forte inhaler 40 µg/dose; Ipravent respirator solution 250 µg/mL, respules 500 µg/2 mL)

Ketotifen

Children > 2 years: 1 mg/day/q OD PO; maximum 2 mg/day div q BID. Not recommended below 2 years of age

S/E: Drowsiness, dry mouth, and dizziness

(Asthafen, Tritofen 1 mg tab, syr 1 mg/5 mL)

Levosalbutamol

Bronchodilator:

A. For bronchial asthma acute exacerbation (status asthmaticus):
   By nebulization
   - 0.075 mg/kg (minimum 1.25 mg) q 20 minutes × 3 doses, then 0.075–1.5 mg/kg up to 5 mg every 1–4 h as needed or 0.25 mg/kg/h by continuum nebulization

B. *Bronchial asthma (as reliever drug in persistent asthma):*
   - *MDI 50 ug puff;* 2–4 puffs as needed
   - Oral 0.05–0.2 mg/kg/dose q BID/TID

S/E: Palpitation, tremor, nervousness, headache, nausea, and hypokalemia

(*Levolin 1 mg tab; syrup 0.5 and 1 mg/5 mL;*)

(*Levolin MDI puff 50 μg/puff*)

(*Duolin MDI: Levosalbutamol 50 μg + ipratropium bromide 20 μg per puff; Duolin respules: levosalbutamol 1.25 mg + ipratropium bromide 500 μg per 2.5 mL*).

Magnesium Sulfate

- *Acute attack of asthma:*

25 mg/kg (maximum 2 g/dose) IV diluted in 30 mL N. saline/5% dextrose infusion over 30 minutes

CI: Heart block, myocardial damage, and severe renal impairment

Precaution: Renal insufficiency and digoxin therapy

S/E: Hypotension, respiratory depression, hypermagnesemia, and diarrhea

Antidote: Calcium gluconate IV

Note: 1 mL of 50% magnesium sulfate solution contains 500 mg = 4.0 mEq of magnesium sulfate

Montelukast

Leukotriene receptor antagonist:
- *Asthma-prophylaxis and treatment of mild or moderate chronic asthma:*
  - 2–5 years: 4 mg/dose OD in the evening PO
  - 6–14 years: 5 mg/dose OD in the evening PO
  - ≥15 years and adults: 10 mg/dose OD in the evening PO

S/E: Headache, dizziness, abdominal pain, fatigue, and elevated liver enzymes

(*Montair, Romilast 4 mg, 5 mg, 10 mg tab*)

Salbutamol

Beta-2 adrenergic agonist:
- *Acute severe attack of asthma:*
  i. *MDI with spacer (100 µg/puff)*: 2-8 puffs every 20 minutes × 3 times as needed, then every 1-4 hr as needed
  ii. OR—Nebulised solution through 0.15 mg/kg/dose (min 2.5 mg; maximum 5 mg) every 20 minutes three times, then 0.15-0.3 mg/kg (maximum 10 mg) every 1-4 h as needed OR 0.1-0.15 mg/kg/h by continuous nebulization (maximum 15 mg/h)
- *Chronic asthma*
  - *MDI (100 µg/puff) or rotacap (200 µg/cap)*: 1-2 puffs/cap q 4-6 h PRN
  - *Nebulizing solution (0.5%)*: 0.1-0.15 mg/kg/dose (min 1.25 mg, maximum 5 mg) q 4-6 h PRN
  - *Oral*: 0.2-0.4 mg/kg/day div q 6-8 h

S/E: Palpitation, tremor, nervousness, headache, and nausea

(*Inhalers*: Asthalin, Ventorlin, Vent, Derihaler inhaler 100 µg/puff; Asthalin, Derihaler 200 ug per Rotacap)

(*Nebulizing solution*: Asthalin 2.5 mg per 2.5 mL respirule and 5 mg per mL-15 mL solution; Salsol 2.5 mg/3 mL solution)

(*Tablets*: Asthalin, Salbetol 2 mg, 4 mg;)

(*Syrup*: Asthalin, Ventorlin 2 mg/5 mL)

Note: Various combination products of salbutamol with bromhexine or theophylline or ambroxol or guaiphenesin also available.

Salmeterol

Long acting beta-2 agonist:
- *Chronic bronchial asthma:*
  - *By inhalation*
    - *Children 4-12 years*: 50-100 µg/day div q BID
    - *> 12 years and adults*: 100 µg/day div q BID (maximum 200 µg/day)

- *Exercise induced asthma:*
  - *> 12 years*: 50 µg/dose, single dose 30–60 minutes before exercise (if patient not already on salmeterol)

(Serobid inhaler 25 µg/puff, rotacap 50 µg/cap; Salmeterol, Solvent inhaler 25 µg/puff)

Terbutaline Sulfate

Beta-2 adrenergic agonist

- For acute severe attack of asthma:

  S/C:
  - *Initial*: 0.005–.01 mg/kg, i.e. 01–0.02 mL/kg (of 0.5 mg/mL solution) stat
  - *Maximum*: 0.3 mg (i.e. 0.6 mL of solution) per dose; may repeat once after 15–20 minutes
  - Subsequently may be given every 2–6 h PRN

  By continuous IV infusion:
  - *Loading dose*: 2–10 µg/kg followed by infusion at the rate of 0.1–0.4 µg/kg/min
  - May increase by 0.1–0.2 µg/kg/min q 30 min PRN. Maximum dose 4 µg/kg/min

  By inhalation:
  - *250 µg/puff*: 2 puffs q 5 minutes for a total of 10–20 puffs

  By nebulization:
  - *< 20 kg*: 2.5 mg
  - *≥ 20 kg*: 5 mg

  For chronic asthma:
  - *PO—< 12 years*: Initial—0.15 mg/kg/day div q TID; increase PRN (maximum 5 mg/day)
  - *PO—12–15 years*: 7.5 mg/day div q TID
  - *PO—> 15 years*: 7.5–15 mg/day div q TID
  - *Inhalation*: 1–2 inhalation q 4–6 h (250 µg/puff)

S/E: Tremor, tachycardia, arrhythmia, headache, and paroxysmal bronchospasm

[Bricanyl 2.5 mg, 5 mg tab; syr 1.5 mg/5 mL; Bricanyl, Terbutaline sulfate (Astra) inj 0.5 mg/mL (1 mL amp) Bricanyl Misthaler 250 µg/puff; Bricanyl Nebulizing solution 10 mg/mL (10 mL)]

(*Note: Various combination products of terbutaline with bromhexine or guaiphensin or ambroxol also available*)

Theophylline

Bronchodilator:
- *Neonate: Apnea, bronchodilation*
  - *Loading dose*: 6 mg/kg PO × once
  - *Maintenance*: 2-4 mg/kg/day div q 12 h PO
- *Infants and children: Bronchodilation—maintenance dose*
  - *6 weeks-6 months*: 10 mg/kg/day PO
  - *6 months-1 year*: 12-18 mg/kg/day PO
  - *1-9 years*: 20-24 mg/kg/day PO
  - *9-12 years*: 16 mg/kg/day PO
  - *12-16 years*: 13 mg/kg/day PO
  - *> 16 years*: 10 mg/kg/day PO
- *Note 1:* The above dosage has been indicated on the basis of theophylline. For the purpose of correct calculation, its true content in different theophylline salts has been given in Table 33.11.
- *Note 2*: Begin therapy initially with two-thirds the usual final dose for that particular age. May later gradually increase dose as per clinical response. *Initial*—maximum dose of theophylline 300 mg/day; maximum final dose 600 mg/day.

  Check the exact theophylline content of the drug preparation before prescribing it.

Some proprietary preparations:
- *Theophylline: Anhydrous preparations*—Theoped syrup (50 mg/5 mL); TR phylline (80 mg/5 mL); Theo PA 100 mg, 300 mg tab; theobid SR tab 200 mg, 300 mg

Table 33.11: Theophylline content and equivalent dose of various theophylline salts.

Theophylline salt	Theophylline %	Equivalent dose
Theophylline anhydrous	100	100 mg
Aminophylline anhydrous	85%	115 mg
Etophylline	80%	120 mg
Choline theophyllinate (oxtriphylline)	64%	156 mg

- *Theophylline salts combination preparations*: Deriphyllin syrup (Etophylline 46.5 mg + theophylline hydrate 14 mg/5 mL); Deriphyllin tab (Etophylline 77 mg + theophylline hydrate 23 mg/tab); Deriphyllin inj (Etophylline 169.4 mg + theophylline hydrate 50.6 mg/2 mL amp) Deriphyllin retard 150 mg, 300 mg, 450 mg tab
- *Aminophylline preparations:* Aminophylline, Minophyl 100 mg tab; 250 mg/10 mL amp

S/E: Nausea, anorexia, abdominal pain, nervousness, tachycardia and at toxic level seizures, arrhythmia, and hypotension

(Theoped syr 100 mg/5 mL; Etophylate syr 125 mg/5 mL; Broncordil 26.67 mg/5 mL; Deriphyllin retard tab 150 mg, 300 mg, 450 mg; Deriphyllin syrup 60.5 mg/5 mL, tab 100 mg)

Zafirlukast

Leukotriene receptor antagonist
- *Prophylaxis and treatment of mild or moderate chronic asthma:*
  - *Children 5–11 years*: 10 mg/dose q BID PO
  - *Children > 12 years and adults*: 20 mg/dose q BID PO

Caution: *Hepatic dysfunction*

S/E: Headache, nausea, abdominal pain, and elevated LFT

(Zuvair 10 mg, 20 mg tab)

GIT DRUGS AND ANTISPASMODICS

Aluminum Hydroxide

Without and with magnesium hydroxide:
- *Peptic ulcer:*
  - *Children*: 5–15 mL/dose q 3–6 h PO
- *Prophylaxis against GI bleeding:*
  - *Neonate*: 1 mL/kg/dose q 4 h PO
  - *Infant*: 2–5 mL/dose q 1–2 h PO
  - *Child*: 5–15 mL/dose q 1–2 h PO

Note: Above doses are based on suspension containing aluminum hydroxide 300 mg/5 mL

Caution: Renal failure

S/E: Constipation, encephalopathy, and phosphorus depletion

(Diovol, Gelusil, Siloxogene tab/susp)

Bethanechol

Cholinergic agent:
- Gastroesophageal reflux (GER) or nonobstructive urinary retention:
  - *Children*: 0.3–0.6 mg/kg/day div q TID/QID PO
  - *Adults*: 10–50 mg/dose q BID/QID PO

S/E: Abdominal cramps, diarrhea, urinary frequency, bronchial constriction, and hypotension

(Urotone 25 mg tab)

Bisacodyl

Stimulant laxative:
- Children 3–12 years
  - *PO*: 5–10 mg; per day once as a single dose
  - *PR < 2 years*: 5 mg; *2–11 years*; 5–10 mg; once as a single dose
- Children > 12 year and adults
  - *PO*: 5–20 mg/day once as a single dose
  - PR: 10 mg/day once as a single dose

Note: Oral tablets act in about 10–12 h; suppositories act in about 20–60 minutes

CI: Intestinal obstruction, acute abdominal condition, acute inflammatory bowel disease, pregnancy, lactation, and vomiting

Precaution: Do not chew or crush tablets. May cause gastric irritation

S/E: Fluid and electrolyte imbalance, abdominal cramps; rectal irritation by suppository

[Dulcolax 5 mg tab, suppository 5 mg (child), 10 mg (adult); Bidlax-5, 5 mg tab]

Cimetidine

Histamine-2 antagonist:
Neonates: PO/IV/IM 5–10 mg/kg/day div q 8–12 h
Infants: PO/IV/IM 10–20 mg/kg/day div q 6–12 h
Children: PO/IV/IM 20–40 mg/kg/day div q 6 h
Adults: PO/IV/IM 300 mg/dose q 6 h

S/E: Diarrhea, rash, neutropenia, and elevated LFT

(Tagamed, Ulcipan, Tymild 200 mg, 400 mg tab; Inj Tagamed 200 mg/mL 2 mL)

Dicyclomine Hydrochloride

Anticholinergic:
Infants > 6 months: *PO*: 5 mg/dose q TID/QID
Children:
   PO: 10 mg/dose q TID/QID
Adults:
   IM: 20 mg/dose q QID PRN
   PO: 20–40 mg/dose q QID

[Colimex, Spasmindon, Clomin, Cyclopam drops (dicyclomine 10 mg + dimethicone 40 mg) per mL; Cyclopam susp (dicyclomine 10 mg + dimethicone 40 mg) per 5 mL; Cyclopam, Clomin (dicyclomaine 20 mg + paracetamol 500 mg) tab; Cyclopam inj 20 mg/2 mL]

Docusate

Stool softener and laxative:
< 3 years: 10–40 mg/day div q OD/QID PO
3–6 years: 20–60 mg/day div q OD/QID PO
6–12 years: 40–150 mg/day div q OD/QID PO
> 12 years: 50–500 mg/day div q OD/QID PO

(Laxicon tab 100 mg, syrup 50 mg/5 mL, enema 0.25% solution; Cellubril cap 100 mg)

Drotaverine HCl

Antispasmodic:
1–6 years: 20 mg/dose q TID PO/IM
> 6–12 years: 40 mg/dose q TID PO/IM
Adults: 40–80 mg/dose q TID PO/IM

CI: Glaucoma

(Drotin, Doverin 40 mg, 80 mg tab, inj. 20 mg/mL (2 mL amp); Drotin-M, DVN-Plus, Drotaverine HCl 80 mg + mefenamic acid 250 mg tab, Drotein susp. 10 mg/5 mL, drotin DS susp. 20 mg/5 mL)

Esomeprazole

Proton pump inhibitor:
- *For gastroesophageal reflux disease (GERD):*
  Child 1–12 years:
  - *10–20 kg*: 10 mg q OD × 8 weeks
  - *> 20 kg*: 10–20 mg q OD × 8 weeks

S/E: As of other proton pump inhibitors, such as omeprazole

(Ezoz, Nexpro, Blocacid, Famocid 20 mg, 40 mg tab; Nexpro, Esoz 40 mg inj)

Famotidine

Histamine-2 receptor antagonist:
- *Gastroesophageal reflux disease:*
  - Neonates and infants < 3 months: 0.5 mg/kg/day div q OD PO
  - *Infants 3 months–1 year*: 1 mg/kg/day div q BD PO
- *Gastroesophageal reflux disease and peptic ulcer:*
  - *Children 1–12 years*:
    - *PO/IV*: 0.5–1 mg/kg/day div q BID (maximum 40 mg/day)
  - *Children > 12 years and adults*:
    - *PO*: 20 mg/day div q HS/BID (maximum 40 mg/day; for esophagitis maximum 80 mg/day)
    - *IV*: 20 mg/dose q 12 h

Caution: Reduce dose in renal dysfunction; watch for thrombocytopenia

[Facid, Topcid 20 mg, 40 mg tab, inj 20 mg/mL (2 mL); Facid AC, Topcid CT chew tab 10 mg tab]

Hyoscine Butylbromide

Antispasmodic:

6–12 years:
    PO: 10 mg/dose q 8 h/6 h
    IM/IV: 10 mg/dose q 8 h/6 h
Adults:
    PO: 10–20 mg/dose q TID/QID
    IM/IV: 20 mg/dose q TID/QID

CI: Glaucoma and GI obstruction

(Buscopan, Belloid 10 mg tab; inj 20 mg/1 mL amp; Buscopan 7.5 mg, 10 mg supp.)

Lactulose

- *Chronic constipation:*
  - *Infant 1 month–1 year*: 2.5 mL/dose q BID PO (adjust according to response)
  - *Child 1–5 years*: 5 mL/dose q BID PO (adjust according to response)
  - *Child 5–10 years*: 10 mL/dose q BD PO (adjust according to response)
  - *Child 10–18 years*: 15 mL/dose q BD PO (adjust according to response)
- *Hepatic encephalopathy*
  - *Child 12–18 years*: 30–45 mL/dose q TID (adjust dose to produce 2–3 soft stools per day

CI: Galactosemia and intestinal obstruction

S/E: Flatulence, cramps, and abdominal discomfort

(Livoluk, Looz, Duphalac 3.325 g/5 mL)

Lansoprazole

Gastric acid secretion inhibitor:

- *Gastroesophageal reflux disease:* Duodenal and benign gastric ulcer
    - *Below 30 kg:* 0.5–1 mg/kg (max 15 mg) OD in the morning
    - *> 30 kg*: 15–30 mg q OD
    - Children > 12 years and adults 30 mg q OD

(Lanzol, Lancus, Lansofast 15 mg, 30 mg cap); Lanzol Jr. 15 mg DT)

Loperamide

- *Acute diarrhea:*
    - *Initial dose during the first 24 h:*
        - PO 2–6 years: 1 mg TID;
        - 6–8 years: 2 mg BID;
        - 9–12 years: 2 mg TID
    - *Subsequently (after 24 h)*: 0.1 mg/kg after each loose stool (not to exceed the initial doses indicated above)
        - *Children 12 years and Adults*: First dose 4 mg followed by 2 mg after every stool up to maximum dose of 16 mg/24 h
- *Chronic diarrhea:* 0.08–0.2 mg/kg/day div q BID/TID maximum dose 2 mg/dose

CI: Children < 2 years

Caution: This drug should be used only after careful consideration in exceptional cases for a limited period when specific treatment fails. Not recommended as a routine therapeutic measure.

(Lopamide, Ridol 2 mg tab; Imodium, Diarlop 2 mg cap)

Omeprazole

Gastric acid proton pump inhibitor:
　> 2 years children: 1.0–3.3 mg/kg/day q OD PO PO
Alternative dosing pattern:
　< 20 kg: 10 mg q OD PO

20 kg or more: 20 mg q OD PO
Adults: 20–40 mg/day once daily PO

S/E: Nausea, vomiting, diarrhea, and headache

Precaution: The capsule should be swallowed as a whole before meals. For smaller doses, open the capsule and administer the intact pellets as required.

(Ocid, Omez, Omizac 10 mg, 20 mg cap)

Oxybutynin

Anticholinergic and antispasmodic:
- *Children 1–5 years*: 0.2 mg/kg/dose q BID/TID PO
  - *> 5 years*: 5 mg/dose q BID/TID PO
- *Adults*: 5 mg/dose q BID-QID PO

Caution: Hepatic and renal disease

(Nocturin, Oxybutynin 2.5 mg, 5 mg tab)

Oxyphenonium Bromide

Antispasmodic:
- *Children*: 2.5 mg/dose q OD-TID
- *Adult*: 5–10 mg/dose q QID

Note: Duplex tablets not recommended for children

(Antrenyl 5 mg tab, Duplex tab 10 mg)

Pantoprazole

Proton pump inhibitor:
- *Gastroesophageal reflux disease and duodenal ulcer:*
  Children:
  - *1–5 years*: 0.3–1.2 mg/kg/day (limited data) q OD PO
  - *> 5 years*: > 15 kg to < 40 kg—20 mg/day q OD PO
  - *≥ 40 kg or more*: 40 mg/day q OD PO

(Eracid, Pan, Pantin 20 mg, 40 mg tab; 40 mg inj)

Pipenzolate Methyl Bromide

Antispasmodic: Dose based on pipenzolate content of 4 mg/mL in prescribed preparation.
- *Infants < 6 months*: 4 drops QID before meals;
- *6 months–1 year*: 8–10 drops before meals
- *Children > 1–3 years*: 10–15 drops QID before meals
- *Children > 3 years*: 20 drops QID before meals

(Piplar, Piptal 5 mg tab; Piptal, Piplar drops: pipenzolate methyl bromide 4 mg + dimethyl polysiloxane 40 mg/mL)

Propantheline Bromide

- *Anticholinergic:*
  Children:
  - 1.5–3 mg/kg/day div q 4–8 h PO and HS
  Adults: 15 mg/dose q TID before meals and 300 mg HS

  S/E: Sedation, dry mouth, tachycardia, and blurred vision

  (Probanthine 15 mg tab)

Ranitidine

Histamine-2 receptor antagonist
- *Gastric and peptic ulcer and GE reflux:*
  Neonates: PO 2 mg/kg/day div q 12 h; IV 1.5–2 mg/kg/day div q 12 h or by continuous infusion
  Children: PO 2–4 mg/kg/day div q 12 h (maximum 300 mg/day);
  IM/IV 2–4 mg/kg/day div q 6–8 h or by continuous
  - IV infusion over 24 h (maximum 200 mg/day)
  Adults: PO 150 mg/dose q BID or 300 mg/dose q HS; IM/IV 50 mg/dose q 6–8 h

Precaution: Reduce dose in renal failure

S/E: Headache, mental confusion, GI upset, sedation, arthralgia, and hepatotoxicity

(Aciloc, Zinetac, Histac 150 mg, 300 mg tab, 50 mg/2 mL inj)

Senna (Sennosides)

Laxative:
Children: 1-2 tab HS PO
Adults: 2-4 tab HS PO

S/E: Abdominal cramps, nausea, and diarrhea

[Senasof, Senade (senna extract, as calcium salt, equivalent to 12 mg sennosides) tab; Pursennid-IN (senna extract 90 mg containing senna glycoside 18 mg) tab]

Simethiconet

Antiflatulent:
Children:
- < 2 years: 20 mg/dose q 4-6 h PO
- 2-12 years: 40 mg/dose q 6 h PO
- > 12 years—adults: 40-120 mg/dose q 6 h PO

Sucralfate

Antiulcer agent:

Children: 40-80 mg/kg/day div q 6-8 h PO (maximum 4 g/day)

Adults: 1 g/dose q QID PO

Precaution: Administer on empty stomach. Do not give antacids within 30 minutes of its administration.

S/E: Constipation, abdominal pain, headache, vertigo, and rash

(Sucrase, Mucogard, Sucramal 1 g tab, Sucramal, Mucrase 1 g/10 mL susp)

DIURETICS

Acetazolamide

Diuretic and carbonic anhydrase inhibitor:
- *Edema:*
    - *Children*: 5 mg/kg/dose q OD PO/IV
    - *Adults*: 250-375 mg/dose q OD PO/IV

- *Raised intracranial pressure; pseudotumor cerebri; refractory seizures; and glaucoma:*
  - *Children*: 50–70 mg/kg/day div q 6–8 h PO (maximum 1 g/24 h)

CI: Hepatic failure and sulfa allergy

Caution: Reduce dose and increase dose interval if renal dysfunction.

S/E: Hyperchloremic metabolic acidosis, hypokalemia, and bone marrow suppression

(Diamox, Synomox 250 mg tab)

Bumetanide

Loop diuretic and antihypertensive:

Neonates: Oral/IV/IM 0.01–0.05 mg/kg/dose every 24–48 h

Children: Oral/IV/IM 0.015–0.1 mg/kg/dose q 6–24 h (maximum 10 mg/day)

Adults:
- *Edema*: PO—0.5–2 mg/dose q OD/BID
- *IM/IV*: 0.5–1 mg/dose, repeat q 3 h up to twice PRN

S/E: Hypotension, electrolyte losses (Na$^+$, K$^+$, Ca$^+$, Cl$^-$), and metabolic alkalosis

(Bumet tab 1 mg; 0.25 mg/mL inj)

Chlorthalidone

Thiazide diuretic
- *Edema and mild hypertension:*

Children: 1–2 mg/kg/day q OD PO

Adults: 25–100 mg/dose/day q OD PO

S/E: Dehydration, electrolyte imbalance, and hypokalemia

CI: Anuria

(Hydrazide 12.5 mg, 25 mg tab; Hythalton 100 mg tab)

Ethacrynic Acid

- *Diuretic:*
  - *PO*: 1-3 mg/kg/day (maximum—50-100 mg/day)
  - *IV*: 0.5-1 mg/kg/dose q 12-24 h (maximum 50 mg/dose)

S/E: Hypotension, fluid and electrolyte disturbance, and ototoxicity

Monitoring: Serum electrolytes closely during therapy

(Ethacrin, Edecrin tab 50 mg; inj Edecrin 50 mg per vial)

Furosemide

Loop diuretic:
- *Neonates*: PO: 1-2 mg/kg/dose q 12-24 h
  - *IM/IV*: 0.5-2 mg/kg/dose q 12-24 h
- *Infants and children*:
  - *PO*: 1-4 mg/kg/dose q 12-24 h
  - *IM/IV*: 1-2 mg/kg/dose q 6-12 h; may be given by continuous infusion at the rate of 0.05 mg/kg/h; titrate to effect
- *Adults*: Oedema, heart failure initial: PO 20-80 mg/dose, later 20-40 mg q 6-8 hour; maximum 600 mg/day; IM/IV 20-40 mg/dose q 6-12 hour; or by continuous IV infusion 10-40 mg/hour; titrate to effect

Caution: Hepatic disease, risk of ototoxicity in renal disease

[Lasix, Frusenex, Salinex 40 mg tab; Lasix inj 20 mg/mL (2 mL)]

Hydrochlorothiazide

Thiazide diuretic:
- *Neonates and infants*: 2-4 mg/kg/day div q BID PO
  - *> 6 months and children*: 2 mg/kg/day div q BID PO
- *Adults*: 25-100 mg/day (maximum 200 mg/day) PO

S/E: Hypokalemia, hypochloremia, hyperuricemia, and marrow suppression

(Esidrex 50 mg tab; Aquazide, Hydride 12.5 mg, 25 mg tab)

Mannitol

Osmotic diuretic:
- *Cerebral edema*: 0.25–1 g/kg/dose IV over 20–30 minutes. Followed by 0.25–0.5 g/kg/dose q 4–6 h PRN. Avoid frequent use.
- *Anuria or oliguria:* Test dose—0.2 g/kg/dose IV over 3–5 minutes. No diuresis within 2 h suggests intrinsic renal dysfunction, discontinue mannitol. If response, give 0.5–1 g/kg/dose followed by 0.25–0.5 g/kg/dose q 4–6 h IV

CI: Severe renal disease, pulmonary edema, active intracranial bleed

S/E: CHF, electrolyte imbalance, headache, seizures, and circulatory overload

[Mannitol 20% (Albert David, Mount Methur, Parenteral Drugs)]

Metolazone

Diuretic:
- *Children:* Edema—0.2–0.4 mg/kg/day div q 12–24 h
- *Adults:* Edema—5–10 mg/dose q 24 h
  - *Hypertension:* 2.5 mg/dose q 24 h

Precautions: Use with caution in patients with severe renal disease, impaired hepatic function, and diabetes mellitus

S/E: Palpitation, orthostatic hypotension, vertigo, headache, rash, hypokalemia, hyponatremia, abdominal bloating, blood dyscrasias, hepatitis, and uremia

CI: Anuria and coma

(Diareon, metiz, metoral, metevix tab 2.5 mg, 5 mg, 10 mg)

Spironolactone

Potassium sparing diuretic:
- *Neonates*: 1–3 mg/kg/day div q 12–24 h PO
- *Children*: 1.5–3.3 mg/kg/day div q 8–24 h PO

CI: Severe acute renal failure

S/E: Lethargy, hyperkalemia, GI distress, rash, and gynecomastia

[Aldactone 25 mg, 100 mg tab; Lasilactone 50 and Fruselac (spironolactone 50 mg + frusemide 20 mg) tab]

Triamterene

Potassium sparing diuretic
- *Oedema and hypertension:*
  PO: 2–4 mg/kg/day div q OD-BID; maximum 6 mg/kg/day or 300 mg/day, whichever is less
  CI: Renal failure, hyperkalemia, and severe liver disease

S/E: Fatigue, headache, constipation, hyperkalemia, and hyponatremia

[Frusemene 20 (triamterene 50 mg + furosemide 20 mg) tab]

ANALGESICS, ANTIPYRETICS AND ANTI-INFLAMMATORY AGENTS

Aspirin

- *Analgesic or antipyretic:*
  - 30–65 mg/kg per day div q 4–6 h PO (maximum 60–80 mg/kg/24 h)
- *Acute rheumatic fever:* 90–120 mg/kg/day div q 6 h PO
- *Rheumatoid arthritis:* 65–130 mg/kg/day div q 4–6 h PO
- *Kawasaki disease:* 80–100 mg/kg/day div q 6–8 h PO × 2 weeks or till child remains afebrile for 48 h, followed by 3–5 mg/kg single dose PO × 6–8 weeks

CI: Chickenpox or flu-like symptoms in children < 16 years of age (risk of Reye's syndrome); peptic ulcer, bleeding disorders, severe renal dysfunction, and asthma

Desired therapeutic level in rheumatic fever 20–25 mg/dL

(Aspirin 350 mg; Colsprin 100 mg, 325 mg, 650 mg; Disprin 350 mg, Ecosprin 75 mg, 150 mg, 325 mg)

Auranofin

- *Juvenile rheumatoid arthritis (JRA) (nonresponsive to first- and second-line drugs):*
  - *Initial dose*: 0.1 mg/kg/day div q OD/BD;
  - *Maintenance*: 0.15 mg/kg/day

Caution: Discontinue if WBC falls < 4000/mm^3, granulocytes less than 1,500/mm^3 or platelets less than 100,000/mm^3

S/E: Rash, proteinuria, hematuria and bone marrow depression.

(Goldar, Ridaura 3 mg tab; inj Aurocris 10 mg, 20 mg, 50 mg per 0.5 mL amp)

Codeine

- *As analgesic*: 0.5–1 mg/kg/dose q 4–6 h PO/IM; maximum 60 mg/dose
- *For cough:* 1–1.5 mg/kg/day div q 4–6 h; maximum 60 mg/day

CI: Children < 2 years, asthma, and diminished respiratory reserve

S/E: Constipation, sedation, CNS and respiratory depression, and hypotension

(Codeine sulfate 10 mg tab; Codeine linctus liquid 15 mg/5 mL)

Diclofenac Sodium

Nonsteroidal anti-inflammatory drug:
- *Children*: 2–3 mg/kg/day (maximum 150 mg/day) div q BID/QID PO
- *Adults*: 100–200 mg/day div q BID/QID PO

S/E: Abdominal pain, peptic ulcer, fluid retention, and renal impairment; suppository may cause rectal irritation

[Voveran, Jonac, Nac 50 mg tab, Voveran, Nac SR 75 mg, 100 mg tab; Voveran, Jonac, Nac inj 25 mg/mL (3 mL inj); Jonac supp 12.5 mg; 100 mg]

Fentanyl

Analgesic, sedative, and narcotic:
- For pain, sedation, and preoperative medication:
  - Children:
    - IM/IV: 1–3 µg/kg/dose (IV given over 3–5 minutes); may repeat q 30–60 minutes PRN or by IV continuous infusion:
    - IV infusion initial: 1 µg/kg/h, titrate as required (maximum 5 µg/kg/h)
- Oral lozenge (transmucosal) for sedation:
  - 5–15 µg/kg/dose (maximum 400 µg/dose)

S/E: Bradycardia, chest wall rigidity, hypotension, and respiratory depression or arrest

[Fendrop, Fenilate 50 µg/mL (2 mL amp); Oralit lozenge 200 µg, 300 µg, 500 µg]

Ibuprofen

Nonsteroidal anti-inflammatory drug:

Children:
- *Analgesic and antipyretic:* 5–10 mg/kg/dose q 6–8 h PO
- *Juvenile rheumatoid arthritis:* 30–50 mg/kg/day div q QID (maximum dose 2,400 mg/day) PO
- For closure of patent ductus arteriosus in preterm/LBW babies 10 mg/kg IV followed by 5 mg/kg IV every 24 h × 2 doses

Adults: 400–600 mg q 8 hr or SOS PO

CI: Peptic ulcer, active GI bleeding; use cautiously in hepatic and renal disease

S/E: Heartburn, abdominal pain, GI bleeding, granulocytopenia, anemia, and acute renal failure

(Brufen, Ibugesic 200 mg, 400 mg, 600 mg tab; Ibugesic, Febrilix susp 100 mg/5 mL; Ibusynth 200 mg, 400 mg tab; Ibugesic plus tab: Ibuprofen 200 mg + paracetamol 325 mg; suspension: ibuprofen 100 mg + paracetamol 162.5 mg per 5 mL)

Indomethacin

Nonsteroidal anti-inflammatory drug:

- *Rheumatoid arthritis or Anti-inflammatory*: 3 mg/kg/day div q BID-QID PO (maximum 4 mg/kg/day or 200 mg/day)
  Adults: 25–50 mg q 8 hr PO
- *For closure of patent ductus arteriosus in neonates*:
  - *Initial*: 0.2 mg/kg by IV infusion over 30 minutes; and then 2 doses at 12–24 h intervals as per postnatal age:
    - *PNA < 48 h*: 0.1 mg/kg/dose × 2 doses
    - *PNA 2–7 days*: 0.2 mg/kg/dose × 2 doses
    - *PNA ≥ 8 days*: 0.25 mg/kg/dose × 2 doses

CI: Impaired renal function (BUN >30 mg/dL, serum creatinine >1.8 mg/dL); active bleeding, platelet count < 60,000/mm^3, coagulation defects, necrotizing enterocolitis

Monitoring: Renal and hepatic function, platelet count

(Microcid, Indocap 25 mg, 75 mg SR cap)

Ketorolac

- *Moderate or severe acute pain especially when oral medication not feasible*:
  - *Children 2–16 years*: IM/IV single dose treatment
    - *IM*: 1 mg/kg single dose (maximum 30 mg)
    - *IV*: 0.5 mg/kg single dose (maximum 15 mg)

Caution: Not recommended for children below 2 years, only single IM/IV dose recommended for children 2–16 years, oral administration of drug in this age group not recommended by some authorities. Use with caution in patients with decreased renal function, hepatic impairment and tendency to bleed.

CI: Hepatic or renal failure, bleeding tendency

S/E: Gastritis, bleeding, impaired platelet aggregation, headache, oliguria, and hypersensitivity reactions

[Ketorol inj 30 mg/mL (1 mL)]

Mefenamic Acid

Nonsteroidal anti-inflammatory drug:
- *Arthritis:*
  - *Children*: 10-25 mg/kg/day div q 6 h PO
- *Pyrexia*: 3 mg/kg/dose PO PRN

CI: Peptic ulcer and porphyria

Caution: Avoid in children with seizures

S/E: Diarrhea, rashes (if so, withdraw treatment), thrombocytopenia, aplastic anemia, and hemolytic anemia

(Ponstan 250 mg, 500 mg tab, 50 mg/5 mL susp; Meftal 250, 500 mg tab; Meftal-P 100 mg tab, susp 100 mg/5 mL)

Methotrexate

- *Juvenile rheumatoid arthritis:* PO 10 mg/m^2/dose once a week
- *Antineoplastic: PO/IM:* 7.5-30 mg/m^2 every 1-2 weeks PO
- *Systemic lupus erythematosus and juvenile dermatomyositis:* 10-20 mg/m^2 weekly PO

S/E: GI toxicity, elevated liver enzymes, stomatitis, and leukopenia

(Imutrex, Neotrexate, Biotrexate, Methotrex 2.5 mg tab; inj Imutrex 30 mg/2 mL; inj Neotrexate, Biotrexate, Methotrex 50 mg/2 mL)

Morphine

- *Analgesia; management of cyanotic spell in Tetralogy of Fallot.*
  - *Neonate*:
    IV, IM, SC: 0.05-0.1 mg/kg/dose; repeat 2-4 h PRN; continuous infusion for analgesia 0.01-0.02 mg/kg/h
  - *Infants and children*:
    - *IV, IM SC*: 0.1-0.2 mg/kg/dose, repeat 2-4 h PRN (maximum dose 15 mg/dose); *continuous infusion* 0.01-0.04 mg/kg/h
    - *Oral*: 0.2-0.5 mg/kg/dose repeat 4-6 h PRN

- *Adults*:
  - IV, IM, SC: 2.5–20 mg/dose repeat 2–6 h PRN;
  - Oral: 10–30 mg, repeat 4 hourly PRN

Monitoring: Respiratory and cardiovascular status; In neonate—bowel sounds, abdominal and bladder distension

S/E: Respiratory and CNS depression, hypotension, bradycardia, vomiting, constipation, sedation, increased ICP

[M-Eslon 30 mg cap; Moreontin (CR) 10 mg, 30 mg tab; Rilimorf (morphine HCl) 10 mg/2 mL oral solution (100 mL); Morphine sulfate inj 10 mg/mL]

Naproxen

Nonsteroidal anti-inflammatory drug:
- *Children > 2 years*: 10–20 mg/kg/day div q 8–12 h PO (maximum 1 g/day) for juvenile rheumatoid arthritis; for analgesia 5–7 mg/kg/per dose q 8–12 h PO
- *Adults*: 250–375 mg/dose q 8–12 h PO

CI: Children below 2 years of age; NSAID sensitive asthma

Caution: GI disease, renal or hepatic dysfunction, and heart failure

S/E: Gastrointestinal intolerance, headache, drowsiness, and pseudoporphyria

(Naprosyn 250 mg, 500 mg tab; Artagen 250 mg tab)

Nimesulide

Nonsteroidal anti-inflammatory drug:
Analgesic/antipyretic
- *Children*: 5 mg/kg/day div q 8–12 h PO
- *Adults*: 100 mg/dose q BID PO

CI: Active peptic ulcer, moderate-to-severe hepatic impairment, pregnant and lactating women

Caution: Cautious use in severe renal impairment, congestive heart failure, and cirrhosis

Warning: Recently safety of this drug has become the subject of intense controversy with some reported instances of fulminant hepatic failure following its use. Each clinician needs to carefully exercise his own judgment in this regard.

(Nimulid 50 mg DT, 100 mg DT, 100 mg EF tab, Nise, Nimica 50 mg DT; Nimset, 100 mg DT, Orthobid 100 mg, Pronim 100 mg tab; Orthobid, Nise, Nimulid, Nimcet, Nimica, Pronim susp 50 mg/5 mL)

Paracetamol (Acetaminophen)

Analgesic and antipyretic (but not anti-inflammatory)
- *Children*
  - *PO/PR:* 10–15 mg/kg/dose q 4–6 h; maximum dose 60 mg/kg/day
  - *IM:* 5 mg/kg IM single dose
- *Adults*
  - *PO/PR:* 0.5–1g/dose q 4–6 h; maximum 4 g in 24 hr
  - *IM:* 5 mg/kg/dose

Caution: Excessive intake causes hepatic necrosis

(Crocin, Calpol, Dolo, Metacin, Pacimol 500 mg, and 650 mg tablets; Crocin advance 500 mg tab; Crocin 120 mg/5 mL susp; 100 mg/mL drops; Calpol 125 mg/5 mL and 250 mg/5 mL; 100 mg/mL drops; Dolo 156.25/5 mL and 250 mg/5 mL susp and 100 mg/mL drops; Inj Aeknil, Agpar, febrinil, Metacin 150 mg/mL; Suppository Anamol, Dunimol 80 mg, 170 mg, 250 mg).

Pentazocine

Analgesic and opiate group:
- *Children > 14 years and adults*:
  - *PO*: 50 mg/dose q 4 h PRN, may increase up to 100 mg/dose
  - *IM/IV*: 30 mg/dose q 4 h (maximum 60 mg/dose or 360 mg/day)

CI: Children below 14 years, head injury, and raised intracranial tension

S/E: CNS depression, vomiting, and respiratory depression

[Fortagesic, Pentazen (pentazocine 15 mg + paracetamol 500 mg) tab, Fortwin, Pentawin 30 mg/mL, 1 mL inj]

Pethidine

Meperidine: Narcotic and analgesic:
- *Children*:
  - IM/IV: 1–1.5 mg/kg/dose q 3–4 h PRN maximum dose 100 mg

CI: Asthma, increased ICP, and cardiac arrhythmias

S/E: Hypotension, respiratory depression, lethargy, vomiting, and dependence

Precaution: Lower dose in renal or hepatic impairment, cautious use in seizure disorder

(Pethidine inj 50 mg/mL, 1 mL inj)

Phenazopyridine HCl

Urinary tract anesthetic:
- *Children*: 12 mg/kg/day div q TID PO
- *Adults*: 100–200 mg/dose q TID–QID PO

CI: Severe renal impairment

S/E: Vomiting, vertigo, headache, hepatitis, methemoglobinemia, and hemolytic anemia. Discolors urine harmlessly orange or red.

(Pyridium 200 mg tab)

Piroxicam

Nonsteroidal anti-inflammatory drug:
- *Children*: 0.2–0.3 mg/kg/day div q OD PO (maximum dose 15 mg/day)
- *Adults*: 20–40 mg/day div q OD PO/IM

CI: Young infants, peptic ulcer, bronchial asthma, and NSAID induced allergy

Caution: Severe impairment of hepatic or renal function

S/E: Nausea, heart burn, tinnitus, dizziness, and skin rash

[Pirox, Dolonex 10 mg, 20 mg cap, 20 mg DT, inj 20 mg (1 mL), 40 mg (2 mL) amp, Brexic 10 mg, 20 mg cap, 20 mg DT]

Tolmetin Sodium

Nonsteroidal anti-inflammatory drug:
- *Juvenile rheumatoid arthritis*
  - *Children > 2 years*: 15–30 mg/kg/day div q TID-QID PO
- *For analgesia*: 5–7 mg/kg/dose PO

S/E: GI irritation, dizziness, peptic ulcer, and platelet dysfunction

(Tolectin tab 200 mg, cap 400 mg)

Tramadol

Analgesic (Non-narcotic)

Immediate release formulation:
- *Children*: 1–2 mg/kg/dose q 4–6 h, maximum 400 mg/day PO
- *Adolescents and adults*: 50–100 mg q 4–6 h, maximum 400 mg/day PO

Caution: Avoid extended release formulation in children; restrict use of immediate release formulation in children below 14 years age

Precaution: Use with caution and reduce dose in patients with history or increased risk of seizures, liver disease, renal impairment, or hypothyroidism

S/E: Seizures, renal and hepatic dysfunction, dizziness, pruritus, rash, bronchospasm

(Trump, Contramal, Nobligan 50 mg tab; Trump, Contramol 50 mg, 100 mg per mL inj)

TRANQUILIZERS, HYPNOTICS, SEDATIVES AND ANTIDEPRESSANTS

Alprazolam

Anxiolytic agent:
- *Children*: 0.005–0.02 mg/kg/dose q TID
- *Adults*: 0.25–0.5 mg/dose q BID-TID (maximum dose—anxiety 4 mg/day; panic 10 mg/day)

Important caution:
- *Safety not established in children*
- *Do not discontinue rapidly, abrupt stoppage may cause seizures, and other withdrawal reactions*

(Alprax, Anxit, Zolax 0.25 mg, 0.5 mg, 1 mg tab)

Amitriptyline

Antidepressant:
- *Chronic pain:*
  - *Initial*: 0.1 mg/kg/day q OD HS; increase slowly to 0.5–2 mg/kg/day PRN
- *Depression*
  - *Initial*: 1 mg/kg/day div q TID X 3 days
  - Later gradually increase dose PRN; maximum 5 mg/kg/day. Maximum dose children 100 mg/day; adolescents 200 mg/day.

CI: Seizures, severe cardiac disorders, narrow angle glaucoma

Monitor: ECG, BP, heart rate and CBC when dose exceeds 3 mg/kg/day

(Amitone, Amilite 10 mg, 25 mg, 75 mg tab)

Chloral Hydrate

- *For sedation*
  - *PO/PR*: 25–50 mg/kg/day div q 6–8 h (maximum 500 mg/dose)
- *Sedation for procedure*
  - *PO/PR*: 25–100 mg/kg/dose 30–60 minutes before procedure (maximum dose: infants 1 g, children 2 g)

CI: Hepatic and renal failure

S/E: Paradoxical excitement, hypotension, and respiratory depression

(Acquachloral, somnos, noctec elixir 250 mg, 500 mg/5 mL)

Chlorpromazine

See under section on "Antiemetics".

Diazepam

See under section on "Anticonvulsants".

Fluoxetine Hydrochloride

Selective serotonin re-uptake inhibitor
- For major depression:
  Children: 8–18 years

  Initial: 10 mg OD PO; increase if necessary after 1–2 weeks maximum 20 mg OD PO

S/E: Headache, nervousness, mania, suicidal thinking, GIT upset, rash, asthenia, dry mouth
(Fludac, Flunil, Nuzac 10 mg, 20 mg cap; Fludac, Flutine susp 20 mg/5 mL)

Haloperidol

Antipsychotic drug:
- *Children 3–12 years*:
  - *PO*: Initial—0.25–0.5 mg/day div q BID-TID
  - Increase weekly by 0.25 mg–0.5 mg per day as needed;
  - *Maximum dose*: 0.15 mg/kg/day
  - Usual maintenance dose 0.01–0.03 mg/kg/day q OD PO (in agitation patients)
- *Children 6–12 years*:
  - *IM*: 1–3 mg/dose q 4–8 h (maximum 0.15 mg/kg/day) IM (as lactate)

Caution: For use preferably by trained specialists only

S/E: Extrapyramidal symptoms, tardive dyskinesia, and blood dyscrasias

(Halopace, Serenace 0.25 mg, 1.5 mg, 5 mg tab; Serenace, Senorm 5 mg/mL 1 mL inj)

Hydroxyzine Hydrochloride

Antihistaminic and anxiolytic:
- *Pruritus, anxiety*:
  - *Children*: 0.6 mg/kg/dose q 6 h PO or 2 mg/kg/day div q 6–8 h PO (maximum 100 mg/day)
  - *IM*: 0.5–1 mg/kg/dose q 4–6 hr as needed (maximum 100 mg/day)
  - *Preoperative sedation:*
    - PO 0.6 mg/kg/dose
    - IM 0.5–1 mg/kg/dose
- *Adults:*
  - *Anxiety*: PO 25–50 mg/dose q 4–6 hr as needed (maximum 200 mg/day)
  - *Pruritus*: PO 25 mg q TID/QID
  - *Preoperative sedation* = IM 25–100 mg

Caution: Avoid in asthma

S/E: Drowsiness, hypotension, urinary retention, and blurred vision

(Atarax 10 mg, 25 mg tab, syr 10 mg/5 mL, drops 6 mg/mL, inj 25 mg/mL-2 mL inj; Prugo 10 mg, 25 mg tab)

Imipramine

- *Enuresis:*
  Children 6 years and above:
  - *Initial*: 10–25 mg q HS; increase 10–25 mg/dose at 1–2 week intervals PRN
  - *Maximum dose*:
    - *6–12 years*: 50 mg HS;
    - *Above 12 years*: 75 mg HS;

Continue for 2–3 months and then taper slowly

- *Depression:*

    Initial:1.5 mg/kg/day div q TID PO; increase by 1 mg/kg/day every 3-4 days as needed, maximum 5 mg/kg/day

    S/E: Sedation, constipation, dry mouth, urinary retention, hypotension, and arrhythmias

(Depsonil 25 mg tab, Depsonil PM 75 mg cap; Depsol, Depsin 25 mg, 75 mg tab)

Ketamine

General anesthetic:
- *Induction of general anesthesia:*
    - *IV*: 0.5-3 mg/kg (maximum rate 0.5 mg/kg/min)
- *Sedation:*
    - *PO/PR*: 4-6 mg/kg once;
    - *IM*: 2-3 mg/kg once

CI: CHF, hypertension, hypotension, elevated ICP, and respiratory depression

(Ketmine 10 mg/mL (10 mL), 50 mg/mL (2 mL, 10 mL), Ketalar 10 mg/mL (20 mL), 50 mg/mL (2 mL, 10 mL)

Lithium

- *Acute mania, depression:*
    - *Children*: 15-60 mg/kg/day div q TID/QID PO
    - *Adolescents*: 600-1800 mg/day (not per kg) div q TID/QID

Note: Start with minimum dose, adjust dose weekly to achieve therapeutic blood level of 0.6-1.2 mEq/L. Blood level exceeding 1.5 mEq/L can be quite toxic

S/E: GIT disturbance, fatigue, hypothyroidism, and nephrogenic diabetes insipidus

(Licab, Lithican, Manicarb 300 mg tab)

Lorazepam

Benzodiazepine, anticonvulsant, and anxiolytic:
- *Status epilepticus*
  - *Neonates, infants, and children*:
    - *IV*: 0.05–0.1 mg/kg/dose over 2–5 min. May repeat 0.05 mg/kg once in 10–15 min, maximum dose 4 mg/dose
    - *PR*: 0.05–0.1 mg/kg, (if IV administration not feasible)
    - *Sublingual*: 0.05–1 mg/kg (home treatment of serial seizures to prevent progress to status epilepticus)
  - *Adults*:
    - *IV*: 4 mg/dose (not per kg) over 2–5 minutes. May repeat in 10–15 minutes. Total maximum dose in 12 h period: 8 mg
- *Anxiety/sedation:*
  - *Children*: 0.05 mg/kg/dose every 4–8 h PO/IV/IM; maximum dose 2 mg/dose
- *Adjunct to antiemetic therapy:*
  - *Children*: 0.04–0.08 mg/kg/dose IV (maximum single dose 4 mg); repeat q 6 h PRN

CI: Severe hypotension

S/E: Respiratory depression, sedation, depression, tachycardia, rash, and diplopia

[Larpose, Calmese, Trapex 1 mg, 2 mg tab; Calmese, Trapex 2 mg/mL (2 mL amp)]

Midazolam

Benzodiazepine

- *Status epilepticus:*
  Infants > 2 months and children:
  - *IV*: *Loading dose*—0.15 mg/kg followed by continuous infusion at the rate of 1 µg/kg/min; titrate dose

upward every 5 minutes until clinical seizure activity is controlled (usual infusion rate around 2.5 µg/kg/min); maximum 12 µg/kg/min

For details, *see* under Anticonvulsants Chapter 15

- *Sedation (Preoperative sedation or conscious sedation for procedure)*
  - *IV*: 0.05–0.2 mg/kg load then continuous infusion at the rate of 1–2 µg/kg/min
  - *IM*: 0.1–0.15 mg/kg 30–60 minutes before surgery or procedure (maximum total dose—10 mg)
  - *Buccal and intranasal*: 0.15–0.3 mg/kg; may repeat in 5–15 minutes once
- *Neonates*
  - *Sedation*: Continuous infusion 0.15–0.5 µg/kg/min

S/E: Respiratory depression, apnea, tonic or clonic movements, muscle tremor, sedation, paradoxical excitement, cardiac arrest, hypotension, and diplopia

[Fulsed, Midaz, Sedeven 1 mg/mL (5 mL, 10 mL vials) 5 mg/mL–1 mL amp]

Nortriptyline Hydrochloride

Tricyclic antidepressant:
- *Nocturnal enuresis:*
  - *6–11 years*: 10–20 mg once HS PO
  - *> 11 years*: 25–35 mg once HS, maximum 40 mg/day PO
- *Depression*: 1–3 mg/kg/day once HS PO or div TID/QID; maximum dose 150 mg/day

CI: Cardiac disease and cardiac conduction abnormalities

S/E: Sedation, urinary retention, dry mouth, tachycardia, and constipation (anticholinergic effects)

(Primox, Sensival 25 mg tab)

Paraldehyde

See under section on "Anticonvulsants"

Pentobarbital

- *Barbiturate; anticonvulsant; and hypnotic; general anesthetic:*
  - *Children:*
    - *Hypnotic*: 2–6 mg/kg/dose IM (maximum 100 mg/dose)
- *Conscious preoperative sedation*:
  - *Children > 18 months:*
    - Initial 2 mg/kg IV; may repeat 1–2 mg/kg q 5–10 minutes until adequate sedation (maximum total dose 6 mg/kg or 150–200 mg)
- *Pentobarbital coma*: Loading dose 10–15 mg/kg IV slowly over 1–2 h; maintenance infusion—initial 1 mg/kg/h; may increase to 2–3 mg/kg/h; maintain burst suppression on EEG

S/E: Drowsiness, CNS excitation or depression, respiratory depression, hypotension, and arrhythmia

(*Nembutal sodium solution 20 mL and 50 mL multiple dose vials 50 mg/mL*)

Phenobarbitone
Barbiturate

- *Neonatal seizures and status epilepticus (neonates and children):*
  - *IV*: Loading dose—IV 15–20 kg IV slowly. May repeat 5 mg/kg q 15 min in neonate to a total maximum dose of 30 mg/kg

  Maintenance dose:
  - *Neonates*: PO/IV 3–5 mg/kg/day div q 12–24 h
  - *Children*: PO/IV 5–6 mg/kg/day div q 12–24 h
- *Sedation*
  - *Children:*
    - *PO/IM/IV*: 2 mg/kg/dose; may repeat q TID PRN

Precautions: IV phenobarbitone to be given slowly at the rate of not more than 1 mg/kg/min. Watch closely for hypotension and respiratory depression. Use cautiously in hepatic and renal disease.

CI: Acute intermittent porphyria and hyperkinetic children

S/E: Drowsiness, cognitive function impairment, paradoxical hyperactivity, rash, and hypotension

(Gardenal, Phenobarb 30 mg, 60 mg tab, Luminal 30 mg tab; Luminalettes 15 mg tab; Gardenal syr 20 mg/5 mL; Phenobarbitone sodium 200 mg/mL 1 mL inj)

Promethazine Hydrochloride

Antihistaminic (phenothiazine):
- *Antihistaminic:*
  - PO: 0.1 mg/kg/dose q6h and 0.5 mg/kg/dose (maximum 25 mg/dose) HS PRN
- *Vomiting:*
  - PO/IM/IV: 0.5 mg/kg/dose (maximum 25 mg) q 4–6 h PRN
- *Sedation:*
  - PO/IM/IV: 0.5–1 mg/kg/dose (maximum 50 mg) q 6 h PRN
- *Motion sickness:*
  - PO: 0.5 mg/kg/dose (maximum 25 mg) q 30–60 minutes before departure and then q 12 h as needed

S/E: As with other phenothiazines (like prochlorperazine and chlorpromazine)

[Phenergan, Promet 10 mg, 25 mg tab, inj 25 mg/mL (2 mL amp); Phenergan syr 5 mg/5 mL]

Thioridazine

Phenothiazine Derivative

- *Psychosis and severe behavior problems:*
  - *Children > 2–12 years*: 0.5–3 mg/kg/day div q BID-TID PO

- *Children > 12 years* and adults:
  - *Initial*: 75-300 mg/day div q TID PO, increase as needed to maximum 800 mg/day

CI: Severe CNS depression

S/E: Sedation, dry mouth, extrapyramidal reactions, and blood dyscrasias

(Melozine, Ridazine, Thioril 10 mg, 25 mg, 50 mg, 100 mg tab)

Triclofos Sodium

- *For sedation:*
  20 mg/kg/dose PO; maximum 1 g/dose
  (Pedicloryl, Tricloryl, Silence 500 mg/5 mL)

Trifluoperazine

Antipsychotic drug:
- *Children 6-12 years*:
  - *PO*: 1 mg/dose q OD/BID, increase dose as required (max—15 mg/24 h);
  - *IM*: 1 mg/dose q BID
- *> 12 years and adults*
  - *PO*: 12 mg/dose q BID
  - *IM*: 1-2 mg/dose q 4-6 h PRN (maximum 10 mg/24 h)

(Neocalm, Trazine tabs 5 mg, 10 mg; Manocalm tab 2 mg, 5 mg, 10 mg)

ANTIHISTAMINICS

Astemizole

Dose according to age:
- *<6 years*: 0.2 mg/kg OD PO
- *≥6-12 years*: 5 mg OD PO
- *>12 years and adult*: 10 mg OD PO

CI: Hepatic disease

Caution: Avoid concomitant use with drugs, which impair hepatic metabolism (e.g. erythromycin, ciprofloxacin, cimetidine, and ketoconazole); can cause serious cardiac arrhythmias

(Stemiz, Histeese 10 mg tab, susp 5 mg/5 mL; Histalong 5 mg, 10 mg tab)

Azatadine Maleate

- *Children > 12 years and adults*: 1–2 mg/dose q BID PO

Caution: Not recommended in children age < 12 years

S/E: Dry mouth, thickened bronchial secretions, and sedation

(Zadine tab 1 mg, syrup 0.5 mg/5 mL)

Cetirizine

- *2–5 yr*: 5 mg/day div q OD-BID PO
- *≥6 yr and above*: 10 mg/day div q OD-BID PO

Caution: Avoid in children below 2 years; reduce dose in hepatic and renal impairment

Adverse effects: Headache, dizziness, dry mouth, and GI upset.

(Alerid, Cetzine, CZ-3, Cetiriz 10 mg tab, syrup 5 mg/5 mL)

Chlorpheniramine Maleate

- *As antihistaminic*:
  0.35 mg/kg/day div q 6 h PO
  According to age:
  2–6 years: 1 mg/dose q 4–6 h PO
  6–12 years: 2 mg/dose q 4–6 h PO
  > 12 years: 4 mg/dose q 4–6 h PO
- *Emergency treatment of anaphylactic reaction, symptomatic relief of allergy*:

  Child below 6 months: 250 µg/kg (max 2.5 mg) IM/IV, repeat upto 4 times in 24 hr

Child 6 months – 6 yr: 2.5 mg per dose IM/IV, repeat up to 4 times in 24 hr

Child > 6–12 yr: 5 mg per dose IM/IV, repeat up to 4 times in 24 hr

Child > 12–18 yr: 10 mg per dose IM/IV, repeat up to 4 times in 24 hr

Caution: Use with caution in asthma

Adverse effects: Dry mouth, blurred vision, urinary retention, and paradoxical excitation

(Cadistin, Piriton 4 mg tab; cipium, CPM tab 2, 4 mg, syrup 2 mg/5 mL inj 10 mg/mL; also as a constituent in several cough syrups)

Clemastine

- *< 6 years*: 0.05 mg/kg/day div q BID/TID PO (maximum 1 mg/day)
- *6–12 years*: 0.5 mg/dose q BID PO (maximum dose 3 mg/day)
- *> 12 years*: 1 mg/dose q BID PO (maximum dose 6 mg/day)

CI: Glaucoma and bladder neck obstruction

S/E: Dry mouth, constipation, dizziness, and drowsiness

(Tavegyl 1.34 mg tab; syr 0.67 mg/5 mL; Clamist 1 mg tab, syr 0.5 mg/5 mL)

Cyproheptadine

- *Children ≥ 2 years*: 0.25–0.5 mg/kg/day div q BID/TID

Maximum dose: *2–6 years*: 12 mg/day;
7–14 years: 16 mg/day

CI: Neonates, asthma, glaucoma, urinary obstruction, and therapy with MAO inhibitors

S/E: Drowsiness and bronchospasm

(Ciplactin, Practin 4 mg tab, syr 2 mg/5 mL; Peritol syr 2 mg/5 mL, drops 1.5 mg/mL)

Dimethindene Maleate

Children > 12 years and adults: 1–2 mg/dose q 8 h or SR tab 2.5 mg q BID

(Foristal tab 1 mg; Foristal lontab 2.5 mg)

Diphenhydramine HCL

- *As antihistaminic:*
  - *Children*: 5 mg/kg/day div q 6 h PO/IM/IV; maximum 300 mg/day
- *As antidote for phenothiazine toxicity and for anaphylaxis:* 1–2 mg/kg IV slowly

CI: Acute asthma, neonates, and glaucoma

(Benadryl 25 mg, 50 mg cap, syr 12.5 mg/5 mL)

Fexofenadine

Children: 6 months to < 2 years: 15 mg BD PO
2–11 years: 30 mg BD PO
> 12 years and adults: 120–180 mg OD PO

S/E: Headache, drowsiness, nausea, dizziness, and fatigue

(Altiva 30 mg, 60 mg, 120 mg, 180 mg tab, syr 60 mg/5 mL; Allegra 30 mg, 120 mg, 180 mg tab)

Hydroxyzine

- *Antihistaminic and anxiolytic:*

Children: 0.6 mg/kg/dose q 6 h PO/IM
Adults: 25–100 mg/dose q TID-QID PO/IM

Caution: Avoid in asthma

S/E: Drowsiness, hypotension, urinary retention, and blurred vision

(Atarax 10 mg, 25 mg tab, syr 10 mg/5 mL, drops 6 mg/mL, inj 25 mg/mL–2 mL inj)

Levocetirizine

Antihistamine

Children 2–6 yr: 1.25 mg OD PO

>6–12 yr: 2.5 mg OD PO

>12 yr-adult: 5 mg OD PO

Precaution: Reduce dose in cases with renal dysfunction

CI: End stage renal disease

S/E: Headache, drowsiness, nausea, myalgia
(Levocet, levorid, lezyncet 5 mg tab; Susp 2.5 mg/5 mL)

Loratadine

- *Children above 3 years.*
  < 30 kg: 5 mg/day q OD PO
  > 30 kg: 10 mg/day q OD PO

S/E: Sedation, headache, dermatitis, and palpitation

(Loridin, Lormeg, Lorin 10 mg tab, syr 5 mg/5 mL Lorfast 10 mg DT)

Methdilazine Hydrochloride

- *Children above 3 years*: 4 mg/dose q BID PO
- *Adults*: 8 mg/dose q BID PO

(Dilosyn 8 mg tab, syr 4 mg/5 mL)

Pheniramine Maleate

- *Children*:
  - ≤14 yr: 0.5 mg/kg/day div q 8 h PO/IM/IV
  - *> 14 years*: 25 mg BID-TID (up to 100 mg/day) PO;

Parenteral (IM/IV): Total daily dose same as oral dose given above, div q BID
- *Adults*:
  - *PO*: 25 mg BID-TID (up to 100 mg/day);
  - *IM/IV*: 22.5–45 mg BID

Note: Vial preparation of Avil inj is for IM use only

CI: Hypersensitivity

[Avil 25 mg, 50 mg tab, syr 15 mg/5 mL, inj 22.75 mg/mL (2 mL amp, 10 mL vial); Avil Retard 75 mg Drag (R)]

Promethazine Hydrochloride

Phenothiazine:
- *Antihistaminic:*
  - *PO*: 0.1 mg/kg/dose (maximum 12.5 mg) q 6 h and 0.5 mg/kg/dose (maximum 25 mg) HS PRN
- *Vomiting:*
  - *PO/IM/IV*: 0.25–1 mg/kg/dose (maximum 25 mg) q 4–6 h PRN
- *Sedation:*
  - *PO/IM/IV*: 0.5–1 mg/kg/dose (maximum 50 mg) q 6 h PRN
- *Motion sickness:*
  - *PO*: 0.5 mg/kg/dose (maximum 25 mg) 30–60 minutes before departure and then q 12 h as needed
  - For parenteral use IM administration is preferable. Do not give S/C as it may cause skin necrosis. Avoid IV use; if given dilute it to a maximum concentration of 25 mg/mL. Maximum infusion rate 25 mg/minute.

S/E: As with other phenothiazines (like prochlorperazine and chlorpromazine)

Promethazine hydrochloride preparations:

[Phenergan, Promit 10 mg, 25 mg tab, inj 25 mg/mL (2 mL amp); Phenergan syr 5 mg/5 mL; Phena syr 5 mg/5 mL; inj 25 mg/mL (2 mL amp)]

Terfenadine

- *3–6 years*: 15 mg/dose q BID PO,
- *> 6–12 years*: 30 mg/dose q BID PO
- *> 12 years and adults*: 60 mg/dose q BID PO

CI: Concomitant administration with erythromycin (and other macrolides); ketoconazole, metronidazole (and other azole type antifungal agents), and cimetidine. It may cause prolonged QT interval and fatal arrhythmias

Caution: Not recommended below 3 years

(Terfed, Trexyl, Zoter 60 mg, 120 mg tab; susp 30 mg/5 mL)

ANTIEMETICS

Chlorpromazine

- *Nausea and vomiting:*
  - *Children > 6 months*:
    - *PO*: 0.5–1 mg/kg/dose q 4–6 h
    - *IM/IV*: 0.5–1 mg/kg/dose q 6–8 h
    - *Maximum IM/IV dose*:
      - « *< 5 years*: 40 mg/24 h;
      - « *5–12 years*: 75 mg/24 h
  - *Adults*:
    - *PO*: 10–25 mg/dose q 4–6 h
    - *IM/IV*: 25–50 mg/dose q 4–6 h
- *Chorea*:
  - *Initial*: 50 mg/day div q BID PO, increase by 25 mg/day till controlled or maximum dose 300 mg/day PO
- *Neonatal tetanus*:
  - 1–2 mg/kg/dose q 2–4 h IM/IV

S/E: Jaundice, hypotension, dystonia, arrhythmia, and agranulocytosis

[Chlorpromazine, Manochlor 10 mg, 25 mg, 50 mg, 100 mg tab; Chlorpromazine, Relitil inj 25 mg/mL (2 mL amp) Largactil 10, 25, 50, 100 mg tab; syr 5 mg/5 mL (ped), inj 50 mg/2 mL ampoule]

Dimenhydrinate

Antihistamine and Antiemetic

- *Motion sickness and vertigo:*
  Children > 2 years: 5 mg/kg/day div q 6 h PO/IM/IV

S/E: Drowsiness, dizziness, hypotension, and tachycardia

[Draminate, Dramamine Gravol 50 mg tab, Dramamine syr 15.625 mg/5 mL, inj 50 mg/mL (1 mL)]

Domperidone

Children: 0.2–0.4 mg/kg/dose q 6–8 h PO
Adults: 10–20 mg/dose q TID/QID PO; maximum dose 80 mg/day PO

S/E: Gynecomastia in males and galactorrhea in females

(Domstal, Dom 5 mg DT; Domstal, Dom, Domperon 10 mg tab, susp 5 mg/5 mL; Domperon 10 mg/mL drops)

Granisetron

Antiemetic:
- For chemotherapy-induced vomiting (prevention and treatment)
  - *Children ≥ 2 years and adults:*
    - 10–20 µg/kg (maximum 1 mg) IV over 15–60 min before chemotherapy; same dose may be repeated 2–3 times following chemotherapy
    - *Alternatively*: 40 µg/kg single dose 15–60 minutes before start of chemotherapy

S/E: Hypertension or hypotension, arrhythmia, agitation, and skin rash

(Granicip, Tapit 1 mg, 2 mg tab; inj 1 mg/mL, 3 mg/3 mL; Grandem syr 1 mg/5 mL; tab 1 mg, inj 1 mg/mL)

Metoclopramide

- *Gastroesophageal reflux:*
  - *Neonates, infants and children:* 0.1–0.2 mg/kg/dose q 6–8 h IV/IM/PO

- *Vomiting:*
  - *Children*: 0.1–0.2 mg/kg/dose q 6–8 h PRN IV/IM/PO
  - *Adults*: 10 mg/dose q 6–8 years PRN IV/IM/PO
- *Chemotherapy-induced emesis:*
  - *Children and adults*: 1–2 mg/kg/dose q 2–4 h; pretreat with diphenhydramine to avoid extrapyramidal reactions

CI: GI obstruction and seizure disorder

Caution: Reduce dose in renal impairment

S/E: Extrapyramidal reaction, anxiety, leukopenia, drowsiness, and diarrhea. Diphenhydramine is the antidote for extrapyramidal reaction

[Perinorm 5 mg DT, Perinorm, Maxeron, Reglan 10 mg tab, syr 5 mg/5 mL, inj 5 mg/mL (2 mL and 10 mL)]

Ondansetron

- *Prevention of chemotherapy or radiotherapy-induced vomiting:*
  - *PO:*
    - *Children < 4 years*: 1–3 mg/dose q TID (1 mg per 0.3 m² body surface area)
    - *Children ≥ 4–11 years*: 4 mg/dose q TID
    - *Children > 11 years and adults*: 8 mg/dose q TID
    - First dose to be given 1–1½ h before chemotherapy, repeat dose q 8 h
  - *IV:*
    - *Children > 3 years*: 0.15 mg/kg/dose IV infusion over 15 minutes, 30 minutes before emetogenic chemotherapy, repeat dose after 4 h and 8 h (maximum 8 mg/dose)
    - *Adults*: 8 mg/dose 30 minutes before chemotherapy, repeat dose after 4 h and 8 h
- *Prevention of postoperative vomiting:*
  - *IV/IM:*
    - *Children > 2 years, below 40 kg*: 0.1 mg/kg IV/IM single dose preoperative or postoperative if patient is symptomatic

- *Children > 40 kg and adults*: 4 mg/dose IV/IM single dose preoperative or postoperative if patient is symptomatic

Note: For IV administration dilute in IV fluid (maximum concentration 1 mg/mL) and administer over 15 minutes; *IM*: Administer as undiluted injection

S/E: Headache, constipation, diarrhea, chest pain, tachycardia or bradycardia, twitching, hypokalemia, and transient increase in liver enzymes

Caution: Reduce dose and increase interval in severe hepatic impairment (maximum 8 mg/dose; q 12-24 h)

[Ondem, Osteron, Emeset 4 mg, 8 mg tab; 2 mg/mL inj (2 mL, 4 mL); suspension Emeset, Glendan 2 mg/5 mL]

Prochlorperazine

Phenothiazine group:
- *Vomiting:*
  - *Children > 10 kg*
    - *Oral, PR*: 0.4 mg/kg/day div TID/QID (maximum 30 mg/day)
    - *IM/IV*: 0.1-0.15 mg/kg/dose q.8-12 h (maximum 30 mg/day)
- *Intractable migraine headache*
  - *IV*: 0.15 mg/kg/dose; single dose

S/E: Extrapyramidal reactions, hypertension, drowsiness, cholestatic jaundice, and blurred vision. Diphenhydramine reverses dystonic reaction

[Stemetil 5 mg, 25 mg tab, inj 12.5 mg/mL(1 mL, 10 mL); Emidoxyn 5 mg tab, inj 12.5 mg/mL (1 mL)]

Promethazine Hydrochloride

Antihistamine (phenothiazine):
- *Antihistaminic:*
  - *PO*: 0.1 mg/kg/dose (maximum 12.5 mg) q 6 h and 0.5 mg/kg/dose (maximum 25 mg) HS PRN

- *Vomiting:*
  - *PO/IM/IV*: 0.25-1 mg/kg/dose (maximum 25 mg) q 4-6 h PRN
- *Sedation:*
  - *PO/IM/IV*: 0.5-1 mg/kg/dose (maximum 50 mg) q 6 h PRN
- *Motion sickness:*
  - PO: 0.5 mg/kg/dose (maximum 25 mg) 30-60 minutes before departure and then q 12 h as needed
  - IM administration of promethazine HCl is preferable. Avoid IV use; if given, dilute it to a maximum concentration of 25 mg/mL with maximum infusion rate of 25 mg/min. Do not give S/C, may cause skin necrosis.

S/E: As with other phenothiazines (like prochlorperazine and chlorpromazine)

[Promethazine hydrochloride preparations: Phenergan, Promit 10 mg, 25 mg tab, inj 25 mg/mL (2 mL amp); Phenergan syr 5 mg/5 mL; Phena syr 5 mg/5 mL; 25 mg/mL (2 mL amp)]

Promethazine Theoclate

- *Motion sickness and vomiting:*

Initial dose: 0.5 mg/kg/dose 2-8 h before travel (maximum 25 mg/dose), then 0.25/kg/dose q 6-8 h PRN (maximum 1 mg/kg/day)

CI: Epilepsy

(Avomine 25 mg tab; Promet 10 mg, 25 mg tab, inj 25 mg/mL; Apizine 5 mg/5 mL)

Triflupromazine

- *Nausea and vomiting associated with chemotherapy and radiation:*

PO: 0.5 mg/kg/day div q 8 h

IM: 0.25 mg/kg/day div q 8 h

CI: Children < 3 years, hepatic damage, coma, and bone marrow depression

[Siquil 10 mg tab, inj 10 mg/mL (1 mL, 10 mL)]

HORMONES AND DRUGS FOR ENDOCRINE DISORDERS

Adrenocorticotropic Hormone

- *Infantile spasms:*
  - *Adrenocorticotropic hormone Gel*: 20 units/dose IM q OD × 2 weeks; if no response, increase dose to 30–40 units/dose IM q OD × additional 4 weeks *Note*: Taper dose over several weeks; Prednisolone 2 mg/kg/day has been found to be almost equally effective
- *Anti-inflammatory:*
  - *Adrenocorticotropic hormone aqueous*: 1.6 units/kg/day div. q 6–8 h IM/SC
  - *Adrenocorticotropic hormone gel*: 0.8 units/kg/day div. q 12–24 h IM

CI: Acute psychosis, CHF, peptic ulcer, and hypertension

S/E: As with other corticosteroids (*see* under prednisolone)

(Acton Prolongatum 60 IU/mL–0.5 mL amp, 5 mL vial)

Betamethasone

- *In pregnant female (suspected premature labor):* 12 mg IM once daily × 2 days or 6 mg IM q 12 h × 4 doses (maximum effectiveness between 24 h after and up to 1 week after its administration)
- *For children with severe attack of bronchial asthma and brain edema:* 0.1–0.2 mg/kg/day div q BID/TID PO

(*Note*: 750 µg of betamethasone equivalent to 5 mg prednisolone)

S/E: As with corticosteroids (*see* prednisone)

Caution: Monitor for development of hypertension and pulmonary edema

(Betnesol, Solubet, Celestone 0.5 mg, 1 mg tab, drops 0.5 mg/mL, inj 4 mg/mL)

Carbimazole

- *Hyperthyroidism and thyrotoxicosis:*
  Neonate: PO Initially 250 ug/kg q TID (maximum 1 mg/kg daily) until enthyroid
  Child 1 month–12 years: Initially 250 µg/kg (maximum 10 mg) q TID until euthyroid then adjusted as necessary
  Child >12–18 years: Initially 10 mg q TID daily until enthyroid, then adjust dose as necessary

S/E: Nausea, headache, fever, malaise, hepatitis, and rash

(Neo-mercazole, thyrocab, Anti-thyrox 5 mg, 10 mg, 20 mg tab)

Chorionic Gonadotropin

- *Prepubertal cryptorchidism*:

  Dose: 500 units three time a week IM × 4-6 weeks
  Hypogonadotropic hypogonadism:
  500–1000 units 3 times a week IM × 3 weeks followed by same dose twice weekly × 3 weeks
  or 4000 units 3 times a week × 6–9 months; then 2000 units 3 times a week × additional 3 months

S/E: Depression, fatigue, precocious puberty, premature closure of epiphysis
(Inj Corion, Fertigyn, Pubergen 1000 IU, 2000 IU, 5000 IU, 10,000 IU)

Cortisone Acetate

- *Anti-inflammatory:*

  PO: 2.5–10 mg/kg/day div q 6–8 hr

  IM: 1-5 mg/kg/day div q 12–24 hr

For physiological replacement (in Adrenocortical insufficiency cases):

PO: 0.5–0.75 mg/kg/day div q 8 hr

IM: 0.25–0.35 mg/kg/dose OD

(Cortin tab 5 mg, 25 mg; cortisyl, Cortelyn 25 mg; Inj cortone 25 mg, 50 mg per mL)

Desmopressin Acetate

Vasopressin analog:
- *Nocturnal enuresis (>6 years):*
  - *Oral*: 0.2–0.6 mg
  - *Intranasal*:
    - *Initial*: 10 µg HS; subsequently may increase up to 40 µg HS (one-half of total dose in each nostril);
- *Hemophilia A and von Willebrand's type I (Mild cases):*
  - *IV*: 0.3 µg/kg/dose diluted in 50 mL N. saline and infused over 15–30 minutes; administer 30 minutes before procedure
- *Diabetes insipidus:*
  - *Intranasal < 2 years*: 0.15–0.5 µg/kg/day div q 12–24 h
  - *Intranasal > 2 years*: 5–10 µg/day (not per kg) div q 12–24 h; titrate to response; maximum dose 30 µg/day
  - *Oral 3 months–12 years*:
    - *Initial*: 0.05 mg/day div q OD, then titrate to response.

Caution: Use with caution in hypertension; ensure sufficient intake of water

Monitor: Activated partial thromboplastin time (APTT), serum electrolytes, and urine output

(Minirin—nasal spray 10 µg per activation (100 µg/mL; intranasal solution 100 µg/mL (2.5 mL bottle); tablet 0.1 mg; inj 4 µg/mL)

Dexamethasone

Corticosteroid:
Neonates:
- *Airway edema or extubation:*
  - *IV*: 0.25 mg/kg 4 h prior to extubation and then 0.75–1 mg/kg/ 24 h div q 8 h/6 h

- *Bronchopulmonary dysplasia:*
  - *IV/PO*: 0.25 mg/kg/dose q 12 h × 6 doses, then taper over 1 to 6 weeks

Children:
- *Cerebral edema:*
  - *Initial*: 0.5 mg/kg/dose (maximum 10 mg) PO/IV/IM once followed by
  - *Maintenance*: 1.5 mg/kg/day div q 4-6 h (maximum 16 mg/24 h) PO/IM/IV; taper over 1-6 weeks
- *Bacterial meningitis due to Hib infection:*
  - *Children > 6 weeks*: 0.6 mg/kg/day div q 6 h × first 2-4 days of treatment; start dexamethasone 15-20 minutes before or along with first dose of antibiotic
- *Croup (viral):*
  - 0.5 mg/kg/dose IV/IM × 1 dose
- *Airway edema or extubation:*
  - 0.5-2 mg/kg/day div q 6 h PO/IM/IV
- *Anti-inflammatory:*
  - 0.08-0.3 mg/kg/day q 6-12 h PO/IM/IV (maximum 9 mg/day)

S/E and precautions: as with prednisolone

[Decadron, Dexona 0.5 mg tab, drops 0.5 mg/mL, inj 4 mg/mL (2 mL), inj 20 mg/mL (5 mL), Wymesone, Decdan 0.5 mg tab, inj 4 mg/mL]

Fludrocortisone Acetate

Adrenal corticosteroid:
- For replacement therapy (as mineralocorticoid) along with glucocorticoid (such as hydrocortisone) in Addison's disease or following adrenalectomy:
  - Children: Initial 0.05-0.1 mg/day; maintenance 0.05-0.3 mg/day q OD PO as per response

S/E: As with other corticosteroids

(Floricort 100 µg tab)

Human Growth Hormone

Somatropin (synthetic human growth hormone)
- *Growth hormone deficiency:*
  - *Genotropin*: 0.16–0.24 mg/kg SC/IM weekly divided into daily dose (6–7 doses)
  - *Humatrope*: 0.18 mg/kg SC/IM weekly div into alternate days or six times/week
  - *Norditropin*: 0.024–0.034 mg/kg/dose SC/IM × 6–7 times per week
- *Idiopathic short stature:*
  - *Humatrope*: 0.037 mg/kg SC/IM weekly divided into daily dose
- *Children small for gestational age at birth*:
  - *Genotropin*: 0.48 mg/kg SC/IM weekly divided into 6–7 doses per week

Precaution: Use with caution in patients with diabetes and active malignancy

S/E: Headache, intracranial hypertension, rash, mild hyperglycemia, reversible hypothyroidism, GIT upset, muscles skeletal pain, and gynecomastia.

(Genotropin 4 μ, 12 μ, 16 μ 36 μ inj; Norditropin inj 5 mg, 10 mg, 15 mg; Humatrope cart and vials each containing somatropin in variable amount; 6 mg, 12 mg, 1.33 mg or 5.33 mg)

Hydrocortisone Sodium Succinate

Corticosteroid:
- *Status asthmaticus:*
  - *Initial*: 4–8 mg/kg/dose (maximum 250 mg dose) followed by 8 mg/kg/day IV div q 6 h
- *Anti-inflammatory:*
  - *PO*: 2.5–10 mg/kg/day div q 6–8 h
  - *IM/IV*: 1–5 mg/kg/day div q OD/BID
- *Acute adrenal insufficiency:*
  - *Load*: 1–2 mg/kg/dose IV bolus;
  - *Maintenance*:
    - *Infants and young children*: 25–150 mg/day div q 6–8 h
    - *Older children*: 150–250 mg/day div 6–8 h

- *Anaphylaxis (as adjunct to other essential treatment):*
  - 5 mg/kg/dose q 6 h IV PRN
- *Shock:*
  - Children IV:
    - *Initial*: 50 mg/kg, may repeat after 4 h and then 50–150 mg/kg/day div q 6 h/24 h for 48–72 h
    - *Adults*: 500 mg–2 g/dose q 2–6 h IV
- *Neonatal hypoglycemia (refractory to glucose infusion):*
  - Neonates: IV; PO—5 mg/kg/day div q 8–12 h or 1–2 mg/kg/dose q 6 h

Note: Use only sodium succinate salt of hydrocortisone for IV/IM use. The acetate salt is meant for intra-articular, intrasynovial or intralesional injection only

S/E: As with prednisolone

[Inj Efcorlin, Hydrocortisone sodium succinate (Lyka, Samarth), (Hydrocortisone sodium succinate 134 mg equivalent to 100 mg hydrocortisone) vial]

Insulin, Regular

- *For diabetic ketoacidosis:*
  - *Initial*: 0.1 U/kg IV bolus; followed by continuous infusion around 0.1 U/kg/h in N. saline to maintain steady decrease of blood glucose level of 80–100 mg/dL/h until blood sugar comes down to 300 mg/dL (Usual range of insulin infusion 0.05–0.2 U/kg/h). At this stage change IV fluid to 5% dextrose in 1/2 N. saline.
  - When acidosis and ketosis are resolved, discontinue insulin drip and start S/C regular insulin 0.1–0.25 U/kg q 6–8 h for 24 h to assess daily insulin need. Subsequently shift to combination of regular and intermediate acting insulins.
  - For more details refer to Chapter 23 "Management of childhood type 1 diabetes and diabetic ketoacidosis"
- *Severe hyperkalemia:*
  - 0.1 U/kg IV with 2 mL/kg of 25% glucose (i.e. 1 unit insulin per 5 g glucose) slowly over 30 minutes

S/E: Hypoglycemia (pallor, sweating, apprehension, trembling, tachycardia, hunger; if severe hypoglycemia–mental confusion, seizures, and coma)

(Insulin regular bovine-Rapidica, Bovine Fastact, Actrapid 40 IU/mL; Insulin regular human-Human Actrapid, Human Rapidica, Human Fastact 40 IU/mL; Insulin lispro–Humalog 40 IU/mL 10 mL vial, 100 IU/mL 3 mL cartridge)

Insulin Intermediate Acting

- For usage refer to Chapter 23 "Management of childhood type 1 diabetes"
- Insulin intermediate acting trade preparations

(NPH insulin, porcine: Iletin N, Prodica 40 IU/mL 10 mL vial; NPH insulin, human: Huminsulin-N, Human Insulatard 40 IU/mL vial; Lente insulin, porcine: Zinulin 40 IU/mL 10 mL vial; Lente insulin, human: Human zinulin, Human Monotard 40 IU/mL vial)

Liothyronine

- *Congenital hypothyroidism (cretinism)*
  - *Initial*: 5 µg/day; ↑ by 5 µg every 3 days (maximum in neonates 20 ug/day; in infants 50 ug/day; in children 1–3 years—50 ug/day)
- *Hypothyroidism*
  - *Children*: Initial 5 µg/day PO ↑ by 5 µg/day every 3–4 days to usual maintenance dose:
  - Infants 20 µg/day; children 1–3 years—50 µg/day; children > 3 years—full adult dose may be necessary
  - *Adults*: 25 µg/day PO; ↑ 15–25 µg/day dose every 1–2 weeks; maximum 100 µg/day
- *Goiter nontoxic*
  - *Children*: 5 µg/day PO; increase by 5 µg/day every 1–2 weeks; usual *maintenance dose*—15–20 ug/day

S/E: As with thyroxine sodium

(Tertroxin 20 µg tab; inj triiodothyronine 20 µg amp)

Methylprednisolone Sodium Succinate

Corticosteroid:
- *Status asthmaticus:*
  - *Initial*: 1 mg/kg/dose q 6 h (maximum 180 mg/24 h) IV/IM × 48 h followed by
  - *Maintenance*: 1–2 mg/kg/day div q 12 h IV/IM (maximum 60 mg/24 h) till peak expiratory flow rate (PEFR) is 70% of the personal best or predicted
- *Anti-inflammatory, immunosuppressive:*
  - PO/IM/IV: 0.5–2 mg/kg/day div q 6–12 h
- *Acute spinal cord injury:*
  - *IV*: 30 mg/kg IV over 15 minutes, followed in 45 minutes by continuous infusion at the rate of 5.4 mg/kg/h for 23 h
  - *IM (acetate)*: 10–80 mg/day q OD

Note: For IV administration use only succinate salt of methylprednisolone. Acetate form can be used by IM but not by IV route

S/E: As with prednisolone

[Methyl prednisolone sodium succinate preparations IV/IM—Solu-medrol, Neo-drol, 40 mg, 125 mg, 500 mg, 1000 mg vials; Methylprednisolone acetate preparation (IM only)—Depo-medrol 40 mg/mL; 1 mL, 2 mL inj]

Potassium Iodide and Iodine (Lugol's Solution)

Antithyroid agent:
- *Neonatal thyrotoxicosis:*
  - *Neonate*: PO 1 drop TID; if response in 48 h; increase dose by 25% per day until control achieved; usual 10–14 days
- *Preoperative thyroidectomy* (for thyrotoxicosis)
  - *Children and adults*: For 10–14 days before surgery
  - Lugol's solution 0.1–0.3 mL (3–5 drops) q TID PO
- *Thyrotoxic crisis:*
  - *Children and adults*: 1 mL q TID PO
  - *Child 1 month–1 year*: 0.2–0.3 mL q TID PO

(Lugol's iodine 5% solution added to 10% potassium iodide freshly boiled and cooled provides iodine 130 mg per mL)

Prednisone or Prednisolone

Corticosteroid:
- *Anti-inflammatory*: 0.1-2 mg/kg/day PO, div q OD-QID
- *Acute asthma:*
  - *Children ≤ 12 years*: 1 mg/kg/dose q 6 h for 48 h; then 1-2 mg/kg/day (maximum 60 mg/day) div q BID until peak expiratory flow (PEF) is 70% of predicted or personal best
  - *Children > 12 years and adults*: 120-180 mg/day div q TID/QID × 48 h then; 60-80 mg/day div q BID till response
- *Nephrotic syndrome:*
  - *Initial*: 2 mg/kg/day or 60 mg/m^2/day (maximum daily dose 80 mg/day) div q BID/TID PO until urine is protein free (i.e. urine trace or negative for protein for 3 consecutive days) × 4-6 weeks followed by
  - *Maintenance*: 1.5 mg/kg/day or 40 mg/m^2/day on alternate days div q OD in morning for next 2-3 months. (Some authorities now advise low dose alternate day therapy for longer period especially in children with tendency to relapse)
  - *For relapse*: Initial dose as given above till child goes into remission, then alternate day dosing once daily; taper over 1-2 months
- *Thrombocytopenic purpura, idiopathic:*
  - 1-4 mg/kg/day div q BID/TID × 2-3 week or until a rise in platelet count above 20,000; taper dose rapidly

S/E: Edema, hypertension, peptic ulcer, psychosis; prolonged use causes cushingoid effects, adrenal (HPA axis) suppression, cataract, acne, skin, and muscle atrophy

Note: see under "Hydrocortisone" for further details regarding corticosteroids

(Prednisolone-prepn: Wysolone, Omnacortil, Nucort 5 mg, 10 mg, 20 mg, 40 mg tab; Predone syr 5 mg/5 mL, Predone Forte syr 15 mg/5 mL)

Propylthiouracil

Antithyroid drug:
- *Neonates*: 5–10 mg/kg/day div q TID PO
- *Children*: 5–7 mg/kg/day div q TID PO
  - *Maintenance*: After the patient becomes euthyroid following initial treatment—one-third–one-half the initial dose

S/E: Hepatitis, arthralgia, skin rash, vertigo, and blood dyscrasias

(Propylthiouracil 50 mg tab)

Thyroxine Sodium (Levothyroxine Sodium)

- *For hypothyroidism:*
  - *0–3 months*: 10–15 µg/kg div q OD PO; adjust dose in steps of 5 µg/kg at 2–4 week intervals to maintain T4 in 10–16 µg/dL range and TSH below 5 MU/L
  - *3–12 months*: 6–10 µg/kg or 25–75 µg/day
  - *1–12 years*: 4–6 µg/kg or 75–125 µg/day
  - *> 12 years*: 2–3 µg/kg or 150 µg/day or more

S/E: Nervousness, palpitation, tachycardia, tremor, diarrhea, and hypertension.

(Eltroxin, 50 µg, 100 µg tab, Thyrox 25 µg, 50 µg, 100 µg, 200 µg tab)

Triamcinolone

Corticosteroid:
- *Children 6–12 years*:
  - *IM*: 0.03–2 mg/kg every 1–7 days
  - *Intra-articular, intrabursal*: 2.5–15 mg; repeat PRN

S/E: Cataracts, fatigue, osteoporosis, and poor growth

Caution: Not recommended below 6 years

(Kenacort, Ledercort, Tricort 4 mg tab, inj Kenacort, Tricort 10 mg/mL, 40 mg/mL)

Vasopressin

- *Variceal hemorrhage due to portal hypertension:*
  - *Initial*: 0.33 units/kg diluted in 25 mL of 5% dextrose by IV bolus over 20 minutes and then continued infusion* 0.33 U/kg/h or 0.2 units/1.73 m^2/min PRN
- *Diabetes insipidus:*
  - *IM/SC*: 2.5–10 U/dose q BID-QID as per response
- *Catecholamine refractory vasodilatory septic shock:*
  - *IV*: 0.3–2 mU/Kg/minute IV infusion

S/E: Tremor, vertigo, anaphylaxis, hypertension, seizures, and cardiac arrhythmia

Caution: IV infusion dose should be tapered slowly

[Vasopin, Petresin inj 20 IU/mL (1 mL amp)]

VITAMINS

Alfacalcidol

Vitamin D preparation:
- *Renal rickets, hypophosphatemic Vit D rickets, and hypoparathyroidism*
  - *< 20 kg*: 0.05 µg/kg/day q OD PO
  - *> 20 kg*: 1 µg/day q OD PO
- *Renal osteodystrophy*: 0.04–0.08 µg/kg/day

S/E: Hypercalcemia and hyperphosphatemia

(Alfacip, Alpha D$_3$, Alphadol 0.25 µg, 1 µg cap)

Ascorbic Acid

See Vitamin C below

Calcitriol

Vitamin D analog:
- *Hypocalcemia in premature infants:*
  - *PO*: 1 µg/day × 5 days
  - *IV*: 0.05 µg/kg/day × 4 days

- *Renal failure:*
    - *PO*: 0.01–0.04 µg/kg/day (no hemodialysis)
    - *IV*: 0.01–0.05 µg/kg three times weekly (hemodialysis)

Note: Adjust dose to maintain normal serum calcium level

S/E: Vitamin D toxicity and hypercalcemia

(Rocaltrol, Bio-D$_3$, Rolsical 0.25 µg cap, Calen, Setcal Mom tab contain calcitriol 0.25 mg + calcium carbonate and zinc)

Vitamin A

- *For severe deficiency with xerophthalmia:*
    - < *6 months*: PO 50,000 U/dose q OD × 2 days; repeat once 2–4 weeks later
    - *6 months–1 year*: PO 100,000 U/dose q OD × 2 days; repeat once 2–4 weeks later
    - *1–6 years*: PO 200,000 U/dose q OD × 2 days; repeat once 2–4 weeks later

Note: IM dose of water miscible preparation of vitamin A is half the oral dose

- *For prophylaxis in patients at risk and during measles*
    - *6 months–1 years*: PO 100,000 U/dose once every 6 months
    - *1–5 years*: PO 200,000 U/dose once every 6 months
    - Child should receive a total of nine oral doses of Vitamin A by 5th birthday when dietary intake is likely to be insufficient and high risk of contracting infections.

S/E (due to over dosage): Anorexia, headache, irritability, pseudotumor cerebri

(Vit A 50,000 IU (NPIL) tab; Vit A 50,000 IU (USV) cap; Rovigon (Vit A 10,000 IU + Vit E 25 mg) tab; Aquasol-A 50,000 IU cap; 100,000 IU in 2 mL inj)

Vitamin B$_1$

Thiamine:
- *Beriberi*
    - *IM/IV*: 10–25 mg/day; or PO 10–50 mg/day × 2 weeks; then 5–10 mg/day × 1 month

- *Wernicke encephalopathy*
  - *IM/IV*: 100 mg/day until patient takes a balanced diet

Caution: IV administration may cause allergic or anaphylactic reaction

[Benalgis 75 mg tab; Berin 50 mg, 100 mg tab, 100 mg/mL inj (10 mL vial)]

Vitamin B$_2$

Riboflavin:
- *Deficiency*: 2.5–10 mg/day div q OD–BID PO

S/E: Hypersensitivity extremely rare

(Lipabol 20 mg tab, Riboflavin 10 mg/mL inj)

Vitamin B$_6$

Pyridoxine:
- *Pyridoxine dependent persistent neonatal seizures:*
  - 100 mg/dose IM (as neurobion inj containing pyridoxine 50 mg per mL; 1 ml injection IM in thigh on both sides)
- *Drug induced neuritis:*
  - *Treatment*: 10–50 mg/day PO/IM/IV q OD
  - *Prophylaxis*: 1–2 mg/kg/day PO q OD
- *Dietary deficiency:*
  - *Initial*: 5–25 mg/day PO/IM/IV q OD × 3 weeks, then
  - *Maintenance*: 2.5 to 10 mg/day PO q OD
- *As antidote for isoniazid poisoning:*
  - 1 mg IV for each 1 mg of isoniazid. If amount of INH taken is unknown, administer 500 mg

S/E: Nausea, allergic reaction, decreased serum folic acid, and elevated LFT

(B-Long 100 mg tab; Benadon 40 mg tab; Ingavit 10 mg, 50 mg tab)

Vitamin B₁₂

Cyanocobalamin:
- *Pernicious anemia:*
  - *Initial*: 30–50 µg/day IM OD to a total dose of 1,000–5,000 µg and then
  - *Maintenance*: 100 µg once per month IM
- *Pernicious anemia (with neurologic involvement):*
  - *Initial*: 1,000 µg IM OD × 2 weeks, then *maintenance*: 100 µg IM once a month
- *Vitamin B₁₂ deficiency:*
  - *Initial*: 100 µg/day IM × OD 10–15 days (to a total dose of 1–1.5 mg), then 100 µg once or twice a week for several months; may taper to 60 µg/month

Note: Oral therapy not recommended due to uncertainty of absorption

S/E: Pruritus and hypersensitivity

[Ingavit B₁₂ 500 µg/mL, 1000 µg/mL (10 mL vial); Mecobar (mecobalamin) tab 500 µg, inj 500 µg/1 mL amp]

Vitamin C

Ascorbic acid:
- *Scurvy*:
  - *Children*: 100–300 mg/day
- *Urinary acidification*
  - *Children*: 500 mg every 6 h

S/E: Vomiting, heartburn, dizziness, and hyperoxaluria

(Limcee, Redoxon, Celin 500 mg tab; Sukcee, Celin, chewable 200 mg; Cecon drops 100 mg/mL)

Vitamin D₃ (Cholecalciferol)

A. *For prevention of rickets and hypocalcemia*:
- *Premature neonates: Vitamin D 400 IU; calcium 150–220 mg/kg per day*
- *Neonates: Vitamin D 400 IU + calcium 200 mg per day*

- > 1 month to 1 year: Vitamin D 400 IU + calcium 250–500 mg/day
- > 1 year to 18 year: Vitamin D 600 IU + calcium 600–800 mg/day

B. **For treatment of rickets:**
   - < 1 month neonates: Vitamin D 1000 IU + calcium 70–80 mg/kg/day
   - > 1 month up to 1 year: Vitamin D 2000 IU + Calcium 500–800 mg/day
   - > 1 year to 18 years: Vitamin D 3000–6000 IU + calcium 600–800 mg/day

   Alternatives:
   i. PO—3 months to 18 year: Vitamin D 60,000 IU per week × 6–10 weeks + calcium: 500–800 mg calcium per day
   ii. IM—Vitamin D_3: Single dose 300,000 IU IM*
   iii. PO—3 lac–6 lac units over 5–10 days PO (60,000 IU per dose)

*Better avoid IM route unless severe malabsorption or doubt about proper compliance to oral therapy.

(Calcirol, Calcibest, Calcitas Calshine K granules 60,000 units per sachet; Biocital, briocal-D_3 D-build 60,000 units per cap; Acicium, Calsma D_3, Vital-CL D_3 60,000 units chew tab; Arachitol 3 lac, 6 lac IU, Devita 6 lac IU, NU-D3 3 lac and 6 lac IU inj; D_3 drops, kid D_3 drops 400 IU/mL)

Vitamin E

Alpha-tocopherol

- *Vitamin E deficiency:*
  - *Neonates and premature infants*: 25–50 IU/day;
  - *Children*: IU/kg/day
- *Beta-thalassemia:* 800 IU/day.
- *Sickle cell anemia:* 400 IU/day

Note: 1 mg of alpha-tocopherol = 1.49 IU of vitamin E

(Evion 100 mg, 200 mg, 400 mg, 600 mg pearls; drops 50 mg/mL, Tocofer, Vit-E, 200 mg, 400 mg cap)

Vitamin K$_1$ (Phytanadione)

- *Hemorrhagic disease of newborn:*
  - *Prophylaxis*: 0.5–1 mg IM (preterm < 34 weeks—0.5 mg; term infants 1 mg)
  - *Treatment*: 1–5 mg by IV infusion

Note: Dilute Vit K$_1$ in 5% dextrose and infuse slowly. In case of active bleeding, 10 mL/kg of fresh frozen plasma (FFP) or whole blood transfusion may also be administered.

Vitamin K$_3$ synthetic preparations-menadione and acetomenaphthone, are not to be employed for prophylaxis or treatment of hemorrhagic disease of newborn.

- *Overdose of anticoagulant:*
  - *Infants and children:* 0.5–2 mg IM/SC/IV;

In case of severe bleeding give up to 5 mg of Vit K$_1$, through slow IV infusion diluted in 5% dextrose, along with other measures, such as, FFP or blood transfusion as needed.

- *Vitamin K deficiency:*
  - *PO:* 2.5–5 mg/day
  - *IM/IV:* 1–2 mg/dose once

S/E: Large doses of Vit K$_1$ (10–20 mg) in newborn may cause hyperbilirubinemia and severe hemolytic anemia. IV administration of vitamin K$_1$ may rarely cause flushing, hypotension, and anaphylactic reaction.

i. *K$_1$ prepn*: Kenadion (phytonadione) inj 1 mg (0.5 mL); 10 mg (1 mL);
ii. *K$_3$ prepn*: Styptindon (menadione sodium sulfite 5 mg + Vitamin C 50 mg + rutin 25 mg) tab; inj 2 mL;
iii. *Acetomenaphthone prepn*: Kapilin (acetomenaphthone) 10 mg tab, inj 10 mg/mL (1 mL); Kalpastic (acetomenaphthone 2 mg + Rutin 20 mg + Vit C 100 mg + Calcium gluconate) tab

HEMATINICS AND MICRONUTRIENTS

Erythropoietin

- *Anemia of prematurity*: 250 units/kg SC three times a week × 2–3 weeks (along with iron 2–3 mg/kg/day div q TID PO)

- *Chronic renal failure:*
  - *Initial*: 50–100 U/kg/day SC/IV three times per week
  - *Maintenance*: 10 U/kg/day SC/IV three times per week

(Human-LG Espogen 2,000 IU, 4,000 IU (prefilled syringe, 10,000 IU, 20,000 IU (vials); Epox, Vintor, Zyrop 2,000 IU, 4,000 IU vials)

Folic Acid

Treatment of folate deficiency anemia (Table 33.12):

Caution: Avoid use in pernicious anemia. Induces deceptive hematologic improvement without beneficial effect on neurologic abnormalities

(Folvite, Ingafol, Sysfol 5 mg tab)

Granulocyte Colony-stimulating Factor; Filgrastim

Reduces duration of neutropenia *(acts by stimulating production, maturation and activation of neutrophils):*

Dose: IV; S/C (refer to individual protocols):
- *Neonates:* 5–10 µg/kg/day OD S/C × 3–5 days
- *Children and adults:* 5–10 ug/kg/day q OD × for up to 14 days or until ANC becomes 10,000/mm^2. Discontinue when ANC over 10,000/mm^3 for 3 consecutive days

S/E: Fever, bone pains, thrombocytopenia, and hematuria

(Neupogen inj 300 µg/vial)

Table 33.12: Treatment of folate deficiency anemia.			
	Infants	1–10 yr	≥11 years
Initial	50 µg/day 1 mg/day	1 mg/day	1–2 mg/day PO/IM/IV/SC
Maintenance	30 µg/day	0.25 mg/day	0.5 mg/day PO/IM/IV/SC

Iron

Oral:
- *Treatment of deficiency*: 3–6 mg/kg/day div q 12 h PO
- *Prophylaxis*: 1–2 mg/kg/day div q 12 h PO

S/E: Constipation, epigastric pain, nausea, and dark stools
- *Total replacement of iron Deficiency IV/IM*
    - Formula for calculating total replacement dose of iron dextran (mL) = 0.0442 × BW (kg) × (desired Hb – patients Hb) + [0.26 × BW (kg)]
    - *IV*: Give a test dose of 10–25 mg of iron dextran IV over 5 minutes. If no untoward reaction over next 1 h, give one-third of the calculated total replacement dose as IV infusion diluted in N. saline (50–100 mL), maximum concentration of 50 mg/mL; over 1–6 h (maximum rate of infusion 50 mg/min). The remainder can be given in two divided doses over the next 2 days
    - *IM*: The total dose may be given in divided doses over several days. Maximum dose per day; < 5 kg: 25 mg; 5–10 kg: 50 mg; children >10 kg and adults: 100 mg
    - Use Z-track technique while injecting the drug into a large muscle

S/E: Anaphylaxis, hypotension, myalgia, and arthralgia

(Oral prepn. The strength of following preparations is given as per their content of elemental iron:

Tab Ferium 50 (50 mg); Tab Ferium 100 mg (100 mg); Hb Fast, Tofe; Fersolate tab (66 mg); Syrup Ferium, Hb Fast, Mumfer, Tofe, Vitcofol com 50 mg/5 mL; Drops Ferium, Hb Fast, Mumfer 50 mg/mL; Tonoferon syrup 250 mg/5 mL, ped syrup 50 mg/5 mL, drops 25 mg/mL)

[Parenteral Iron prepn (Iron dextran complex)]:

Inj Imferon (iron dextran equivalent to 50 mg elemental iron per mL) 2 mL amp; Inj Jectofer, Inj Jectocos 50 mg elemental iron per mL) 1.5 mL amp

Zinc Supplements

- *Zinc deficiency:*
  - *PO*: 0.5–1 mg/kg/day (elemental zinc) div q OD-TID
- *As adjunct in acute and persistent diarrhea treatment:*
  - *< 6 months*: 10 mg/day × 14 days
  - *> 6 months*: 20 mg/day × 14 days
- *Acrodermatitis enteropathica treatment 6 mg/kg/day.*

Note: Zinc sulfate 4.4 mg = 1 mg elemental zinc

[Zevit syrup (elemental zinc 10 mg + multivitamins) per 5 mL; Becozinc syrup (elemental zinc 4 mg + multivitamins) per 5 mL; Drops Zevit (elemental zinc 3 mg + multivitamin) per 1 mL; Drops Becozinc (elemental zinc 3 mg + multivitamin) per 1 mL; Capsules Zevit, Cobadex-Z, Polyzee (elemental zinc 22.5 mg + multivitamins) per cap; Syrup Zinconia (zinc acetate equivalent to elemental zinc 20 mg/5 mL)]

MISCELLANEOUS DRUGS

Acetylcysteine

See under "Antidote for acetaminophen poisoning"

Albumin (Human)

- *Hypovolemia and shock:*
  - *Neonates*: 0.5 g/kg/dose (10 mL/kg/dose of 5% albumin) IV rapid infusion
  - *Infants and children*: 0.5 to 1 g/kg/day (10–20 mL/kg of 5% albumin) IV rapid infusion (maximum 6 g/kg/day, 120 mL/kg/day of 5% albumin)
  - *Adults*: 25 g/dose (maximum 250 g/within 48 h)
- *Hypoproteinemia and nephrotic syndrome*

Children: 0.5–1 g/kg/dose (20% albumin) IV over 2–4 h; repeat q 1–2 days PRN

CI: CHF, and severe anemia

Caution: Watch for pulmonary edema, CHF, hypertension, hypersensitivity reaction. In preterm infants use 5% albumin solution (risk of IVH with 20% albumin). Dilute 20% albumin with NS or 5% dextrose.

[Human albumin (Paviour) 5% 50 mL, 250 mL, 20% 10 mL, 50 mL, 100 mL; Albumed 5% and 10% 100 mL infn; Albudac 20% 10 mL, 50 mL, 100 mL]

Allopurinol

Uric Acid Lowering Agent

- *Prevention of hyperuricemia during cancer chemotherapy:*
  Children ≤ 10 years: 10 mg/kg/day div q BD/TID PO
  Children > 10 years: 200-600 mg/day div q BID/TID PO

Caution: Reduce dose in renal impairment. Discontinue if skin rash develops

S/E: Rash, hepatic and renal toxicity, and peripheral neuropathy

(Zyloric, Aloric 100 mg tab; Aloric 300 mg tab)

Antihemophilic Factor

Factor VIII Concentrate

Bleeding in Hemophilia A:
- *Hemarthrosis:* 50-60 units/kg stat; then 20-30 U/kg, on day 2, 3, and 5 and then repeat same dose on alternate days PRN × 1 week-10 days.
- *Muscle or significant subcutaneous hematoma*: 50 units/kg stat; repeat daily or on alternate days till well resolved
- *Mouth bleeding, tooth extraction, epistaxis:* 20 U/kg stat + antifibrinolytic therapy + topical treatment
- *Major surgery, life-threatening hemorrhage (e.g. CNS, airway):* 50-75 U/kg stat and then continuous infusion at the rate of 2-3 U/kg/h for 5-7 days and then 1.5-2 U/kg/h × 5-7 days

- *Iliopsoas hemorrhage:* 50 U/kg stat, then 25 U/kg/dose every 12 h until asymptomatic, then 20 U/kg/dose on alternate days for total 10–14 days
- *Hematuria:* 20 U/kg if it persists for 1–2 days (despite bed rest and extra oral fluids)

Note: May use desmopressin 0.3 µg/kg instead of Factor VIII in mild to moderate hemophilia

> *For more details, refer to consensus statement of the Indian Academy of Pediatrics in Diagnosis and Management of Hemophilia 2018, outlined in Chapter 26*

[Factor VIII (Paviour Pharma) 250 IU/vial; Emoclot DI 250 IU, 500 IU vial; Monoclate P 250 IU, 500 IU, 1000 IU vial]

Antivenin Serum Polyvalent

Generally recommended dose against venoms of cobra, common krait, Russel's viper, and saw scaled viper (Table 33.13)

To prepare the vaccine for administration, reconstitute each vial of antivenin with 10 mL of diluent (isotonic saline or distilled water) and roll the vial between your hands to prepare the solution.

According to earlier recommendations, the patient's sensitivity to the anti-venin serum was to be checked by doing skin or conjunctival sensitivity test before administering it to the patient. However, according to the 'management of snake bite, quick reference guide, issued by Ministry of

Table 33.13: Severity and amount of antivenin serum polyvalent.

Severity of envenomation	Amount of antivenin to be given
Mild	5 vials
Moderate	5–15 vials (50–150 mL)
Severe	15–20 vials (150–200 mL)
Children may need additional 50%	

Health, Government of India, 2016; no ASV test doses are to be administered for checking ASV reactions.

The readers are further advised to study and follow other instructions laid out in this guide for management of snakebites in our country.

Dilute reconstituted antivenin with three volumes of glucose saline and administer as a continuous IV infusion beginning at a slow rate of 1 mL/min, increasing the rate slowly as tolerated. The total dose can usually be completed in about 2 hours. Thereafter depending upon clinical response, more antivenin (5–10 vials) may be given every 2 hours till all the systemic signs and symptoms disappear and progressive swelling on the bitten part ceases.

In patients with hypersensitivity to antivenin serum, desensitization should be done slowly and the antivenin administered with much caution and prompt management of any anaphylactic reactions.

(Serum Institute, Haffkine, Bharat Serums, 10 mL vial)

Atomoxetine

Norepinephrine Reuptake Inhibitor

- *Selective treatment of attention deficit hyperactivity disorder (ADHD):*
  Children 6 years and above and adolescents < 70 kg:
  - *Initial:* 0.5 mg/kg/day PO; increase after a minimum of 3 days slowly to 1.2 mg/kg/day (maximum 1.4 mg/kg/day or 100 mg/day) div q OD/ BID PO

Precautions:
- *Reduce dose to 50% in cases with moderate and to 25% in cases with severe hepatic impairment. No dose adjustment in renal impairment*
- *Use with caution in patients with hypertension, cardiovascular, or cerebrovascular disease.*

CI: Concurrent use or within 14 days of monoamine oxidase (MAO) inhibitors, narrow angle glaucoma

S/E: Orthostatic hypotension, hypertension, tachycardia, decreased appetite, headache, dizziness, sleep disturbance, mood swings, lethargy, urinary retention, tremor, and mydriasis

(Tomexetin tab 10 mg, 18 mg, 25 mg, 40 mg)

Atorvastatin Calcium

- *Antilipemic agent for cases of hypercholesterolemia:*
  - *Children 10–17 years*: 10 mg/dose q OD; maximum 20 mg/dose q OD
  - *> 17 yr and adults*: 10–80 mg/day div q OD

Caution: Avoid use in active liver disease

(Arpitor, Atchol, Atocor 10 mg, 20 mg tab)

Atropine Sulfate

- *Cardiopulmonary resuscitation, sinus bradycardia:*
  - *IV*: 0.02 mg/kg/dose (min dose 0.1 mg; maximum dose 0.5 mg) stat; may repeat q 5 minutes × 1–2 times PRN (maximum total dose 1 mg)
- *Antidote to organophosphorus and carbonate poisoning:*
  - *IV*: 0.02–0.05 mg/kg every 5–10 minutes until full atropinization effect (when all secretions become dry), then every 1–4 h for 24 h, taper in the next 24 h
- *As preanesthetic:*
  - *SC/IV/IM*: 0.01 mg/kg/dose (min 0.1 mg/dose; maximum 0.4 mg/dose) may repeat q 4–6 h

Precaution: Avoid in very hot weather; may initiate hyperpyrexia

S/E: Dry mouth, blurred vision, urinary retention, constipation, dizziness, tachycardia, and hallucination

CI: Tachycardia, GI obstruction, glaucoma, and thyrotoxicosis

(Inj Atropt, Tropine 0.6 mg/mL, 1 mL amp; Inj Tropine 0.6 mg/mL, 10 mL vials)

Azathioprine

- *Immunosuppressant:*
  Initial: 3–5 mg/kg/day q OD PO/IV
  Maintenance: 1–3 mg/kg/day q OD PO/IV

Caution: Monitor CBC, platelets, LFT, and renal functions for toxicity

(Zymurine, Transimune, Imuran, Azaprin 50 mg tab; inj 100 mg vial)

Baclofen

- *Muscle relaxant:*
    - *Children ≥2 yrs and older:*
        - *Initial*: 10–15 mg/day div q 8 h PO. Increase dose at 3 days interval until desired effect or maximum dose reached
        - *Maximum dose < 8 years*: 40 mg/day;
    - *> 8 years*: 60 mg/day

Caution: Patients with renal impairment, seizures; avoid abrupt withdrawal

(Lofen, Lioresal 10 mg, 25 mg tab)

British Anti-Lewisite (BAL)

Dimercaprol: See under "Lead, arsenic and mercury poisoning antidotes".

Caffeine Citrate

- *Apnea of prematurity:*
  Loading dose: IV 10 mg/kg caffeine base (20 mg/kg of caffeine citrate) × 1 dose
  Maintenance: PO/IV 2.5–5 mg/kg caffeine base, q 24 h (start 24 h after the loading dose)
  Loading IV dose of caffeine citrate should be infused over at least 30 minutes; maintenance dose over at least 10 minutes (without dilution or diluted with D_5W to 10 mg caffeine citrate/mL)

Note: Injectable caffeine citrate can be administered for oral use.

Monitor: Heart rate; if heart rate more than 180/min withhold and then reduce dose

S/E: Tachycardia, restlessness, and vomiting; overdosage may cause seizures.

(*Inj cafirate, primicef 20 mg/mL in 3 mL vial; Cafirale, primicef oral solution in 1.5 mL vial*)

Calcium Chloride 10% (100 mg/mL)

- *Cardiac arrest (especially with hypocalcemia):*
  - *Infants, children*: 0.2 mL/kg/dose IV (maximum 10 mL/dose) stat; may repeat q 10 minutes PRN
  - *Adults*: 2.5–5 mL/dose (maximum dose 10 mL), may repeat q 10 minutes PRN

Important: Maximum rate of IV bolus—1 mL/min. Monitor heart rate, stop if bradycardia occurs. Avoid extravasation as it may lead to severe local tissue necrosis.

Note: Elemental calcium content per mL of 10% calcium chloride solution—27.2 mg

Calcium Gluconate 10%

- *Neonatal symptomatic hypocalcemia (tetany):*
  - *Emergency treatment*: 1–2 mL/kg/dose IV slow push, maximum rate 0.5–1 mL/min. Monitor heart rate and stop infusion if heart rate falls below 100/min
  - *Maintenance therapy:*
    - *IV*: 2–8 mL/kg/day as continuous infusion or div q QID or
    - *PO*: 5–10 mL/kg/day diluted with feeds in divided doses
- *Hypocalcemia in infants and children*:
  - *PO*: 5–7.5 mL/kg/day div q 6 h
  - *IV*: 2–5 mL/kg/day as continuous infusion or div q 6 h;

Note: Maximum IV infusion rate: 1.2–2.4 mL/kg/h with a maximum concentration of 0.5 mL calcium gluconate/mL

- *Cardiac arrest:*
  - *Neonates, infants and children*: 0.5–1 mL/kg/dose IV; may repeat once q 10 minutes PRN (maximum 30 mL/dose)
  - *Adults*: 5–8 mL/dose IV; may repeat once after 10 minutes PRN
    - *Maximum dose*: 30 mL/dose (3 g/dose)
- *Hyperkalemia:*
  - *IV*: 0.5 mL/kg/dose over 10 minutes

Precaution: Do not allow mixture with sodium bicarbonate as it would precipitate. Use with caution in digitalized patients as it may cause arrhythmia.

Note: 1 mL of 10% calcium gluconate solution contains 9 mg of elemental calcium.

Calcium Supplements

- *Carbonate, glubionate, or lactate salts:*
  - *Neonates*: Elemental calcium 20–80 mg/kg/day PO div q QID
  - *Infants and children*: 20–40 mg/kg/day PO div q QID

Carnitine

- *Carnitine deficiency:*
  PO: 50–100 mg/kg/day div q BID/TID (maximum 3 g/day)
  IV:
  - *Initial*: 50 mg/kg;
  - *Maintenance*: 50 mg/kg/day div q 4–6 h; maximum 300 mg/kg/day

S/E: Vomiting, abdominal cramps, and body odor

(Carnivit 500, cap 500 mg; oral solution 500 mg/5 mL; Carnit inj 500 mg/1 g for IV use)

Cyclizine

- *Anti-emetic especially for vomiting associated with vestibular disorder (motion sickness):*
  Dose:
    - *Children 6-12 years:* 25 mg/dose q TID PO
    - *>12-18 years*: 50 mg/dose q TID PO

S/E: Drowsiness, dry mouth, headache, diplopia, and urinary retention

(Medazine 50 mg tab)

Cholestyramine Resin

- *Antilipemic:*

Children: 240 mg/kg/day div q TID PO after meals; maximum 8 g/day

Adults: 4 g/dose q BID-QID PO

S/E: Constipation, GI upset, Vit A, D, E, K deficiencies, and rash

(Questran 4 g sachet, 378 g tin; 9 g questran contains 4 g cholestyramine)

Chlorzoxazone

- *Skeletal muscle spasm relaxant (symptomatic relief):*
  Dose:
    - *Children*: 20 mg/kg/day div q TID/QID PO
    - *Adults*: 250-750 mg/dose q TID/QID PO

S/E: Drowsiness, headache, rash GIT upset, and hepatic dysfunction

(Mobizox and Diclonac-MR tab contain chlorzoxazone 500 mg + diclofenac sodium 50 mg + paracetamol 500 mg)

Citrate Solutions

- *Chronic metabolic acidosis:*
  Children: 2-3 mEq/kg/day div q TID/QID PO

Adults: 15–30 mL/dose q QID (of citrate solution containing citrate 10 mEq/5 mL)

CI: Severe renal impairment and acute dehydration

S/E: Metabolic alkalosis, hyperkalemia, hypernatremia, and hypocalcemia

Cyclophosphamide

- For treatment of (1) various cancers, including Hodgkins disease, malignant lymphomas, multiple myeloma, and others; (2) steroid resistant nephrotic syndrome; (3) lupus erythematosus; (4) severe rheumatoid arthritis; and (5) rheumatoid vasculitis.
- *Dose:* Children:
    - *Nephrotic syndrome (steroid resistant):* 2–3 mg/kg/day OD PO × for up to 12 weeks
    - *Systemic lupus erythematosus*: 500–750 mg/m^2 IV every month (maximum dose 1 g/m^2)
    - *Juvenile rheumatoid arthritis or vasculitis*: 10 mg/kg IV every 2 weeks
    - *Bone marrow transplant conditioning:* 50 mg/kg/day IV OD × 3–4 days
    - *Cancers; different types:* Dose and administration as per individual protocols

Warning and precautions: Cyclophosphamide is potentially carcinogenic and mutagenic; it may impair fertility and cause birth defects. Use with caution and modify dosage in patients with bone marrow suppression, renal, or hepatic impairment (refer to drug literature for details)

S/E: Cardiotoxicity with high dosage, hemorrhagic cystitis, leucopenia, thrombocytopenia, hemolytic anemia, jaundice, renal toxicity, secondary malignancy, alopecia, rash, oligospermia, sterility, nausea and vomiting.

(Cycloxan, Endoxan–Asta, Ledoxan 50 mg tab; 200 mg, 500 mg, 1 g inj.)

Deferiprone

See "Iron poisoning antidotes".

Deferoxamine

See "Iron poisoning antidotes"

Dextran 40/70

Plasma Volume Expander (Like Albumin)

- *Shock or impending shock:*
  Children: IV dose and infusion rate to be adjusted according to individual patient's fluid status. Total dose during first 24 h—maximum 20 mL/kg; then 10 mL/kg/day × maximum 5 days

S/E: Bleeding due to impaired platelet function and pulmonary edema

Dextromethorphan

Antitussive:
- *2–6 years*: 2.5–7.5 mg/dose q 6 h PO
- *> 6–12 years*: 10–15 mg/dose q 6 h PO
- *12 years and adults*: 10–30 mg/dose q 6 h PO

S/E: Drowsiness, blurred vision, constipation, and GI upset

(As a constituent in several cough syrups along with other constituents, e.g. in Respi, Triatussic, and Grilinctus. Check content of dextromethorphan before prescribing)

Dimercaptosuccinic Acid

Succimer: See under "Arsenic, mercury and lead poisoning antidotes".

Doxapram Hydrochloride

Respiratory Stimulant

- *Neonatal apnea refractory to aminophylline:*

Loading dose: 2.5-3 mg/kg over 15 minutes followed by continuous infusion at the rate of 1 mg/kg/h diluted in 5% glucose solution; stepwise increase in dosage at the rate of 0.5 mg/kg/h at 24-48 h intervals until control of apnea or maximum dose of 2.5 mg/kg/h reached, whichever earlier. Taper dose after apnea controlled. Do not mix with fluid containing sodium bicarbonate

S/E: Tachycardia, hypertension, seizures, vomiting, and hyperpyrexia

[Caropram 20 mg per mL (5 mL) inj]

Ethylenediaminetetraacetic Acid (EDTA)

See under "Antidotes for lead poisoning".

Ergotamine

- *Migraine*:
  Older children and adolescents:
  - *Initial*: 1 mg sublingual or oral at onset of attack, then (if needed) 1 mg q 30 min till relief: maximum 3 mg per attack

CI: Patients with history of hemiplegic episode; use with caution in renal and hepatic disease

S/E: Vomiting, leg cramps, and paresthesia

[Migranil (ergotamine tartrate 1 mg, caffeine 100 mg) tab; Migranil inj—dihydroergotamine mesylate 1 mg/1 mL inj; Vasograin (ergotamine tartrate 1 mg, paracetamol 250 mg, prochlorperazine 2.5 mg, caffeine 100 mg tab)]

Epsilon Aminocaproic Acid

- *Hemostatic*:
  Initial load IV/PO: 100-200 mg/kg (maximum 12 g)
  Maintenance: 100 mg/kg/dose (maximum 5 g/dose) q 4-6 h or continuous infusion at the rate of 33.3 mg/kg/h (maximum dose 30 g/24 h)

CI: DIC and hematuria

Monitor: Activated clotting time (target 180–200 seconds) and serum potassium

S/E: Headache, diarrhea, hypotension, and arrhythmia

[Hamostat inj 500 mg amp, 5 g in 20 mL vial; Hemocid 5 g (20 mL) inj]

Ethanol

See under "Antidotes for ethylene, glycol and methanol poisoning".

Flumazenil

See under "Antidotes for benzodiazepines poisoning".

Flunarizine

Calcium Channel Blocker

- *Prophylaxis of migraine:*
    - *Children*: 5 mg/dose PO OD HS, increase dose to 10 mg OD HS SOS

S/E: Drowsiness, constipation, dry mouth, hypotension, flushing, and rarely extrapyramidal symptoms

(Migrid, Migazin, Migon, 5 mg, 10 mg tab)

Granulocyte Colony-stimulating Factor; (G-CSF) Filgrastim

Reduces duration of neutropenia (acts by stimulating production, maturation and activation of neutrophils):
- *Dose*: IV; S/C (refer to individual protocols)
    - *Neonates*: 5–10 µg/kg/day OD S/C × 3–5 days
    - *Children and adults*: 5–10 µg/kg/day q OD × for up to 14 days or until ANC becomes 10,000/mm^2. Discontinue when ANC over 10,000/mm^3 for 3 consecutive days.

S/E: Fever, bone pains, thrombocytopenia, and hematuria

(Neupogen inj 300 µg/vial)

Glucagon

- *As adjunct in hypoglycemia control IM/IV/SC:*
  - *Neonates, infants*: 0.025–0.3 mg/kg/dose q 30 min PRN (maximum 0.5 mg/dose)
  - *Children*: 0.03–0.1 mg/kg/dose q 20 minutes PRN (maximum 1 mg/dose)

S/E: Vomiting, urticaria, respiratory distress, and hypersensitivity reactions

- *As antidote:* See under "Antidotes for benzodiazepines poisoning"

[Glucagon (Torrent, Knoll, Novo Nordisk) 1 mg/mL vial]

Glycopyrrolate

Anticholinergic:
- *Control of upper airways secretion and hypersalivation:*
  - *Children*: PO 40–100 ug/kg/dose q TID/QID
  - *IM/IV*: 4–10 ug/kg/dose q 3–4 h
- *Preoperative:*
  - *IM*:
    - < 2 *years*: 4–9 µg/kg 30–60 minutes before procedure; may repeat 4 µg/kg in intervals of 2–3 minutes (maximum 0.1 mg/day)
    - > 2 *years*: 4 µg/kg 30–60 min before procedure; may repeat intraoperatively 4 µg/kg in intervals of 2–3 minutes (maximum 0.1 mg/day)

S/E: Tachycardia, orthostatic hypotension, headache, nervousness, xerostomia, constipation, urinary retention, and blurred vision

(*Glyco-P, Pyrolate, Vagolate 1 mL inj*)

Heparin Sodium

Anticoagulant:
- *Thrombosis:*
  - *Initial*: 50 IU/kg IV bolus, then continuous infusion at the rate of 15–25 IU/kg/h (or 75–125 IU/kg/dose IV q 4 h)

- Dose adjusted to maintain patient's APTT 1.5–2.5 times control. In case of overdosage, use protamine sulfate as antidote-1 mg per 100 IU heparin in previous 4 h
- *For catheter patency in peripheral vein*
  - Inject 1–2 mL of heparin 10 units/mL solution every 4 h

CI: Severe thrombocytopenia, intracranial hemorrhage, and bacterial endocarditis

[Heparin, Caprin, Declot 5,000 IU/5 mL, 25,000/5 mL; Heplock, cath flush 10 U/mL (2 mL amp) Lomorin inj 2,000, 4,000, 6,000, 8,000, 20,000 IU/mL amp]

Interferon Alfa-2A

Infants and children:
- Hemangiomas of infancy, pulmonary hemangiomatosis: 1–3 million units/m^2 q OD S/C
- *Philadelphia chromosome-positive chronic myeloid leukemia:* 2.5–5 million units/m^2 q OD SC/1M

S/E: Flu-like symptoms, tachycardia, arrhythmias, hypotension, depression, psychiatric symptoms, GIT disturbance, skin rash, and pancytopenia

(Zavinex, 3 mil i, u and 5 mil i, u inj; Alferon 3 mil i, u inj)

Ipecac Syrup

Emetic

To induce vomiting in some poisoning cases:
- < *6 months*: Not recommended
- *6–12 months*: 5–10 mL PO followed by 10–20 mL/kg or 120–240 mL of water
- *1–12 years*: 15 mL PO followed by 10–20 mL/kg or 120–240 mL of water
- > *12 years and adults*: 30 mL PO followed by 240 mL of water

Note: May repeat dose once if emesis does not occur within 30 minutes.

Precaution: Do not administer with carbonated beverage or milk

CI: Ingestion of kerosene oil, strong alkalies, or acids; unconscious patient and absent gag reflex

Ketotifen

- *For prophylaxis of bronchial asthma:*
  Children > 2 years: 1 mg/day/q OD PO; maximum 2 mg/day div q BID; not recommended below 2 years of age

S/E: Drowsiness, dry mouth, and dizziness

(Asthafen, Tritofen 1 mg tab, syr 5 mg/5 mL)

Lactase

Beta-D-galactosidase
Lactose intolerance:

Nolac-12 drops to be added to 0.5 L of milk 3 h before consumption.

Magnesium Sulfate

- *Severe hypomagnesemia (<1.2 mg/dL) or symptomatic hypomagnesemia:*
  - *Initial*: 0.1–0.2 mL of magnesium sulfate 50% (i.e. 50–100 mg)/kg IV slowly over 10 min or IM; repeat q 4–6 h until serum Mg level normalized or symptoms resolved. Maximum single dose 2 g (4 mL of 50% solution)
  - May give later doses PO (instead of IV/IM) 100–200 mg/kg/ dose q 6 h
  - *Maintenance*: 30–60 mg/kg/day or 0.25–0.4 mEq/kg/24 h (i.e. 0.06–0.12 mL/kg/day of 50% magnesium sulfate solution) added to 24 h maintenance IV infusion

Note: Magnesium sulfate 50% solution 1 mL contains—magnesium sulfate 500 mg = 4.0 mEq

- *Acute attack of asthma:* 25 mg/kg (maximum 2 g/dose) IV diluted in 30 mL N. saline/5% glucose infusion over 30 minutes

CI: Heart block, myocardial damage, severe renal impairment

Precaution: Renal insufficiency, and digoxin therapy

S/E: Hypotension, respiratory depression, hypermagnesemia, and diarrhea

Antidote: Calcium gluconate IV

Mannitol

Osmotic diuretic:
- *Cerebral edema*: 0.25–0.5 g/kg/dose IV over 20–30 minutes; may increase gradually to 1 g/kg/dose if needed. Avoid frequent use.
- *Anuria or oliguria:*
  - *Test dose*: 0.2 g/kg/dose IV over 3–5 minutes. No diuresis within 2 h suggests intrinsic renal dysfunction, discontinue mannitol. If response give 0.5–1 g/kg/dose followed by 0.25–0.5 g/kg/dose q 4–6 h IV

CI: Severe renal disease, pulmonary edema, high CVP, and active intracranial bleed

S/E: CHF, electrolyte imbalance, headache, seizures, and circulatory overload

[Mannitol 20% (Albert David, Mount Mettur, Parenteral Drugs)]

Meclizine

- *For motion sickness, prevention of vertigo:*
  Children over 12 years and adults:
  - *Motion Sickness*: 25–50 mg 1 h before travel PO: Repeat every 24 h PRN
  - *Vertigo*: PO 25–100 mg/day div q BID/QID

S/E: Hypotension, tachycardia, drowsiness, hallucinations, restlessness, urticaria, diplopia, tinnitus, bronchospasm, and hepatitis

(PNV tab 25 mg, Diligan 12.5 mg, Pregnidoxin 25 mg tab)

Mefenamic Acid

Nonsteroidal anti-inflammatory drug:
- Arthritis:
    - *Children*: 10–25 mg/kg/day div q 6 h PO
- *Pyrexia*: 3 mg/kg/dose PO PRN

CI: Peptic ulcer and porphyria

Caution: Avoid in children with seizures

S/E: Diarrhea, rashes (if so, withdraw treatment), thrombocytopenia, aplastic anemia, and hemolytic anemia

(Ponstan 250 mg, 500 mg tab, 50 mg/5 mL susp; Meftal 250, 500 mg tab; Meftal-P 100 mg tab, susp 100 mg/5 mL)

Metformin

Hypoglycemic agent:
- Type 2 diabetes:
    - ≥10–16 years:
    - *Initial*: 500 mg/dose q BID with meals, later 500 mg weekly increments as required. Maximum 2,000 mg/day

CI: Renal dysfunction (serum creatinine >1.5 mg/dL)

S/E: GIT disturbance (nausea, vomiting, and diarrhea)

(Bigomet, Xmat 250 mg, 500 mg, 850 mg tab, Glyciphage, Glumet 500 mg, 850 mg tab)

Methocarbamol

Skeletal muscle relaxant:
- *Supportive therapy in tetanus management:*
  IV: 15 mg/kg/dose (or 500 mg/m^2/dose); may repeat PRN q 6 h (for 3 days only)

S/E: Hypotension, dizziness, headache, and syncope

[Robinax 500 mg tab, inj 100 mg/mL (10 mL), Robiflam, Ibugesic-M (methocarbamol 750 mg + ibuprofen–200 mg); Ibugesic-M (methocarbamol 750 mg + ibuprofen–400 mg)]

Methylene Blue

See under "Antidote for methemoglobinemia".

Methylphenidate

- *For attention-deficit hyperactivity disorder (ADHD):*
  Children ≥6 yr:
  - *Initial*: 0.3 mg/kg/dose or 2.5 mg–5 mg/dose q BID empty stomach before breakfast and lunch or sustained release 5 mg tab OD PO
  - *Later*: Increase by 0.1 mg/kg/dose or 5–10 mg/day at weekly intervals (maximum 2 mg/kg/day or 60 mg/day)

CI: Glaucoma, motor tics, substance abuse disorder, use of MAO inhibitors within 14 days (may cause hypertensive crisis)

Caution: Long-term use may cause suppression of growth, avoid use in psychotic children; reduce dose to 40% if concurrent use with clonidine (fatality reported); and cautious use in patients with hypertension and seizures

S/E: Tachycardia, hypertension, hypotension, insomnia, drowsiness, dizziness, rash, growth retardation, GIT upset, and thrombocytopenia

(Addwize tab 10 mg, addwize OD 18 mg; inspiral OD tab 10 mg and 20 mg sustained release tab)

Naloxone

See under "Antidote for morphine and other narcotic poisoning".

Neostigmine or Prostigmine

Cholinergic agent (cholinesterase inhibitor):
- *Myasthenia gravis treatment:*
  Children:
  - *IV, IM, SC*: 0.01–0.04 mg/kg/dose q 2–3 h PRN
  - *PO*: 0.4 mg/kg/dose q 4–6 h PRN

Caution: Asthma

S/E: Excess dosage may cause cholinergic overactivity (bronchospasm, profuse tracheal secretion, diarrhea, bradycardia, and hypotension)

Antidote: Atropine 0.01 mg–0.04 mg/kg/dose

[Prostigmine, Tilstigmin 15 mg tab; 0.5 mg/mL inj (1 mL amp)]

Nortriptyline Hydrochloride

Tricyclic antidepressant:
- *Nocturnal enuresis:*
  - *6–11 years:* 10–20 mg once HS PO
  - *> 11 years:* 25–35 mg once HS, maximum 40 mg/day PO
- *Depression:*
  - 1–3 mg/kg/day once HS PO or div q TID/QID (maximum dose 150 mg/day)

CI: Cardiac disease and cardiac conduction abnormalities

S/E: Sedation, urinary retention, dry mouth, tachycardia, and constipation (anticholinergic effects)

(Primox, Sensival 25 mg tab)

Octreotide

Antisecretory antidiarrheal agent; somatostatin analog
Secretory diarrhea:

1–10 µg/kg/dose q 12 h IV/SC

Note: IV administration may be done either through infusion over 15–30 minutes (after dilution in NS or D_5W) or over 24 h as a continuous infusion; or in an emergency situation by direct IV push over 3 minutes.

S/E: Flushing, hypo/hyperglycemia, dizziness, and skin rashes

(Octride, Sandostatin 50 µg, 100 µg/1 mL inj.)

Pancuronium

Skeletal muscle relaxant:
- *Neonates and infants*: 0.1 mg/kg q 30–60 minutes SOS or as continuous infusion 0.02–0.04 mg/kg/hour

- *Children*: 0.15 mg/kg q 30-60 min SOS or as continuous infusion 0.03-0.1 mg/kg/hr
- *Adolescents and adults*: 0.15 mg/kg q 30-60 min SOS or as continuous infusion 0.02-0.04 mg/kg/hr

Caution: Ensure ventilatory support while drug is administered

S/E: Tachycardia, hypertension, excessive salivation, and bronchospasm

[Enemar, Ancomium, Pavulon 2 mg/mL (2 mL inj)]

Penicillamine

Metal chelating agent:
- Wilson disease: 20 mg/kg/day div q 6-12 h (maximum 1 g/day) PO
- *Arsenic poisoning:* 100 mg/kg/day div q 6 h; (maximum dose 1 g/day) PO × 5 days
- *Lead intoxication (3rd line drug):* 30-40 mg/kg/day div q 8 h (maximum 1.5 g/day) PO × 3-6 months until body lead burden is depleted
- *Rheumatoid arthritis:* 3 mg/kg/day div q 12 h PO. May increase by 3 mg/kg/day every 2 months. Maximum 10 mg/kg/day

S/E: Rash, fever, nausea, bone marrow suppression, nephrotic syndrome, and polymyositis

(Artin 150 mg, 250 mg tab, Cilamin 250 mg cap)

Phenazopyridine

Urinary anesthetic:
- *Children*: 12 mg/kg/day div q TID PO × 2 days
- *Adults*: 100-200 mg/dose q TID PO

S/E: Orange or red discoloration of urine, headache, vertigo, GI distress, methemoglobinemia, hemolytic anemia, and renal insufficiency

(Pyridium 200 mg tab)

Physostigmine

See under "Antidote for anticholinergic poisoning/toxicity"

Piracetam

- *Psychomotor retardation, learning problems, and psychomotor reactions:*
    - *Children*: 40 mg/kg/day div q 8 h PO; reduce dose to half once desired effect is obtained
    - *Adults*: 800 mg/dose q TID PO

S/E: Excitement and sleep disturbance

(Normabrain, Cetam 400 mg cap, 800 mg tab, syr 500 mg/5 mL, Alcetam 400 mg, 800 mg tab, inj 100 mg, 200 mg amp)

Potassium Chloride

- *Children*: 1–2 mEq/kg/day div q 8 h PO
    - *IV*: 1–2 mEq/kg/day by IV infusion (maximum 4 mEq/100 mL of IV solution). Potassium chloride inj (15%) provides 2 mEq of K^+ per mL

Caution: Do not administer until urine flow is established.

[Potklor, Keylyte, syr (20 mEq of elemental potassium per 15 mL) 200 mL; inj (2 mEq of elemental potassium per mL); 10 mL ampoules)]

Pralidoxime

See "Antidote for organophosphates poisoning".

Prochlorperazine

Phenothiazine Group
- *Vomiting:*
    - *Children > 10 kg*
        - *Oral, PR*: 0.4 mg/kg/day div TID/QID (maximum 30 mg/day)
        - *IM/IV*: 0.1–0.15 mg/kg/dose Q. 8–12 h (maximum 30 mg/day)
- *Intractable migraine headache*
    - *IV*: 0.15 mg/kg/dose; single dose

S/E: Extrapyramidal reactions, hypertension, drowsiness, cholestatic jaundice, blurred vision Diphenhydramine reverses dystonic reaction

[*Stemetil 5 mg, 25 mg tab; inj 12.5 mg/mL (1 mL, 10 mL); Emidoxyn 5 mg tab, inj 12.5 mg/mL (1 mL)*]

Promethazine Theoclate

- *Motion sickness and vomiting:*
  Initial dose: 0.5 mg/kg/dose 2–8 h before travel (maximum 25 mg/dose), then 0.25/kg/dose q 6–8 h PRN (maximum 1 mg/kg/day)

CI: Epilepsy

(*Avomine 25 mg tab; Promet 10 mg, 25 mg tab, inj 25 mg/mL; Apizine 5 mg/5 mL*)

Prostaglandin-E1

- *Maintenance of patent ductus in ductus dependent congenital heart disease:*
  - *Initial*: 0.05–0.1 µg/kg/min continuous IV infusion. Titrate dose as per infant's response; after response reduce to lowest effective dose
  - *Usual maintenance dose*: 0.01–0.4 µg/kg/min

Note: Infuse through a large vein or umbilical artery catheter placed near ductus arteriosus opening

CI: Coagulation abnormalities

S/E: Apnea, bradycardia, hypotension, cardiac arrest, bleeding, and seizures

[*Inj Alpostin, Prostin VR 500 µg (1 mL inj)*]

Protamine Sulfate

See "Antidote for heparin poisoning".

Pseudoephedrine

- *Sympathomimetic nasal decongestant:*
  Children: 4 mg/kg/day div q BID-QID PO
  Adults: 60 mg/dose q TID-QID; maximum 240 mg/day

Caution: Cautious use in cardiac disease, hypertension, and hyperthyroidism

S/E: Nervousness, insomnia, tachycardia, and headache

[Sudafed 60 mg tab, 30 mg/5 mL susp; Sinarest AF tab (pseudoephedrine HCl 60 mg, chlorpheniramine maleate 2 mg, caffeine 30 mg); susp (pseudoephedrine HCl 30 mg, CPM 2 mg 5 mL) and drops (pseudoephedrine HCl 15 mg, CPM 1 mg per mL); Recofast tab (pseudoephedrine 60 mg, triprolidine 2.5 mg); susp (pseudoephedrine 15 mg, triprolidine 0.625 mg per 5 mL)]

Pyridostigmine

Cholinesterase inhibitor
- *Myasthenia gravis:*
  PO: 7 mg/kg/day div q 5–6 doses
  IM/IV: 0.05–0.15 mg/kg/dose (maximum 10 mg) q 4–6 h

Caution: In patients with asthma, cardiac dysfunction, epilepsy, and peptic ulcer

S/E: Bradycardia, diarrhea, headache, muscle cramps, and excessive secretions

(Distinon, Mustone, Myestin 10 mg tab)

Pyritinol

- *Infants*: 50–100 mg/dose q OD-TID
- *Children*: 100–200 mg/dose q BID
- *Adults*: 100–200 mg/dose q TID

(Encephabol 100 mg, 200 mg tab, 100 mg/5 mL susp, 200 mg infusion)

Sodium Bicarbonate

- *Severe acidosis in acute renal failure* (when arterial pH <7.15; serum bicarbonate < 8 mEq/L)
  – Administer IV sodium bicarbonate as per following correction formula: mEq NaHCO$_3$ (or mL of 7.5%

solution of sodium bicarbonate) = 0.3 × weight (kg) × 12-patient's serum bicarbonate (mEq/L)
- *Aim of therapy*: To raise arterial pH to 7.20 (approximately serum $NaHCO_3$ level 12 mEq/L). Correction of remainder of acidosis to be done later by oral administration of $NaHCO_3$ tablets or sodium citrate solution
- *Severe cyanotic spells in TOF unresponsive to initial management* (for correction of metabolic acidosis): 1 mEq/kg IV
- *Cardiac arrest*
  - After establishment of effective ventilation
    □ *Initial dose*: 1 mEq/kg/dose (1 mL of 7.5% $NaHCO_3$ solution = 0.9 mEq bicarbonate). Administer at the rate of less than 1 mEq/min. May repeat half dose after 10 minutes PRN (In neonates, dilute 7.5% $NaHCO_3$ solution 1:1 with distilled water before administration)
- *Correction of hyperkalemia* (as adjunct to other measures): 1-2 mEq/kg IV slowly over 10-20 minutes for induction of metabolic alkalosis (moves K^+ into cells)

CI: Alkalosis, hypocalcemia, and inadequate ventilation

Warning: Do not mix with calcium gluconate, atropine, or catecholamines (dopamine and epinephrine)

Caution: Too rapid correction of acidosis by IV sodium bicarbonate can cause tetany, hypokalemia, and cerebral hemorrhage

Note: Inj sodium bicarbonate 7.5% solution provides 0.9 mEq bicarbonate per mL

[Sodium bicarbonate inj 7.5%, inj (2.5 mL)]

Sodium Polystyrene Sulfonate

- *Potassium removing resin:*
  Children: PO 4 g/kg/day div q 6 h; PR 4-12 g/kg/day div q 2-6 h as rectal enema in 20-30% sorbitol

Precaution: Do not give orally with antacids containing Mg or Al

Succinylcholine

- *Neuromuscular blocking agent:*
  Children
  Initial dose:
  IV: 1–2 mg/kg

Maintenance: 0.3–0.6 mg/kg IV every 5–10 minutes as needed

Caution: In patients with major trauma, hyperkalemia, renal and hepatic failure, elevated ICP

(Scoline, Midarine 100 mg per 2 mL inj, Entubate 100 mg/2 mL and 500 mg/10 mL inj)

Sulfasalazine

Anti-inflammatory agent
- *Ulcerative colitis:*
  Children > 2 years:
  - *Initial*: 40–75 mg/kg/day PO div q 4–6 h (maximum 6 g/day)
  - *Maintenance*: 30–50 mg/kg/day PO div q 6–8 h (maximum 2 g/day)

S/E: Rash, headache, dizziness, blood dyscrasias, GIT upset, and nephrotoxicity.

(Salazopyrin 500 mg tab)

Surfactant Pulmonary

- *For rescue therapy of RDS in neonate*

In preference to earlier first generation artificial surfactants, natural surfactants derived from animal sources are now recommended for administration through endotracheal tube for early rescue therapy in RDS cases in neonates. The surfactant preparations now available in India and their dosages are indicated below:

1. Bovine mixed (Survanta, by Abbott): Dosage 4 mL/kg (100 mg/kg);

Interval between dosages—6 hr
Maximum doses—2
2. Bovine lavage (Neosurf, Cipla) Dose 5 mL/kg (135 mg/kg)
   Interval—12 hours
   Maximum doses—3
3. Porcine mixed (Curosurf, Abbott) Dose 1.25 mL – 2.5 mL/kg (100–200 mg/kg)
   Interval—12 hr
   Maximum doses—2

Monitoring: Due to improved lung performance within minutes after administration of lung surfactants, there is danger of overventilation, pneumothorax and oxygen toxicity. As such, close watch should be kept on pulse oximetry and $PaCO_2$. Volume—targeted ventilation is better than pressure-targeted ventilation

(*Survanta by Abbott, Neosurf by Cipla, Curosurf by Abbott, Nicholas*)

Thiopental Sodium

Pentothal:
- *Cerebral* edema: 1.5–5 mg/kg/dose IV, repeat PRN
- *Status epilepticus:*
  - *IV loading dose*: 5–10 mg/kg over 5 minutes followed by 2–10 mg/kg/h continuous infusion for uncontrolled status epilepticus. Patient will need mechanical ventilation.
- *Anesthesia induction:* 5–8 mg/kg IV

Tranexamic Acid (Antifibrinolytic Agent)

- *For pre and post-tooth extraction in hemophilics:*
  - *Children and adults*: 10 mg/kg immediately before surgery IV; then PO 25 mg/kg/dose q TID/QID × 2–8 days.

Caution: Reduce dose in renal impairment

S/E: Hypotension, thromboembolic complications (deep vein thrombosis, pulmonary embolism, acute cortical necrosis), GIT upset, thrombocytopenia, and visual abnormalities.

(*Cyclocapron, Dubatran, TX 500 mg tab, 500 mg/5 mL amp*)

Ursodiol and Ursodeoxycholic Acid

Ursodiol:
- *Biliary atresia*: 10–15 mg/kg/day q OD PO
- *Cystic fibrosis*: 30 mg/kg/day div q OD/BID PO
- *Cholestasis*: 30 mg/kg/day div q BID/TID PO

S/E: Diarrhea, biliary pain, rash, and headache

Note: Drug generally ineffective in dissolving cholesterol gallstones in children

(Urso, Udca tab 150 mg)

Vasopressin

- *Variceal hemorrhage due to portal hypertension:*
    - *Initial*: 0.33 units/kg diluted in 25 mL of 5% dextrose by IV bolus over 20 minutes and then continued infusion 0.33 U/kg/h or 0.2 units/1.73 m^2/min PRN
      Caution: IV infusion dose should be tapered slowly
- *Catecholamine refractory shock:* 0.3–2 units/kg/min
- *Diabetes insipidus:*
    - IM/SC: 2.5–10 U/dose q BID–QID as per response

S/E: Tremor, vertigo, anaphylaxis, hypertension, seizures, and cardiac arrhythmia

Caution: IV infusion dose should be tapered slowly
[Vasopin, Petresin inj 20 IU/mL (1 mL amp)]

Warfarin

Anticoagulant:
- *Initial*: 0.1–0.3 mg/kg/dose PO (maximum 10 mg) on day 1, then
- *Maintenance*: 0.1 mg/kg/day (usual); titrate according to prothrombin time (range 0.05–0.34 mg/kg/day); target prothrombin time—2–3 INR

CI: Severe liver or kidney disease, GI ulcers

S/E: Bleeding, hemoptysis, fever, skin necrosis, and GI upset

(Warf, Uniwarfin 1 mg, 2 mg, 5 mg tab)

34. Dosage of Antimicrobial Agents in Neonates

ANTIMICROBIAL AGENTS IN NEONATES (TABLES 34.1 AND 34.2)

Table 34.1: Dosages of antimicrobial agents in neonates in mg/kg or units/kg per 24 hours.

Weight	<1,200 g	1,200–2,000 g	1,200–2,000 g	>2,000 g	>2,000 g
Age	0–4 weeks	0–7 days	>7 days	0–7 days	>7 days
Ampicillin IV, meningitis	100 div q 12 h	100 div q 12 h	150 div q 8 h	150 div q 8 h	200 div q 6 h
Other infections IV, IM	50 div q 12 h	50 div q 12 h	75 div q 8 h	75 div q 8 h	100 div q 6 h
Aztreonam IV, IM	60 div q 12 h	60 div q 12 h	90 div q 8 h	90 div q 8 h	120 div q 6 h
Cefazolin IV, IM	40 div q 12 h	40 div q 12 h	40 div q 12 h	40 div q 12 h	60 div q 8 h
Cefotaxime IV, IM	100 div q 12 h	100 div q 12 h	150 div q 8 h	150 div q 8 h	150 div q 8 h
Ceftazidime IV, IM	100 div q 12 h	100 div q 12 h	150 div q 8 h	150 div q 8 h	150 div q 8 h
Ceftriaxone IV, IM	50 div q 24 h	50 div q 24 h	50 div q 24 h	50 div q 24 h	75 div q 24 h
Cephalothin IV	40 div q 12 h	40 div q 12 h	60 div q 8 h	60 div q 8 h	80 div q 6 h

Contd...

Contd...

Weight	<1,200 g	1,200–2,000 g	1,200–2,000 g	>2,000 g	>2,000 g
Age	0–4 weeks	0–7 days	>7 days	0–7 days	>7 days
Chloramphenicol IV, PO	25 div q 24 h	25 div q 24 h	25 div q 24 h	25 div q 24 h	50 div q 12 h
Clindamycin IV, IM, PO	10 div q 12 h	10 div q 12 h	15 div q 8 h	15 div q 8 h	20 div q 6 h
Erythromycin PO	20 div q 12 h	20 div q 12 h	30 div q 8 h	20 div q 12 h	30 div q 8 h
Methicillin IV, IM meningitis	100 div q 12 h	100 div q 12 h	150 div q 8 h	150 div q 8 h	200 div q 6 h
Other diseases	50 div q 12 h	50 div q 12 h	75 div q 8 h	75 div q 8 h	100 div q 6 h
Nafcillin IV	50 div q 12 h	50 div q 12 h	75 div q 8 h	75 div q 8 h	100 div q 6 h
Oxacillin IV, IM	50 div q 12 h	50 div q 12 h	75 div q 8 h	75 div q 8 h	100 div q 6 h
Penicillin G IV meningitis	100,000 U div q 12 h	100,000 U div q 12 h	150,000 U div q 8 h	150,000 U div q 8 h	200,000 U div q 6 h
Other infections	50,000 U div q 12 h	50,000 U div q 12 h	75,000 U div q 8 h	75,000 U div q 8 h	100,000 U div q 6 h
Penicillin G					
Benzathine IM	–	50,000 U (one dose)	50,000 U (one dose)	50,000 U (one dose)	50,000 U (one dose)
Procaine IM	–	50,000 U q 24 h	50,000 U q 24 h	50,000 U q 24 h	50,000 U q 24 h
Ticarcillin IV, IM	150 div q 12 h	150 div q 12 h	225 div q 8 h	225 div q 8 h	300 div q 6 h
Vancomycin IV	15 div q 24 h	15 div q 12–18 h	15 div q 8–12 h	30 div q 12 h	45 div q 8 h

(IM: intramuscular; IV: intravenous)

Table 34.2: Dosages of antimicrobial agents in neonates in mg/kg or units/kg per dose.

Weight	<1,200 g	1,200–2,000 g	1,200–2,000 g	>2,000 g	>2,000 g
Age	0–4 weeks	0–7 days	>7 days	0–7 days	>7 days
Amikacin IV, IM	7.5 q 18–24 h	7.5 q 12–18 h	7.5 q 8–12 h	10 q 12 h	10 q 8 h
Gentamicin IV, IM	2.5 q 18–24 h	2.5 q 12–18 h	2.5 q 8 h	2.5 q 12 h	2.5 q 8 h
Imipenem IV, IM	20 q 18–24 h	20 q 12 h	20 q 12 h	20 q 12 h	20 q 8 h
Kanamycin IV, IM	7.5 q 18–24 h	7.5 q 12–18 h	7.5 q 8–12 h	10 q 12 h	10 q 8 h
Meropenem IV, IM	– –	20 q 12 h	20 q 12 h	20 q 12 h	20 q 8 h
Metronidazole IV, PO	7.5 q 48 h	7.5 q 24 h	7.5 q 12 h	7.5 q 12 h	15 q 12 h
Netilmicin IV, IM	2.5 q 18 h	2.5 q 12–18 h	2.5 q 8–12 h	2.5 q 12 h	2.5 q 8 h
Tobramycin IV, IM	2.5 q 18–24 h	2.5 q 12–18 h	2.5 q 8–12 h	2.5 q 12 h	2.5 q 8 h

(IM: intramuscular; IV: intravenous)

35 Drugs in Renal Failure

INTRODUCTION

Drugs primarily eliminated from the body through the kidney and the potentially nephrotoxic drugs, need careful modification in dosing pattern in patients with renal insufficiency, so as to prevent toxicity while maintaining their adequate therapeutic levels.

This is achieved by either:
- Extension of interval (I) between individual doses while keeping the dosage quantity normal or
- Reduction of dose (D) wherein the amount of dose is reduced, keeping the interval between the doses normal
- In some cases (DI method), the dose needs to be reduced along with the extension of interval.

In Table 35.1, D and I listed separately indicate that either the dose or interval modification method can be employed. DI indicates that both dose and interval adjustments need to be made for that particular drug.

Table 35.1: Dose and intervals of drug in renal failure.					
Drug	Normal dose interval	Method interval: I* dose: D**	Adjustment for renal failure GFR (mL/min)		
			>50	10–50	<10
Aminoglycosides					
Amikacin	8–12 h	D	60–90	30–70	20–30
		I	8–12	12–18	24–48

Contd...

Contd...

Drug	Normal dose interval	Method interval: I* dose: D**	Adjustment for renal failure GFR (mL/min)		
			>50	10–50	<10
Gentamicin	8–12 h	D	60–90	30–70	20–30
		I	8–12	12–18	24–48
Kanamycin	8 h	D	60–90	30–70	20–30
		I	8–12	12	24
Tobramycin	8–12 h	D	60–90	30–70	20–30
		I	8–12	12–18	24–48
Cephalosporins					
Cefazolin	8 h	I	8	12	24–48
Cefotaxime	6–12 h	I	8	12	24
Cefoxitin	8 h	I	8	12	24
Cefuroxime	8–12 h	I	8–12	12	24
Cephalothin	4–6 h	I	4–6	8	8–12
Ceftriaxone	8–12 h	D	100	100	100
Ceftazidime	8–12 h	D	50–75	50	25
		I	12	24	48
Penicillins					
Ampicillin	6 h	I	6	6–12	12–16
Carbenicillin	6 h	I	8–12	12–24	24–48
Methicillin	4–6 h	I	4	4–8	8–12
Nafcillin	6 h	D	100	100	100
Penicillin G	4–6 h	I	6–8	8–12	12–16
Piperacillin	4–6 h	I	4–6	6–8	8
Ticarcillin	6 h	I	6	8–12	12
Piperacillin-tazobactam	6 h	I	6	8	12
Ticarcillin-clavulanate	6 h	I	6	8	12

Contd...

Contd...

Drug	Normal dose interval	Method interval: I* dose: D**	Adjustment for renal failure GFR (mL/min)		
			>50	10–50	<10
Other Antibacterial Agents					
Chloramphenicol	6 h	D	100	100	100
Ciprofloxacin	12 h	D	100	50–75	30–50
Clindamycin	6–8 h	D	100	100	100
Imipenem	6–8 h	DI	75–100 q 8	50 q 8	25 q 8
Metronidazole	6 h	D	100	100	50
Trimethoprim–sulfamethoxazole	6–12 h	D	100	50	Avoid
Vancomycin	6–12 h	I	6–12	24–48	48–96
Antituberculous agents					
Ethambutol	24 h	I	24	36	48
Isoniazid	24 h	D	100	100	50–100
Pyrazinamide	24 h	D	100	100	50
Rifampin	24 h	D	100	100	25–50
Antifungal					
Amphotericin B	24 h	I	24	24	24–36
Ketoconazole	24 h	D	100	100	100
Itraconazole	OD-BD	D	100	100	100
Fluconazole	24 h	I	24	24–48	48–72
		D	100	25–50	25
Antivirals					
Acyclovir	Variable	I	8	12–24	24
		D	25–50	25–50	25–50
Non-narcotic drugs					
Acetaminophen	4 h	I	4	6	8
Narcotics					
Codeine	4–12 h	D	100	75	75

Contd...

Contd...

Drug	Normal dose interval	Method interval: I* dose: D**	Adjustment for renal failure GFR (mL/min)		
			>50	10–50	<10
Fentanyl	30 min–1 h	D	100	75	50
Meperidine	4 h	D	100	75	50–75
Morphine	Variable	D	100	75	50–75
Anticonvulsants					
Carbamazepine		D	100	100	75
Phenobarbital	8–12 h	I	8–12	8–12	12–16
Diazepam	Variable	D	100	100	100
Lorazepam	Variable	D	100	100	75
Midazolam	Variable	D	100	100	50
Gabapentin	TID	I	TID	BID-OD	q OD
Antihypertensives					
Methyldopa	6–12 h	I	6	9–18	12–24
Propranolol	6–12 h	D	100	100	100
Captopril	6–24 h	D	100	75–100	50
Enalapril	Variable	D	100	50	25
Hydralazine	6–12 h	I	8	8–12	8–16
Nitroprusside	Variable	D	100	100	100
Diltiazem	TID-QID	D	100	100	100
Nifedipine	Variable	D	100	100	75
Verapamil	Variable	D	100	100	100
Atenolol	q OD	D	100	50	25
Cardiac glycosides					
Digoxin	q 24 h	D	100	25–75	10–25
Diuretics					
Acetazolamide	6–24 h	I	6–8	12	Avoid
Furosemide	Variable	D	100	100	100
Spironolactone	6–12 h	I	6–12	12–24	Avoid

Contd...

Contd...

Drug	Normal dose interval	Method interval: I* dose: D**	Adjustment for renal failure GFR (mL/min)		
			>50	10–50	<10
Triamterene	12–24 h	I	12	12	Avoid
Antiarrhythmic agents					
Bretylium	q 1 min –8 h	D	100	25–50	Avoid
Lidocaine	Variable	D	100	100	100
Procainamide	4–6 h	I	4–6	6–12	8–24
Quinidine	Variable	I	100	100	100
Phenytoin	Variable	D	100	100	100
Flecainide	8–12 h	D	100	50	25
Other drugs					
Chloroquine	q 6 h–7 d	D	100	100	50
Cimetidine	6–12 h	D	100	75	50
Insulin (regular)	Variable	D	100	75	25–50
Metoclopramide	6–8 h	D	100	50–75	25–50
Midazolam	Variable	D	100	100	50
Ranitidine	8–12 h	D	100	75	50

*I: Interval adjustment in hours between dose administration.
**D: Dose adjustment in percentage of usual dose

Appendices

Appendix 1

AGENTS WHICH MAY CAUSE HEMOLYSIS IN G-6-PD DEFICIENT CASES

Analgesics

Aspirin
Antipyrine
Phenacetin

Antibacterials

Sulfonamides
Trimethoprim-sulfamethoxazole
Nitrofurantoin
Nalidixic acid
Furazolidone
Chloramphenicol (in large doses)
Para-amino salicylic acid (PAS)

Antimalarials

Primaquine
Pamaquine
Chloroquine
Quinacrine
Quinine

Other Agents

Vitamin K analogs (water soluble)
Methylene blue
Napthalene
Benzene

Fava beans
Probenecid
Phenazopyridine

Diseases

Hepatitis
Diabetic acidosis

Appendix 2

COMMON DRUGS WHICH MAY PRECIPITATE/AGGRAVATE ACUTE PORPHYRIAS

Barbiturates
Chloramphenicol
Chloroquine
Imipramine
Meprobamate
Pentazocine
Primidone
Estrogens
Oral contraceptives
Sulfonamides
Theophylline
Valproic acid (and others)

Appendix 3

HEMATOLOGIC ADVERSE EFFECTS OF DRUGS

Drug	Red Cell Aplasia	Thrombo-cytopenia	Neutro-penia	Pancy-topenia	Hemo-lysis
Acetazolamide		+	+	+	
Allopurinol			+		
Amiodarone	+				
Amphotericin B				+	
Amrinone		++			
Asparaginase		+++	+++	+++	++
Barbiturates		+		+	
Benzocaine					++
Captopril			++		+
Carbamazepine		++	+		
Cephalosporins			+		++
Chloramphenicol		+	++	+++	
Chlordiazepoxide			+	+	
Chloroquine		+			
Chlorothiazides		++			
Chlorpropamide	+	++	+	++	+
Chlortetracycline				+	
Chlorthalidone			+		
Cimetidine		+	++	+	
Codeine		+			
Cyclophosphamide		+++	+++	+++	+
Dapsone					+++
Digitalis		+			

Contd...

Contd...

Drug	Red Cell Aplasia	Thrombocytopenia	Neutropenia	Pancytopenia	Hemolysis
Digitoxin		++			
Erythromycin		+			
Ethacrynic acid			+		
Furosemide		+	+		
Gold salts	+	+++	+++	+++	
Heparin		++		+	
Ibuprofen			+		+
Imipramine			++		
Indomethacin		+	++	+	
Isoniazid		+		+	
Meperidine		+			
Methimazole			++		
Methyldopa		++			+++
Methotrexate		+++	+++	+++	++
Methylene blue					+
Metronidazole			+		
Nalidixic acid					+
Naproxen				+	
Nitrofurantoin			++		+
Penicillamine		++	+		
Penicillins		+	++	+	+++
Phenazopyridine					+++
Phenothiazines		+	++	+++	+

Appendix 4

FEVER DUE TO DRUGS

Most Common		
Atropine	Cephalosporins	Procainamide
Amphotericin B	Interferon	Quinidine
Asparaginase	Methyldopa	Salicylates (high doses)
Barbiturates	Penicillins	Streptomycin
Bleomycin	Phenytoin	Sulfonamides
Less Common		
Allopurinol	Hydralazine	Nitrofurantoin
Antihistamines	Hydroxyurea	Pentazocine
Azathioprine	Imipenem	Procarbazine
Carbamazepine	Iodides	Propylthiouracil
Cimetidine	Isoniazid	Rifampin
Cisplatin	Mercaptopurine	Streptokinase
Colistimethate	Metoclopramide	Triamterene
Diazoxide	Nifedipine	Vancomycin
Folic acid	NSAIDs	

BIBLIOGRAPHY

1. Cunha BA. Antibiotic side effects. Med Clin North Am. 2001:85(1):149-85.
2. Mackowiak PA, LeMaistre CF. Drug fever: a critical appraisal of conventional concepts. An analysis of 51 episodes in two Dallas Hospitals and 97 episodes reported in the english literature, Ann Intern Med. 1987:106(5):728-33.
3. Tabor PA. Drug-induced fever. Table 2, Drugs implicated in causing a fever, Drug Intell Clin Pharm. 1986:20(6):416.

Appendix 5

DISCOLORATION OF STOOLS DUE TO DRUGS

Black
Acetazolamide
Alcohols
Alkalies
Aluminum hydroxide
Aminophylline
Aminosalicylic acid
Amphetamine
Amphotericin
Antacids
Anticoagulants
Aspirin
Betamethasone
Bismuth
Charcoal
Chloramphenicol
Chlorpropamide
Clindamycin
Corticosteroids
Cortisone
Cyclophosphamide
Cytarabine
Dicumarol
Digitalis
Ethacrynic acid
Ferrous salts
Floxuridine
Fluorides
Fluorouracil
Halothane
Heparin
Hydralazine
Hydrocortisone
Ibuprofen
Indomethacin
Iodine drugs
Iron salts
Levarterenol
Levodopa
Manganese
Melphalan
Methylprednisolone
Methotrexate
Methylene blue
Oxyphenbutazone
Paraldehyde
Phenacetin
Phenolphthalein
Phenylbutazone
Phenylephrine
Phosphorous
Potassium salts
Prednisolone
Procarbazine
Pyrvinium
Reserpine
Salicylates
Sulfonamides
Tetracycline
Theophylline
Thiotepa
Triamcinolone
Warfarin
Red
Anticoagulants
Aspirin
Heparin
Oxyphenbutazone
Phenolphthalein
Phenylbutazone
Pyrvinium
Salicylates
Tetracycline syrup
Pink
Anticoagulants
Aspirin
Heparin
Oxyphenbutazone
Phenylbutazone
Salicylates
Red-Brown
Oxyphenbutazone
Phenylbutazone
Rifampin

Contd...

Contd...

Tarry	Rifampin	Oxyphenbutazone
Ergot preparations	**Blue**	Phenylbutazone
Ibuprofen	Chloramphenicol	**White/Speckling**
Salicylates	Methylene blue	Aluminum
Warfarin	**Green**	hydroxide
Light Brown	Indomethacin	Antibiotics (oral)
Anticoagulants	Iron	**Yellow**
Dark Brown	Medroxyprogesterone	Senna
Dexamethasone	**Greenish Gray**	**Yellow-Green**
Orange-Red	Oral antibiotics	Senna
Phenazopyridine		

Adapted from: Drugdex® — Drug Consults, Micromedex, Vol 62, Denver, CO: Rocky Mountain Drug Consultation Center, 1998.

Note: A drug may cause different types of discoloration. For example, use of anticoagulants may result in change of stools color to black, tarry, red, pink or light brown.

Appendix 6

ANTIMICROBIALS AND OTHER AGENTS IN HEPATIC DISEASE

In the presence of hepatic disease, dosage adjustment may be indicated for several drugs which are chiefly excreted/metabolized by the liver.

A list of some of these drugs is given below

A. Antibacterials:
   - Cefoperazone
   - Ceftriaxone
   - Chloramphenicol
   - Clindamycin
   - Indinavir
   - Isoniazid
   - Metronidazole
   - Nafcillin
   - Nevirapine
   - Rifabutin
   - Rifampin
   - Rimantadine
   - Trovafloxacin
   - Voriconazole

B. Other drugs:
   - Morphine (reduce dose or avoid)
   - Pentobarbitone (reduce dose or avoid)
   - Lidocaine (reduce dose or avoid)
   - Propranolol (reduce dose or avoid)

C. Use of lorazepam is preferable in place of diazepam on account of its shorter t½

D. Prednisone is less effective in hepatic disease as it needs hepatic metabolism for activation

E. Hepatotoxic drugs should be avoided in liver disease

Note: While prescribing the above named drugs in hepatic disease, drug literature should be carefully consulted.

Appendix 7

IMPORTANT INTERACTIONS BETWEEN ANTIBIOTICS AND OTHER DRUGS

Antibiotic	Interacting drug	Effect
AMINOGLYOSIDES (amikacin, gentamicin, kanamycin, netilmicin, streptomycin, tobramycin, capreomycin)	Amphotericin B Cyclosporine, Vancomycin Loop diuretics (Furosemide, bumetanide, ethacrynic acid) NSAIDs Neuromuscular blocking agents	↑ nephrotoxicity ↑ nephrotoxicity ↑ nephrotoxicity ↑ ototoxicity ↑ nephrotoxicity ↑ apnea or respiratory paralysis
AMPHOTERICIN B	Aminoglycosides Digitalis	↑ nephrotoxicity ↑ digitalis toxicity
AMPICILLIN, AMOXICILLIN	Allopurinol	↑ frequency of rash
CEPHALOSPORINS	Furosemide Ethacrynic acid	↑ nephrotoxicity
CHLORAMPHENICOL	Phenytoin Rifampin	↑ toxicity of phenytoin ↓ chloramphenicol effect
CIPROFLOXACIN (and most other quinolones)	Antacids, sucralfate, iron, diadenosine Theophylline, cyclosporine, warfarin NSAIDs	↓ ciprofloxacin (and other quinolones) absorption ↑ effect of theophylline, cyclosporine, and Warfarin ↑ risk of CNS stimulation seizures

Contd...

Contd...

Antibiotic	Interacting drug	Effect
CLINDAMYCIN	Erythromycin	Mutual antagonism
ERYTHROMYCIN, CLARITHROMYCIN	Carbamazepine	↑ serum levels of carbamazepine (nystagmus, ataxia, vomiting, better AVOID THIS COMBINATION)
	Cisapride, astemizole	↑ risk of cardiac arrhythmias
	Theophylline	↑ level of theophylline and its toxicity (vomiting, seizures, apnea)
	Digoxin, phenytoin, valproic acid, warfarin, protease inhibitors	↑ serum level of digoxin and others
ISONIAZID	Carbamazepine, phenytoin Rifampin	↑ levels and toxicity of carbamazepine and phenytoin ↑ hepatotoxicity
LINEZOLID	Adrenergic agents	Risk of hypertension
MEFLOQUINE	Valproic acid Halofantrine Quinine, β-adrenergic blockers, calcium channel blockers	↓ level of valproic acid (seizures may develop) QT prolonged (avoid) ↑ arrhythmias
MEROPENEM	Valproic acid	↓ level of valproic acid (to sub-therapeutic level in some cases)
METRONIDAZOLE	Anticoagulants Phenobarbitone, hydantoins	↑ anticoagulant effect ↓ effect of metronidazole
NALIDIXIC ACID	Oral anticoagulants	↑ anticoagulant effect

Contd...

Contd...

Antibiotic	Interacting drug	Effect
PIPERAZINE	Chlorpromazine	Convulsions (can be life-threatening)
QUININE	Digoxin	↑ digoxin levels and toxicity
	Mefloquine	↑ arrhythmias
SULFONAMIDES	Phenytoin, oral anticoagulants, sulfonylureas	↑ levels of phenytoin and others, toxicity
	Phenobarbitone, rifampin, cyclosporine	↑ levels of phenobarbitone and others
TETRACYCLINES	Antacids, iron, sucralfate	↓ tetracycline effect
	Digoxin	↑ toxicity of digoxin (may persist for several months in about 10% patients)

Appendix 8

A. MATERNAL DRUGS CONTRAINDICATED DURING BREASTFEEDING

Drug	Possible adverse effect on breastfed infant
Amphetamines	Significant amount secreted in milk may affect infant
Azathioprine	Immunosuppression
Anticancer agents	Anemia, immunosuppression, diarrhea
Bromocriptine	Reduces lactation
Chloramphenicol	Diarrhea, bone marrow suppression
Cyclosporine	Immunosuppression
Ergot compounds	Ergotism, may suppress lactation
Gold salts	Rashes and other reactions
Immunosuppressants	Immunosuppression in infants
Iodine/Iodides	Hypothyroidism, goiter
Lithium	Cardiac arrhythmias, intoxication
Metformin	Hypoglycemia, lactic acidosis
Methimazole	Hypothyroidism
Oral contraceptives	Avoid until 6 months after birth, estrogens may cause gynecomastia in male infant
Tetracycline	Tooth discoloration, growth retardation
Radioactive iodine	After diagnostic dose do not give breast-feeding for 24 hr and for long period after therapeutic dose

The maternal use of following drugs is also contraindicated during breastfeeding on account of possible adverse effects on the suckling infant:
- Cimetidine
- Clemastine
- Cocaine

- Diethylstilbestrol
- Doxorubicin
- Meprobamate
- Phencyclidine
- Phenindione

B. MATERNAL DRUGS TO BE AVOIDED OR USED WITH GREAT CAUTION DURING BREAST-FEEDING

Drug	Possible adverse effect on infant
Amiodarone	Hypothyroidism
Anthraquinones (senna, etc.)	Diarrhea
Aspirin	Avoid high dose, bleeding, Reye's syndrome
Calciferol	Avoid high doses, risk of hypervitaminosis
Estrogens	Gynecomastia in male infants
Metoclopramide	Diarrhea, dystonia
Metronidazole	Suspend breastfeeding for 12 hr after single dose as it is secreted in large amount in breast milk
Narcotics (morphine, etc.)	May cause lethargy; withdrawal symptoms in infants of dependent mothers
Phenobarbitone (and other sedatives)	Sedation

Appendix 9

MATERNAL USE DRUGS AND OTHER AGENTS HARMFUL FOR FETUS AND NEWBORN

Drug	Possible adverse effect on fetus and newborn
Antibiotics	
Streptomycin	Deafness
Tetracycline	Teeth pigmentation, enamel hypoplasia, cataract, skeletal growth retardation
Anti-cancer drugs	
Busulfan	Stunted growth, corneal opacities, hypoplasia of thyroid and ovaries
Cyclophosphamide	Multiple malformations
Mercaptopurine	Abortion
Azathioprine	Abortion
Anticonvulsants	
Carbamazepine	Spina bifida
Phenytoin	Congenital anomalies, IUGR, bleeding (due to vitamin K deficiency)
Valproate	Spina bifida, impaired neurologic function
Antimalarials	
Chloroquine	Deafness
Quinine	Abortion, thrombocytopenia, deafness
Hormones	
Danazol (androgens)	Virilization
Methyltestosterone	Masculinization of female fetus
Norethindrone	Masculinization of female fetus
Progestrone	Masculinization of female fetus
Progestoral	Masculinization of female fetus

Contd...

Contd...

Drug	Possible adverse effect on fetus and newborn
Stilbestrol	Vaginal adenocarcinoma in adolescence
Miscellaneous agents and drugs	
Alcohol	Congenital cardiac, CNS, limb anomalies, developmental delay, attention deficits, autism
Amphetamines	Congenital heart disease, IUGR
Cocaine	Microcephaly, IUGR, behavior disturbances
Cigarette smoking	Small for gestational age
Lithium	Macrosomia, Ebstein's anomaly
Thalidomide	Phocomelia, other malformations
Vitamin D	Aortic stenosis (supravalvular), hypercalcemia

Appendix 10

THERAPEUTIC AND TOXIC RANGE OF SERUM DRUG LEVELS

Drug	Serum therapeutic level	Serum toxic level	Desired duration of therapy before serum sampling	Timing of serum sampling (*see notes)
ANTIBIOTICS				
Amikacin	Peak 20–30 mg/L Trough 5–10 mg/L	> 40 mg/L	Before and after the 3rd consecutive dose	D
Chloramphenicol	Peak 10–25 mg/L Trough 5–15 mg/L	> 30 mg/L	Newborn: 3 days Children: 1 day	E
Gentamicin	Peak 6–10 mg/L Trough < 2 mg/L	> 12 mg/L	Before and after 3rd consecutive dose	D
Isoniazid	2–10 μg/mL	> 15 μg/mL	When steady-state achieved	B
Kanamycin	Peak 15–25 mg/L Trough < 5–10 mg/L	> 30 mg/L	When steady-state achieved	D

Contd...

Contd...

Drug	Serum therapeutic level	Serum toxic level	Desired duration of therapy before serum sampling	Timing of serum sampling (*see notes)
Streptomycin	Peak 15–40 mg/L Trough < 5 mg/L	> 40 mg/L	Before and after the 3rd consecutive dose	D
Tobramycin	Peak level 6–10 mg/L Trough level < 2 mg/L		Before and after the 3rd consecutive dose	D
Vancomycin	Peak: 25–40 mg/L Trough: < 10 mg/L		Before and after the 3rd consecutive dose	D
ANTICONVULSANTS				
Carbamazepine	6–12 µg/mL	>12 µg/mL	1 month	B
Clonazepam	20–80 ng/mL	> 80 ng/mL	8 days	B
Ethosuximide	40–100 µg/mL	> 150 µg/mL	5–10 days	B
Phenobarbitone	15–40 mg/L	> 40 mg/L	10–14 days	B
Phenytoin	10–20 mg/L	> 25 mg/L	5–10 days	B
Valproic acid	50–100 µg/mL	> 100 µg/mL	2–3 days	B
MISCELLANEOUS DRUGS				
Aspirin	250–400 µg/mL	> 400 µg/mL	2 days	A

Contd...

Contd...

Drug	Serum therapeutic level	Serum toxic level	Desired duration of therapy before serum sampling	Timing of serum sampling (*see notes)
Digoxin	0.8–2 µg/mL	> 2 µg/mL	2 weeks	C
Theophylline	10–20 µg/mL (for asthma) 6–15 µg/mL (for neonatal apnoea)	> 20 µg/mL	1–2 days	F

Note:

A—For trough level just prior to dose; for toxicity monitoring: 2 hr after a dose

B—Serum sampling to obtain trough level: within 30 minutes prior to next scheduled dose

C—At least 6–8 hours postdose to just before the next scheduled dose

D—For trough level within 30 minutes prior to; and for peak 30–60 min after administration of 3rd consecutive dose

E—For trough level (PO/IV) within 30 min before dose; for peak level 2 hr after oral and 30 min after end of IV infusion

F—Guidelines for obtaining blood samples for serum theophylline concentration

PO: Peak—1 hr after dose; Trough—Just before dose

IV bolus: 30 min after infusion

IV continuous: 12–24 hr after beginning of infusion

Appendix 11

DOSE EQUIVALENCE OF COMMONLY USED STEROIDS*

Drug	Glucocorticoid effect equivalent to 100 mg cortisol PO	Mineralocorticoid (mg): Na retention effect equivalent to 0.1 mg florinef**
Cortisone	125	20
Cortisol (Hydrocortisone)	100	20
Prednisone	25	50
Prednisolone	20–25	50
Methylprednisolone	15–20	No effect
Triamcinolone	10–20	No effect
9α-Fluorocortisol	6.5	0.1
Dexamethasone	1.5–3.75	No effect

*The doses give approximately equivalent clinical effects.
**Total physiologic replacement for salt retention is usually 0.1 mg Florinef regardless of size.

Appendix 12

COMPARISON OF ACTION OF NARCOTIC ANALGESICS

Drug	Onset (min)	Duration (h)	Equianalgesic IM Dose (mg)	Equianalgesic PO Dose* (mg)	Parenteral Oral Ratio
Codeine	PO: 30–60 IM: 10–30	IM: 4–6	120	200	1/2–2/3
Fentanyl	IM: 7–15 IV: Immediate	IM: 1–2 IV: 0.5–1	0.1–0.2	–	–
Meperidine	PO, IM, SubQ: 10–15 IV: ≤5	PO, IM, SubQ: 2–4 IV: 2–3	75–100	300	1/3–1/2
Methadone	PO: 30–60 IV: 10–20	Acute: 4–6 Chronic: >8	Acute: 10 Chronic: 2–4	Acute: 20 Chronic: 2–4	1/2; ratio decreases to 1/1 upon chronic dosing

Contd...

Contd...

Drug	Onset (min)	Duration (h)	Equianalgesic IM Dose (mg)	Equianalgesic PO Dose* (mg)	Parenteral Oral Ratio
Morphine	PO: 15–60 IV: ≤5	PO, IV, IM, SubQ: 3–5 Extended release tablets: 8–12	10	Acute: 60 Chronic: 30	1/6; ratio decreases to 1/1.5–2.5 upon chronic dosing
Pentazocine	PO, IM, SubQ: 15–30 IV: ≤2–3	PO: 4–5 IV, IM, SubQ: 2–3	50	150	1/3
Propoxyphene	PO: 30–60	PO: 4–6	–	HCl salt: 130 Napsylate salt: 200	–

*Based on acute, short-term use. Chronic administration may alter pharmacokinetics and change parenteral oral ratio.
Note: Values are based on adult studies. Duration may be shorter in children due to faster elimination (in general) compared to adults.

Appendix 13

COMPOSITION OF FREQUENTLY USED PARENTERAL FLUIDS

Liquid	Na$^+$ (mEq/L)	K$^+$ (mEq/L)	Cl$^-$ (mEq/L)	HCO$_3^{-b}$ (mEq/L)	Ca^{2+} (mEq/L)	CHO (g/100 mL)	Protein^a (g/100 mL)	Cal/L
D$_5$w	–	–	–	–	–	5	–	170
D$_{10}$w	–	–	–	–	–	10	–	340
NS (0.9% NaCl)	154	–	154	–	–	–	–	–
1/2 NS (0.45% NaCl)	77	–	77	–	–	–	–	–
D$_5$ (0.2% NaCl)	34	–	34	–	–	5	–	170
3% saline	513	–	513	–	–	–	–	–
8.4% sodium bicarbonate (1 mEq/mL)	1000	–	–	1000	–	–	–	–

Contd...

Contd...

Liquid	Na⁺ (mEq/L)	K⁺ (mEq/L)	Cl⁻ (mEq/L)	HCO₃⁻ᵇ (mEq/L)	Ca²⁺ (mEq/L)	CHO (g/100 mL)	Proteinᵃ (g/100 mL)	Cal/L
Ringer's	147	4	155.5	–	4	0–10	–	0–340
Lactated Ringer's	130	4	109	28	3	0–10	–	0–340
Albumin 25% (salt poor)	100–160	–	<120	–	–	–	25	1000
Intralipidᶜ	2.5	0.5	4.0	–	–	2.25	–	1100

Note: Following equivalent have been shown in the above table

a Protein or amino acid equivalent

b Bicarbonate or equivalent—citrate, acetate, lactate

c Approximate composition

Appendix 14

CALCULATION FOR INTRAVENOUS DRUG INFUSIONS

1. The following formula enables preparation of appropriate infusate for administration of a particular drug in a specific dose/kg/min through intravenous infusion of fluid at a desired rate

   $$\frac{6 \times \text{child's weight (kg)} \times \text{desired dose in mg/kg/min}}{\text{desired fluid rate (mL/hr)}}$$

   = mg of drug to be added per 100 mL of infusate solution

   For example; for infant weighing 5 kg, desired dose of dopamine 10 µg/kg/min, desired fluid rate 30 mL/hr
   Calculation:

   $$\frac{6 \times 5 \,(\text{Wt. in kg}) \times 10 \,(\text{desired dose rate/min})}{30 \,\text{mL/hr (fluid rate desired)}} = 10$$

   i. e. Add 10 mg dopamine per 100 mL fluid

2. The following table provides ready information about drug concentration in infusate, IV infusion rate/dose/kg/min achieved of some commonly employed emergency drugs.

Drug	Usual dose (µg/kg/min)	Dilution in 100 mL, D_5W	IV infusion rate = drug dose per kg/min achieved
Dopamine	2–20	6 mg/kg	1 mL/hr = 1 µg/kg/min
Dobutamine	2.5–15	6 mg/kg	1 mL/hr = 1 µg/kg/min
Epinephrine	0.1–1	0.6 mg/kg	1 mL/hr = 0.1 µg/kg/min
Lidocaine	20–50	6 mg/kg	1 mL/hr = 1 µg/kg/min
Terbutaline	0.1–0.4	0.6 mg/kg	1 mL/hr = 0.1 µg/kg/min
Prostaglandin E_1	0.05–0.1	0.3 mg/kg	1 mL/hr = 0.05 µg/kg/min

Appendix 15

BURN SURFACE AREA ESTIMATION AND FLUID REPLACEMENT FORMULA

The total body surface area of burn involvement is determined by the sum of the percentages of each site.

Site*	0–1 years	1–4 years	5–9 years	10–14 years	15 years	Adult
Head	9.5	8.5	6.5	5.5	4.5	3.5
Neck	0.5	0.5	0.5	0.5	0.5	0.5
Trunk	13	13	13	13	13	13
Upper arm	2	2	2	2	2	2
Forearm	1.5	1.5	1.5	1.5	1.5	1.5
Hand	1.5	1.5	1.5	1.5	1.5	1.5
Perineum	1	1	1	1	1	1
Buttock (each)	2.5	2.5	2.5	2.5	2.5	2.5
Thigh	2.75	3.25	4	4.25	4.5	4.75
Leg	2.5	2.5	2.75	3	3.25	3.5
Foot	1.75	1.75	1.75	1.75	1.75	1.75

*Percentage for each site is only for *a single extremity with* anterior OR posterior involvement. Percentage should be *doubled if both anterior and posterior* of a single extremity is involved.

Adapted from: Coren CV. "Burn Injuries in Children." *Pediatric Annals.* 1987:16(4):328-39.

Parkland Fluid Replacement Formula

A guideline for replacement of deficits and ongoing losses
(*Note:* For infants, maintenance fluids may need to be added to the below mentioned calculation)

Administer 4 mL/kg/% burn of Ringer's lactate (glucose may be added but beware of stress hyperglycemia) over the first 24 hours; half of this total is given over the first 8 hours *calculated from the time of injury*; the remaining half is given over the next 16 hours. The second 24-hour fluid requirements average 50% to 75% of first day's requirement. Concentrations and rates best determined by monitoring weight, serum electrolytes, urine output, NG losses, etc.

Colloid may be added after 18–24 hours (1 g/kg/day of albumin) to maintain serum albumin >2 g/100 mL.

Potassium is generally withheld for the first 48 hours due to the large amount of potassium that is released from damaged tissues. To manage serum electrolytes, monitor urine electrolytes twice weekly and replace calculated urine losses.

Appendix 16

BODY SURFACE AREA NOMOGRAM AND EQUATION

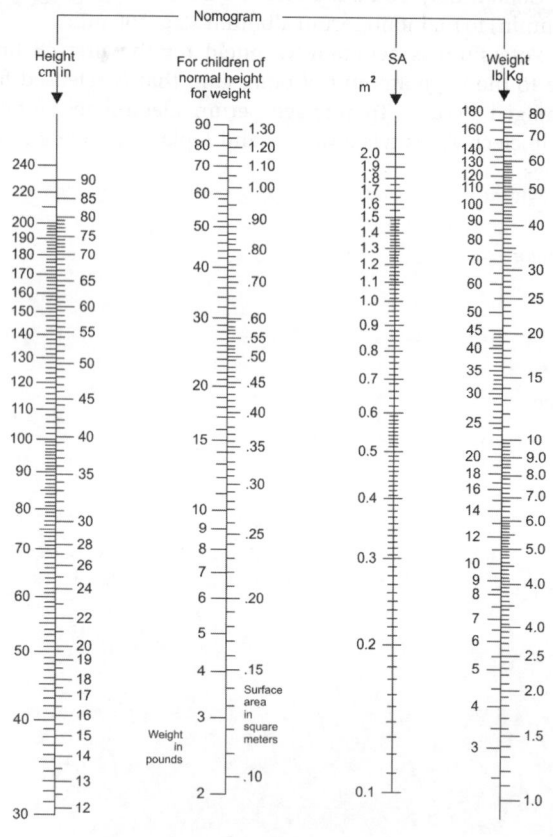

Alternative (Mosteller's formula):

$$\text{Surface area (m}^2) = \sqrt{\frac{\text{Height (cm)} \times \text{Weight (Kg)}}{3600}}$$

Body surface area nomogram and equation

AVERAGE WEIGHTS AND SURFACE AREAS

Average weight and surface area of preterm infants, term infants, and children

Age	Average weight (kg)*	Approximate surface area (m$_2$)
Weeks Gestation		
26	0.9–1	0.1
30	1.3–1.5	0.12
32	1.6–2	0.15
38	2.9–3	0.2
40 (term infant at birth)	3.1–4	0.25
Months		
3	5	0.29
6	7	0.38
9	8	0.42
Years		
1	10	0.49
2	12	0.55
3	15	0.64
4	17	0.74
5	18	0.76
6	20	0.82
7	23	0.90
8	25	0.95
9	28	1.06
10	33	1.18
11	35	1.23
12	40	1.34
Adults	70	1.73

*Weights from age 3 months and over are rounded off to the nearest kilogram.

Appendix 17

CONVERSION FORMULA OF mg TO MEq/L

mEq/L = mg/L per equivalent weight

Equivalent weight = $\dfrac{\text{Atomic weight}}{\text{Valency of element}}$

Factors for Conversion

	A			B		
Element or radical	mEq/L	to	mg/dL	mg/dL	to	mEq/L
Na^+	1	→	2.30	1	→	0.4348
K^+	1	→	3.91	1	→	0.2558
Ca^{++}	1	→	2.005	1	→	0.4988
Mg^{++}	1	→	1.215	1	→	0.8230
Cl^-	1	→	3.55	1	→	0.2817
Bicarbonate (HCO_3^-)	1	→	6.10	1	→	0.1639
Phosphorus valence 1	1	→	3.10	1	→	0.3226
Phosphorus valence 1.8	1	→	1.72	1	→	0.5814

Appendix 18

AVERAGE BODY WEIGHT OF CHILDREN AT DIFFERENT AGE

Age	Weight in kg 50th percentile for boys	Weight in kg 50th percentile for girls
At birth	2.98	2.76
1 month	3.92	3.82
3 months	5.63	5.25
6 months	7.14	6.83
9 months	8.05	7.37
1 year	8.90	8.45
1.5 years	10.05	9.55
2 years	11.53	10.30
2.5 years	11.80	10.92
3 years	12.50	11.90
3.5 years	13.26	13.15
4 years	15.10	14.60
4.5 years	15.22	15.20
5 years	17.60	17.00
6 years	18.90	18.50
7 years	21.00	20.50
8 years	23.90	22.80
9 years	25.50	24.00
10 years	27.50	27.50
11 years	31.00	31.00
12 years	34.30	34.80
13 years	41.50	42.50
14 years	44.00	46.00
15 years	48.40	46.30

Index

Page numbers followed by *f* refer to figure,
fc refer to flowchart, and *t* refer to table

A

Abacavir 324*t*
Acellular pertussis 216
Acetaminophen 399, 472
  poisoning 249
Acetazolamide 389, 473
Acetone 248
Acetylcysteine 439
Acidosis
  correction of 166
  metabolic 102
  severe 462
Acquired immunodeficiency syndrome, management of 93*t*
Activated partial thromboplastin time 423
Acyclovir 318, 472
Adenosine 157, 350
Adrenaline 334, 337, 370, 373
  injection subcutaneous 114
  tartrate 374
Adrenergic
  agonist 132, 335, 339
  blocking agents 138
Adrenocorticotropic hormone 356, 421
  aqueous 356, 421
  gel 356, 421
Airway, breathing and circulation 153, 174, 188
Alanine aminotransferase 293
Albendazole 309

Albumin 439
Alcohol 248
Aldosterone antagonists 130
Alfacalcidol 431
Allergy, symptomatic relief of 411
Allopurinol 440
Alprazolam 402
Aluminum hydroxide 381
Amantadine hydrochloride 320
Amantrel 320
Amebiasis 88, 314, 318
  metastatic 88, 314
  severe intestinal 318
Amebicidal drug 313
Amikacin 48, 469, 470
  sulfate 265
Aminoglycoside 48, 67, 284, 295, 300, 470, 486
  antibiotic 265, 283, 288, 289, 297
Aminopenicillin 266-268
Aminophylline 114, 370
  preparations 381
Amiodarone 156, 157, 350
Amitriptyline 261, 402
Amlodipine 138, 341
Amoxicillin 25, 39, 40, 266, 486
Amphotericin B 313, 472, 486
  deoxycholate 329
  lipid complex 96, 330
Ampicillin 39, 40, 267, 268, 467, 471
Amrinone 133, 166, 335
Amyl nitrite 252
Anaerobic infection 33, 314
Analgesia 188, 397

Analgesics 393, 395, 399, 477
Anaphylactic reaction, emergency treatment of 411
Anaphylaxis 374, 375
Ancylostoma braziliense 86
Anemia
   chronic 196
   pernicious 434
Anesthesia induction 368
Angiotensin-converting enzyme 141, 142
   inhibitor 129, 130, 137, 340*t*, 342, 344, 346
Angiotensin-receptor blocker 129, 130, 137, 340*t*, 343, 346, 348, 350
Anidulafungin 330
Anorexia 369
Antiallergic agent 373
Antiarrhythmic 260, 355, 366
   agent 350, 352, 353, 474
Antibacterial 477
   chemoprophylaxis 70
   drugs 265
Antibiotic 39, 40, 168, 289, 486, 491
   choice of 31
   fluoroquinolone group 285
   initial choice of 10
   role of 17
   therapy 31
      duration of 30, 34
   treatment 7
Anti-cancer drugs 491
Anticholinergic 383
   bronchodilator 376
   poisoning 249
Anticoagulant 452, 466
   overdose of 436
Anticonvulsant 359, 362, 366, 406, 408, 473, 491
   drug 356
   therapy 117

Antidepressant 402
   tricyclic 259, 261, 407, 458
Antidote 249, 251-259
Antiemetic 416, 417
   therapy 362, 406
Antiepileptic drugs 115*t*
Antifibrinolytic agent 465
Antiflatulent 389
Antifungal 333, 472
   agent 333
   drugs 329
Antihelminthics 309
Antihemophilic factor 440
Antihistamines 249, 414, 417, 419
Antihistaminic 404, 409, 410, 413
Antihypertensive 390, 473
   agent 346
   drug 137, 141, 141*t*, 340
      contraindications of 142*t*
Anti-immunoglobulin E 108, 111
Anti-inflammatory 421, 422, 425, 428, 429
   agents 393, 464
   controller drugs, long-term 107
Antileprosy drugs 303
Antimalarial 260, 477, 491
   drugs 304, 305
      therapy 81, 82
Antimicrobial 485
   agents 467
      dosages of 467*t*, 469*t*
   therapy, guidelines for 3
Antimycobacterial drug 299, 304
Antineoplastic 397
Antiparasitic drugs 313
Antiprotozoal 313
   drug 305
Antipseudomonal penicillins 40

Antipsychotic 261
    drug 403, 410
Antipyretics 393
Antiretroviral drug 92-94, 327
    therapy, principle of 94
Antispasmodics 249, 384, 385, 387
Antistaphylococcal penicillin 40, 290
Antithyroid agent 428
Antithyroid drug 430
Antitoxins 239
Antituberculosis drugs 75t, 295, 300, 301
    dosages of 77t
    first line 298
    second-line 284, 301-303
Antituberculous agents 472
Antiulcer agent 389
Antivenin serum polyvalent 441
    amount of 441t
Antiviral 472
    agent 321
    drugs 318
Anuria 392, 455
Anxiety 362, 404, 406
Anxiolytic 362, 404, 406, 413
    agent 402
Apnea, neonatal 370
Arrhythmias 347, 349, 354
    digoxin-induced 366
    life-threatening 349, 354
Arsenic poisoning 250, 459
    mild 250
    moderate 250
Artemether 83, 304
Artemisinin combination therapy 81
Arterial vasodilator 347
Artesunate 82, 304
Arthritis 20, 397
Arthropod infestations 89
Ascariasis 86, 311
Ascorbic acid 431, 434
Aspartate aminotransferase 293
Aspergillosis 96
    allergic bronchopulmonary 96
    invasive pulmonary 96
Aspirin 393
Asplenia 205
Astemizole 410
Asthma 370, 371, 458
    acute 429
        attack of 377, 378, 455
    bronchial 371, 372, 374, 377
    chronic 378
        bronchial 371, 378
    drugs for 370
    exacerbation, severe 113
    exercise induced 379
    intermittent 108, 109
    management of 107
    mild persistent 108, 109
    moderate persistent 108, 109
    nocturnal 371
    severe persistent 108, 109
    severity of 107
    stepwise treatment of 109
    various categories of 108t
Ataxia 369
Atenolol 139, 342, 473
    poisoning 251
Atomoxetine 442
Atorvastatin calcium 443
Atovaquone 84, 307
Atresia, biliary 466
Atrial fibrillation 148, 352, 355
Atrial flutter 148, 352, 355
Atrioventricular block, third-degree 149
Atropine 157, 257
    sulfate 443

Attack
    acute 370
    termination of 147
Attention-deficit hyperactivity disorder 457
    selective treatment of 442
Auranofin 394
Azatadine maleate 411
Azathioprine 444
Azithromycin 25, 49, 268
Azlocillin 40
Aztreonam 52, 269, 467

B

Bacillus calmette-guérin 204
    vaccine 79, 204, 205, 207
Baclofen 444
Bacteremia 24
Bacteroides fragilis 58
    meningitis 33
Balantidiasis 88
Balantidium coli infection 88
Bambuterol hydrochloride 371
Barbiturate 365, 408
Basic life support 151
Beclomethasone dipropionate 371
Beef tapeworm 87
Benadryl 258
Benazepril 137
Benzathine 468
Benzodiazepine 362, 406
    poisoning 251
Benztropine 258
Beriberi 432
Beta-lactamase inhibitor 41, 266, 268, 272, 294
Betamethasone 421
Beta-nonselective adrenergic blocker 345
Bethanechol 382

Bisacodyl 382
Bisoprolol 131, 342
Bites 4
    animal 238t
Bleeding tendency 396
Blood 168
    component therapy 196
    loss, acute 196
    pressure 161
        diastolic 135, 136
        levels 135, 136
        systolic 135, 136, 174
    urea nitrogen 256
Body surface area nomogram and equation 504
Bone marrow
    suppression 320
    transplant 448
Bordetella pertussis 58
Brain abscess 17
Breast abscess 35
Bretylium 157, 474
British anti-Lewisite 250, 255, 256, 444
Broad spectrum 278, 368
    antibiotic 284
Bronchitis, acute 9
Bronchodilator 370, 376, 380
    inhalation 185
    inhaled short-acting 113
Brugia malayi 86
Brugia timori 86
Budesonide 371
Bumetanide 390

C

Caffeine citrate 444
Calcitriol 431
Calcium
    channel blocker 138, 251, 260, 341, 341t, 345, 348, 355, 451

chloride 157, 251, 445
disodium
ethylenediaminetetraacetic acid
    255, 256
gluconate 251, 445
leucovorin 317
salts 251
supplements 446
Campylobacter jejuni 58
Candesartan 137, 343
Candidiasis 96
  neonatal 97
  oral 96, 333
  systemic 97
Capreomycin 301
Captopril 130, 342, 473
Carbamazepine 356, 473
Carbapenem 51, 66
  resistant enterobacteriaceae,
    treatment of 69
Carbenicillin 269, 471
Carbimazole 422
Carbon monoxide poisoning 252
Carbonate 446
Carbonic anhydrase inhibitor
    389
Carboxyhemoglobin 252
Carboxypenicillin 269
Cardiac arrest 445, 446, 463
Cardiac arrhythmias
  drugs for 350
  management of 147
Cardiovascular system 120, 145
Carnitine 446
Carvedilol 131, 343
Caspofungin 96, 331
Catecholamine refractory
    shock 466
  vasodilatory septic shock
    431
Cefaclor 42, 270
Cefadroxil 41, 270

Cefazolin 41, 270, 467, 471
Cefdinir 271
Cefepime 46
  hydrochloride 271
Cefixime 25, 44, 272
Cefoperazone 46, 272
Cefotaxime 26, 43, 273, 467, 471
Cefotetan 42
  disodium 273
Cefoxitin 42, 471
  sodium 273
Cefpirome 46, 274
Cefpodoxime 43
  proxetil 274
Cefprozil 42, 274
Ceftaroline 275
  fosamil 275
Ceftazidime 4, 45, 275, 467, 471
Ceftibuten 44, 276
Ceftizoxime 45, 276
Ceftriaxone 26, 43, 467, 471
  sodium 276
Cefuroxime 42, 277, 471
  axetil 42
Cellulitis 3, 4, 35
  retropharyngeal 6
Central nervous system 87, 119,
    143, 161
  infections of 13, 98
Central venous pressure 161,
    163
Cephalexin 41, 277
Cephalosporin 41, 471, 486
  fifth-generation 275
  first-generation 270, 277
  fourth-generation 271, 274
  second-generation 270, 273,
    274, 277
  third-generation 271-276
Cephalothin 471
Cerebral
  edema 187, 368, 392, 424,
    455
  perfusion pressure 187

Cerebrospinal fluid 187
Cervical adenitis 5
Cetirizine 411
Chancroid 22
Chelation, drugs for 250
Chemoprophylaxis
   against malaria 84
   antimicrobial 70
   antiviral 72
   indications for 78
Chemotherapy 420
   prevention of 418
Chlamydia trachomatis 23, 34, 58
Chloral hydrate 402
Chloramphenicol 25, 50, 278, 468, 472, 486
Chloroquine 80, 84, 260, 305, 313, 474
   resistant *Plasmodium falciparum* malaria 304, 306
Chlorpheniramine maleate 411
Chlorpromazine 258, 261, 403, 416
Chlorpropamide 260
Chlorthalidone 390
Chlorzoxazone 447
Cholecalciferol 434
Cholera 18
   vaccine 232
Cholestasis 466
Cholestyramine resin 447
Cholinergic agent 382, 457
Cholinesterase inhibitor 457, 462
   insecticides 257
Chorea 416
Chorionic gonadotropin 422
Chorioretinitis 36
Ciclesonide 372
Cilastatin 66, 284
Cimetidine 383, 474

Ciprofloxacin 26, 47, 278, 472, 486
Citrate solutions 447
Clarithromycin 49, 279, 487
Clavulanate 40, 41, 296, 471
Clavulanic acid 266
Clemastine 412
Clindamycin 4, 51, 279, 468, 472, 487
Clobazam 357
Clofazimine 303
Clofazine 303
Clonazepam 357
Clonidine 139, 344
Clostridium difficile 59
Clostridium tetani 59
Clotrimazole 331
Cloxacillin 40, 280
Coccidioidomycosis 97
Codeine 260, 394, 472
Colistimethate 54
   sodium 280
Colistin 54, 67, 69, 280
Colitis 88, 318
   amebic 314
   pseudomembranous 314
Common poisoning, antidote for 249
Community-acquired
   infection 24
   pneumonia 9
Complete heart block 149
Complex partial seizures, adjunctive therapy for 368
Congenital syphilis, asymptomatic 292
Congestive heart failure 127, 141, 142, 351*t*
   management of 128
   pathophysiology of 127
   pharmacotherapy in 127

Conjunctivitis, gonococcal 23
Conscious sedation 363
Constipation, chronic 385
Continuous ambulatory peritoneal dialysis 67
Corticosteroid 205, 371, 375, 425, 430
   administration 185
   adrenal 424
   inhaled 107, 110
   role of 189
   systemic 112, 113
   therapy, daily inhaled 110
Cortisone acetate 422
Corynebacterium diphtheriae 59
Cosmetics 247
Cotrimoxazole 281
Cough 372
Cromolyn 373
Cryoprecipitate 199
Cryptococcosis 98
Cryptorchidism, prepubertal 422
Cryptosporidiosis 88, 315
Cutaneous larva migrans 86
Cyanide poisoning 252
Cyanocobalamin 434
Cyanotic spell 349
   management of 397
   severe 463
Cyclizine 447
Cyclophosphamide 448
Cycloserine 302
Cyproheptadine 412
Cystic fibrosis 466
Cysticercosis 86, 87
Cystitis, acute 21
Cytomegalovirus 90, 320

D

Dapsone 303
Daptomycin 52, 53, 282
Datura 249
Deep sedation 188
Deferiprone 255, 449
Deferoxamine 255, 449
   mesylate 253, 254
Dehydration 99, 100
   assessment of 99
   grade of 100
   hypotonic 103
   prevention of 178
   prompt treatment of 178
   severe 102
   status, assessment of 100t
Dehydroemetine hydrochloride 313
Demeclocycline 282
Dengue
   management of 171
   mild 171
   moderate 171, 172fc
   severe 173
   shock syndrome 170
Depression 405, 458
Desmopressin acetate 423
Dexamethasone 423
Dextran 449
Dextromethorphan 449
Diabetes
   insipidus 423, 431, 466
   mellitus 144, 219, 227, 346, 392
Diabetic ketoacidosis 179, 426
   diagnostic features of 181
   management of 181
Diaper dermatitis 96
Diarrhea 99
   acute 386
   chronic 386
   secretory 458
Diazepam 121, 358, 403, 473
   intravenous 120
Diclofenac sodium 394

Dicloxacillin 40
Dicyclomine hydrochloride 383
Didanosine 325
Dietary deficiency 433
Diethylcarbamazine 310
Digitalis 131
    poisoning 252
Digoxin 131, 335, 351, 473
Diloxanide furoate 313
Diltiazem 260, 473
Dimenhydrinate 417
Dimercaptosuccinic acid 250, 255, 449
Dimethindene maleate 413
Diphenhydramine 258, 413
Diphtheria 6, 70, 233
    antitoxin 239
    pertussis and tetanus 233
        vaccine 212, 213
    tetanus
        and acellular pertussis 204
        and pertussis combined vaccines 216
        and whole-cell pertussis 204
        toxoid vaccine 214
    toxoid 214
Diphyllobothrium latum 87
Directly observed treatment short-course strategy 74
Disopyramide 260, 352
Disseminated intravascular coagulation 198
Diuretics 129, 138, 389, 473
Dizziness 369
Dobutamine 132, 157, 165, 336
Docusate 383
Domperidone 417
Dopamine 132, 157, 165, 336
Doxapram hydrochloride 449
Doxycycline 4, 49, 84, 282
D-penicillamine 256
Drug
    guidelines for choice of 86
    hematologic adverse effects of 480
    regimen 75
    therapy 1, 74, 80, 115, 136, 142, 164, 184
    principles of 108
Dysentery 18
Dysplasia, bronchopulmonary 424
Dyspnea 253
Dystonic reaction, acute 258

E

Echinococcosis 86
Echinococcus granulosus, intermediate stage infection of 87
Ectopic tachycardia, postoperative junctional 148
Edema 393
Efavirenz 325
Eikenella corrodens 59
Electrocardiogram 106, 153, 156
    monitor 104
Electrocardiography 161
Electroencephalogram 115
Electrolytes 99
Emergency drugs 156t
Emesis, chemotherapy-induced 418
Emetic 453
Empyema 12
Enalapril 130, 137, 344, 473
    maleate 344
Enalaprilat 137, 344

Encephalitis 17
Encephalopathy, hepatic 385
Endocarditis 27
    bacterial 72
    gonococcal 23
    prosthetic value 67
Endocrine disorders, drugs for 421
Enteric fever, uncomplicated 25
Enterobius vermicularis 86, 87
Enteroviral infections 33
Enuresis 404
    nocturnal 407, 423, 458
Envenomation, severity of 441
Eosinophilia, tropical pulmonary 86, 310
Epididymitis 22
Epiglottitis 8
Epilepsy 115
    partial 369
Epinephrine 132, 156, 165, 185, 337, 373
Epistaxis 372
Eplerenone 138
Epsilon aminocaproic acid 450
Eptoin 367
Equine rabies immunoglobulin 242
Ergotamine 450
Ertapenem 66
Erysipelas 3
Erythromycin 49, 282, 468, 487
Erythropoietin 436
Escherichia coli 31, 59
Esmolol 344
Esomeprazole 384
Ethacrynic acid 391
Ethambutol 76, 77, 301, 472
Ethanol 451
Ethionamide 302
Ethosuximide 359
Ethylene glycol poisoning 252
Ethylenediaminetetraacetic acid 256, 450
Etrapenem 51
Extended-spectrum penicillin 293, 296

F

Fab antibodies, digoxin-specific 252
Famotidine 384
Fatal hepatic failure 369
Fatigue 369
Febrile seizure 124, 363
    types of 124*t*
Felbamate 359
Felodipine 138
Fentanyl 395, 473
Fever 320
    acute rheumatic 393
    severe enteric 26
Fexofenadine 413
Filariasis 86
    lymphatic 310
Fixed drug combination 75
Flecainide 474
    acetate 352
Fluconazole 331, 472
Flucytosine 332
Fludrocortisone acetate 424
Fluid 99
    choice of 163
    overload 173
    therapy 162, 166
Flumazenil 251, 451
Flunarizine 451
Fluoroquinolone 47, 278
Fluoxetine hydrochloride 403
Fluticasone propionate 374
Folate deficiency anemia, treatment of 437, 437*t*

Folic acid 437
Fomepizole 252, 256
Foot-puncture wound,
	osteomyelitis
	of 20
Formoterol fumarate 374
Foscarnet 320
Fosfomycin 54
Fosinopril 137
Fosphenytoin
	intravenous 121
	sodium 359
Fulminant intestinal disease 88
Fungal infections 29
	serious systemic 329
	severe 329
Furazolidone 283, 314
Furosemide 158, 391, 473
Fusidic acid 55
Fusion inhibitor 94

G

Gabapentin 360, 473
Ganciclovir 321
Gastric acid
	proton pump inhibitor 386
	secretion inhibitor 386
Gastric ulcer 388
Gastritis 19, 19t
Gastroenteritis, acute 17, 99
Gastroesophageal reflux 382, 417
	disease 384, 386
Gastrointestinal infections 17
Gastrointestinal tract 258
Gatifloxacin 48
Genitourinary infections 21
Genotropin 425
Gentamicin 48, 283, 469, 471
Giardiasis 88, 314, 315, 318
Gingivostomatitis 6

Glaucoma 384, 390
Glibenclamide 260
Glipizide 260
Glubionate 446
Glucagon 251, 452
Glucose
	6-phosphate dehydrogenase
	deficiency 80
	infusion 426
Glucostix 123
Glycopeptide 51
	antibiotic 297
Glycopyrrolate 452
Glycosides, cardiac 473
Glycylcycline 53
Goiter, nontoxic 427
Gonococcal infection,
	disseminated 23
Gonorrhea 23
Gram-negative enteric bacteria 33
Granisetron 417
Granulocyte colony-stimulating
	factor 437, 451
Griseofulvin 332
Group A streptococcal infection,
	treatment of 292
Growth hormone deficiency 425

H

Haemophilus ducreyi 22, 60
Haemophilus influenzae 3, 60, 125
	type B 204, 216, 218
		vaccine 217, 218
Hallucinations 258
Haloperidol 403
Havrix vaccine 222
Heart
	disease, congenital 128, 461
	rate 152, 153, 156

Helicobacter pylori 19, 19*t*, 60
Helminthic infection 86
    treatment of 86
Hemarthrosis 440
Hematinics 436
Hematocrit 172
Hematoma, significant subcutaneous 440
Hematuria 441
Hemochromatosis, primary 254
Hemophilia
    A 191-193, 423, 440
        bleeding in 440
    management of 191
    mild 191
    moderate 191
    severe 191
Hemorrhage
    iliopsoas 441
    life-threatening 440
    variceal 431, 466
Hemorrhagic disease 436
Heparin
    poisoning 253
    sodium 452
Hepatic disease 485
Hepatitis
    A 204, 236
        pre-exposure prophylaxis 237*t*
        vaccine 206, 222, 223
        virus 222
    B 204, 206, 218, 236
        chronic 90, 321
        immunization 209
        immunoglobulin 204, 240
        vaccine 204, 209, 210, 217, 223
        virus 209
    C, chronic 90
        active 321, 322

Heroin 257
Herpes meningoencephalitis 33
Herpes simplex 90, 318, 320
    infection 24
    virus 17, 318
        infection 318
Herpes zoster 319
Histamine-2 receptor antagonist 185, 383, 384, 388
Histoplasmosis 98
    mildly symptomatic acute pulmonary 98
Hookworm 87, 309, 311, 312
Hormones 421, 491
Hospital-acquired pneumonia 12
Human bovine pentavalent rotavirus live vaccine RV5 211
Human growth hormone 425
Human immunodeficiency virus 10, 92
    drug 324, 328
        antiretroviral 326
    immunization of 205
    infection 327
        antiviral drug for 326
        treatment of 328
    management of 93*t*
    treatment
        guidelines for 92
        NACO guidelines for 92
Human monovalent rotavirus live vaccine RV1 211
Human normal immunoglobulin 241
Human papillomavirus 204
    vaccine 207, 225
Human rabies immunoglobulin 229, 242

Humatrope 425
Hydatid cyst 309
Hydatid disease 87
Hydralazine 345, 473
Hydration status 100
Hydrochlorothiazide 391
Hydrocortisone sodium succinate 375, 425
Hydroquinone 248
Hydroxyzine 413
   hydrochloride 404
Hymenolepis nana 87
Hyoscine butylbromide 385
Hyperbilirubinemia 366
Hypercalcemia 256
Hypercyanotic attacks, management of 177, 177t
Hyperkalemia 446
   acute 104
   correction of 463
   mild-to-moderate 104
   severe 104, 426
Hypernatremia 103
Hypersensitivity 253
Hypertension 134, 135, 141, 141t, 343, 347-349, 393
   choice of drugs in 140
   chronic 348
   classification of 134
   intracranial 187
   pharmacotherapy in 134
   portal 431, 466
   stages of 134, 135
Hypertensive crisis, preoperative management of 348
Hypertensive emergency 134, 142, 143, 348
   drugs for 144t

Hypertensive urgency 142, 146
Hyperthyroidism 422
Hypertonic saline 189
Hypnotics 402
Hypocalcemia 166, 431, 445
   neonatal 426, 445
   prevention of 434
Hypoglycemia 123, 179
Hypoglycemic
   agent 456
   oral 260
Hypogonadism, hypogonadotropic 422
Hypokalemia 102, 105
   acute 104
   asymptomatic 106
   management of 106
Hypomagnesemia
   severe 454
   symptomatic 454
Hyposplenia 205
   anatomic 217
   functional 217
Hypotension 253, 339
   orthostatic 258
   severe 362
Hypothyroidism 427
   congenital 427
Hypovolemia 439

I

Ibuprofen 395
Idiopathic thrombocytopenic purpura 240
Imipenem 51, 66, 284, 469, 472
Imipramine 261, 404
Immunization
   active 203
   regime, primary 212
   schedule 203, 215

Immunoglobulin 239
   intravenous 240
Impetigo 35
Indian Academy of Pediatrics Immunization Schedule 204*t*
Indinavir 326
Infantile spasms 356, 421
Influenza 72
   A 91
   B 91
   vaccine 227
      inactivated 206, 227
Inorganic mercury poisoning 250
Insulin 252, 426, 474
   therapy, alternative regimens of 180
   types of 180*t*
Integrase strand transfer inhibitors 94
Intensive care unit 114, 132, 145
Intestinal disease, mild-to-moderate 318
Intestinal infection, adult 87
Intestinal luminal amebiasis, asymptomatic 88
Intestinal nematodes 312
Intracranial pressure 187
Invasive intestinal disease, mild-to-moderate 88
Iodine 428
Ipecac syrup 453
Ipratropium 113
   bromide 376
   inhalation 114
Iron 438
   deficiency, total replacement of 438
   oral 178
   overload, chronic 254
   poisoning 253

Isoniazid 77, 298, 472, 487
   poisoning 255
      antidote for 433
Isoprinosine 321
Isoproterenol 132, 158, 166, 338
Isradipine 138, 345
Itraconazole 96, 332, 472

J

Japanese encephalitis 231
   vaccine 231
      inactivated vero cell-derived 231

K

Kanamac 303
Kanamycin 284, 302, 469, 471
Kawasaki disease 241, 393
Ketamine 405
Ketoconazole 333, 472
Ketolide 56
Ketorolac 396
Ketotifen 376, 454

L

Labetalol 345
Lactase 454
Lactate salts 446
Lactulose 385
Lamivudine 326
Lamotrigine 360
Lansoprazole 386
Lead
   intoxication 459
   poisoning 255
Leishmaniasis 88, 329
Lennox-Gastaut syndrome 357
Leprosy 303

Leukotriene receptor antagonist 108, 110, 377, 381
Levalbuterol nebulized 113
Levetiracetam 124, 361
Levocetirizine 414
Levofloxacin 48, 285
Levosalbutamol 112, 376
Levothyroxine sodium 430
Lice 89
Lidocaine 124, 156, 353, 474
Lincomycin 285
Lincosamide 51
    antibiotic 279, 285
Linezolid 52, 53, 66, 286, 487
Liothyronine 427
Lipoglycopeptide 51
Lipopeptide 52
Lisinopril 137, 346
Listeria monocytogenes 33, 61
Lithium 405
Liver abscess 314
    amebic 88, 318
Löffler pneumonia 310
Long QT syndrome 149, 349
Loop diuretics 130, 138, 390, 391
Loperamide 386
Lopinavir 326
Loratadine 414
Lorazepam 120, 124, 362, 406, 473
    intravenous 120
Losartan 137, 346
Low dose infusion 336
Loxapine 261
Ludwig's angina 5
Lugol's solution 428
Lung abscess 13

M

Macrolide 49
    antibiotic 268, 279, 282

Magnesium sulfate 114, 377, 454
Malaria 70, 80, 89, 305
    chemoprophylaxis 80
    treatment 80
        complicated 307
        severe 307
    uncomplicated 304
Malarone 84
Mania, acute 405
Mantoux test 78
Mast cell stabilizer 373
Mastoiditis, acute 8
Measles 206, 233
    mumps, and rubella 204
        vaccine 220
    prophylaxis 241
    vaccine 220
Mebendazole 311
Meclizine 455
Mediastinal disease, mild 98
Mefenamic acid 397, 456
Mefloquine 84, 306, 487
Meningitis 31, 70, 468
    bacterial 13, 15t, 424
    gonococcal 23
    neonatal 17, 32, 34, 292
Meningococcal vaccines 227
Meperidine 400, 473
Mercury poisoning 250, 256
Meropenem 51, 66, 286, 469, 487
Metformin 456
Methanol poisoning 252, 256
Methdilazine hydrochloride 414
Methemoglobinemia 256
Methicillin-resistant staphylococcus
    aureus 56, 66, 67
        infection 32
        treatment of 68
    epidermidis 66

Methocarbamol 456
Methotrexate 397
Methyldopa 139, 473
Methylene blue 256, 457
Methylphenidate 457
Methylprednisolone sodium
succinate 428
Metoclopra 474
Metoclopramide 417
toxicity 258
Metolazone 392
Metoprolol 131, 139, 347
Metronidazole 52, 314, 469, 472, 487
Mezlocillin 40
sodium 287
Micafungin 96
Miconazole 333
Micronutrients 436
Midazolam 121, 124, 362, 406, 473, 474
infusion 122
intravenous 120
Migraine 450
headache, intractable 419, 460
prophylaxis 349
Milrinone 133, 338
Miltefosine 315
Minimal potential fatal dose 260
Minocycline 49, 287
Minoxidil 347
Monobactam 52
antibiotic inhibitor 269
Moraxella catarrhalis 61
Morphine 257, 397, 473
Motion sickness 417, 420
Mouth bleeding 440
Moxifloxacin 48
Multidrug-resistant
bacterial pathogens,
treatment of 68
tuberculosis, second-line
drug in 302
Muscle 440
relaxant 444
Myasthenia gravis 462
treatment 457
Mycoplasma pneumoniae 61

N

N-acetylcysteine 249
Nafcillin 40, 468, 471
sodium 287
Nalidixic acid 288, 487
Naloxone 158, 257, 457
Naproxen 398
Narcotics 260, 395, 472
analgesics 497
overdose poisoning 257
Nasal irritation 372
National AIDS Control
Organisation 92
Nausea 416, 420
Necrotizing funisitis 35
Neisseria gonorrhoeae 61
Neisseria meningitidis 62
Nelfinavir 327
Neomycin 288
Neonatal intensive care unit 31
Neonatal seizures 115, 363, 408
management of 122
Neonatal sepsis
early-onset 32
late-onset 32
Neostigmine 457
Nephrotic syndrome 429, 448
Nephrotoxicity 320
Nervousness 258
Netilmicin 48, 289, 469
Neuritis, drug induced 433
Neurocysticercosis 309
Neuromuscular blocking agent 464

Neurosyphilis 24
Neutral protamine Hagedorn 180
Neutropenia, reduces duration of 437
Nevirapine 327
Nicardipine 138
Nifedipine 138, 251, 260, 348, 473
Nimesulide 398
Nitazoxanide 315
Nitrazepam 363
Nitrofurantoin 55, 289
Nitroprusside 473
Nondigitalis inotropic agents 132
Non-nucleoside reverse transcriptase inhibitor 94, 325-327
Nonselective beta-adrenergic blocker 349, 354
Nonsteroidal anti-inflammatory agents 108
    drug 111, 171, 394-398, 400, 401
Norditropin 425
Norepinephrine 165, 339
    reuptake inhibitor 442
Norfloxacin 47, 289
Nortriptyline hydrochloride 407, 458
Nucleoside reverse transcriptase inhibitor 93, 324, 328
Nystatin 333

O

Octreotide 458
Ofloxacin 26, 47, 290
Oliguria 392, 455
Olmesartan 137, 348
Omalizumab 111
Omeprazole 386
Omphalitis 35
Ondansetron 418
Oral corticosteroids
    systemic 108
    use of 112
Oral poliovirus vaccine 204
Oral rehydration solution, administration of 99
Orbital cellulitis 8
Organophosphate poisoning 257
Oropharyngeal candidiasis 97
Oseltamivir 322
Osteomyelitis 20, 35
    acute 20
    chronic 20
Otitis media 7, 35
Oxacillin 40, 290, 468
Oxazolidinone 52
    antibiotic 286
Oxcarbazepine 363
Oxybutynin 387
Oxygen administration 113, 162
Oxyphenonium bromide 387
Oxytetracycline 291

P

Packed red blood cell
    transfusion 196
    volume of 196
Pain
    moderate acute 396
    severe acute 396
Pancuronium 458
Pantoprazole 387
Para-aminosalicylic acid 303
Paracetamol 399

Paraldehyde 364, 408
Parasitic infection, treatment of 86
Parenteral therapy 26, 250
Parkland fluid replacement formula 502
Paromomycin 315
Pasteurella multocida 4, 62
Pediatric
 advanced life support 150
 antiretroviral therapy 95
 basic life support 151*fc*
 bradycardia advanced life support 153*fc*
 drug formulary 265
 life support 150
 pulseless cardiac arrest advanced life support 154*fc*
 tachycardia advanced life support 155*fc*
Pediculosis 89
Pefloxacin 47, 291
Peginterferon 322
Penicillamine 255, 459
Penicillin 4, 39, 40, 296, 468, 471
 allergy 72
 G 39, 468, 471
  aqueous 291
  benzathine 292
  procaine 292
  penicillinase resistant 280, 287
 V 39
  potassium 293
Pentamidine isothionate 316
Pentazocine 257, 399
Pentobarbital 365, 408
 coma 408
Peptic ulcer 384, 388
Pericarditis
 purulent 28
 tuberculous 28

Perinephric abscess 22
Perirectal abscess 19
Peritonitis 27
 acute
  primary 27
  secondary 27
Pertussis 13, 70, 234
 antimicrobial prophylaxis of 235*t*
Pethidine 257, 400
Pharmacotherapy 123
 guidelines for 107
Pharyngitis 5, 372
Phenazopyridine 400, 459
Pheniramine maleate 414
Phenobarbital 473
Phenobarbitone 365, 408
 high dose 122
Phenothiazine 258, 409, 415, 419
 derivative 409
 group 419, 460
Phentolamine mesylate 348
Phenylephrine 166, 353
 hydrochloride 339
Phenytoin 353, 366, 474
 intravenous 121
Pheochromocytoma 347
 diagnosis 348
 surgery 348
Phosphodiesterase inhibitors 133
Physostigmine 249, 459
Phytonadione 259, 436
Pinworm 87, 309, 312
Pipenzolate methyl bromide 388
Piperacillin 4, 40, 294
 sodium 293
Piperazine 488
 citrate 311
Piracetam 460

Pirbuterol 112
Piroxicam 400
Plasma
    transfusion 198
    volume expander 449
Plasmodium falciparum 81
    malaria, uncomplicated 81
        chloroquine resistant 308
Plasmodium ovale malaria 306
Plasmodium vivax malaria 306
    uncomplicated 80
Platelet
    rate of transfusion of 198
    transfusion 197
        role of 173
Pneumococcal conjugate vaccine 204, 218
Pneumococcal polysaccharide vaccine 219
Pneumococcal vaccine 206, 218
Pneumocystis carinii 89
Pneumocystis jirovecii pneumonia 89
Pneumonia 9, 34
    diffuse 97
    necrotizing 13
    neonatal 34
    nosocomial 34
    severe 10
Polio vaccine 203, 206, 207
Poliovirus vaccine, inactivated 204
Pork tapeworm 87
Posaconazole 96
Potassium
    chloride 106, 460
    iodide 428
    level, serum 104
    removing resin 463
    sparing diuretic 138, 392, 393

Pralidoxime 257, 460
Praziquantel 312
Prednisolone 114, 429
    intramuscular 113
    intravenous 113
    oral 113
Prednisone 429
Prehypertension 134
Prematurity
    anemia of 436
    apnea of 370, 444
Primaquine 306
Primidone 367
Procainamide 156, 157, 260, 353, 474
Procaine 468
Prochlorperazine 258, 419, 460
Proguanil 84, 307
Promethazine 258
    hydrochloride 409, 415, 419
        preparations 415
    theoclate 420, 461
Propafenone 355
Propantheline bromide 388
Propofol 367
    infusion 122
Propranolol 349, 354, 473
    oral 178
    poisoning 251
Propylthiouracil 430
Prostigmine 457
Protamine sulfate 253, 461
Protease inhibitor 94, 326, 327
Proteus mirabilis 62
Proton pump inhibitor 384, 387
Protozoal infection 88
    treatment of 86
Pruritus 404
Pseudoephedrine 461
Pseudomonas 20, 31, 33, 34
    aeruginosa 3, 62, 66
        infection 36

Pseudotumor cerebri 390
Pulseless electrical activity 154
Pyelonephritis, acute 21
Pyoderma 5
Pyrantel pamoate 312
Pyrazinamide 76, 77, 300, 472
Pyrexia 397
Pyridostigmine 462
Pyridoxine 124, 255, 433
    dependent persistent neonatal seizures 433
Pyrimethamine 309, 316
Pyritinol 462

Q

Quinapril 137
Quinidine 260, 474
    phenylethyl-barbiturate 355
    sulfate 355
Quinine 260, 488
    dihydrochloride 307
    intramuscular 83
    intravenous 83
    sulfate 308
Quinolone 486
    antibiotic 290
    first-generation 288
    group antibiotic 291, 294

R

Rabies 237
    exposure, categories of 230t
    immunoglobulin 242
    vaccine 229
Radiation 420
Raised intracranial pressure 390
Ramipril 137
Ranitidine 388, 474
Rapid diagnostic test 81
Rash 320
Rat-bite fever 5
Red blood cell 172, 174
Renal abscess 22
Renal disease 391
Renal failure 396, 432, 470
    acute 254, 462
    chronic 437
Respiratory syncytial virus 34, 91
    monoclonal antibody against 242
Respiratory tract infections, lower 8
Resuscitation
    cardiopulmonary 151, 154
    neonatal 152fc
Retinitis 320
Revised National Tuberculosis Control Program 74, 77, 77t
Rheumatic fever 71
    prophylaxis 292, 293
Rheumatoid arthritis 393, 396, 459
    juvenile 394, 397
Rhinitis, allergic 372
Ribavirin 323
Riboflavin 433
Ribonucleic acid 92
Rickets
    prevention of 434
    treatment of 435
Rickettsial infection 29
Rifampicin 67, 76, 77, 299, 303, 304
Rifampin 52, 472
Rimantadine 323
Ritonavir 326
Rotavirus vaccine 206, 211
Roundworm 87, 309
Roxithromycin 49, 294

S

Salbutamol 112, 113, 378
  nebulization 114
Salicylates 258
Salmeterol 378
Salmonella gastroenteritis 18
Scabies 89, 310
Schistosomiasis 87
Scurvy 434
Sedation 358, 362, 363, 368, 406, 408, 420
  preoperative 363, 404
Sedatives 402
Seizures
  multiple types of 363
  myoclonic 363
  partial 359, 363, 366
  persistent 121
  refractory 390
  termination of 120
  types of 115, 116, 124
Selective serotonin re-uptake inhibitor 403
Semisynthetic macrolide antibiotic 294
Senna 389
Sennosides 389
Sepsis 24, 30
  neonatal 31, 34
  nosocomial 24
Septic shock 28, 166, 167*fc*
  syndrome 28, 168
Sexually transmitted infections 21
Shigella infection 18
Shock 159, 169, 375, 426, 439, 449
  anaphylactic 169
  cardiogenic 169
  cardiovascular drugs for 165*t*
  compensated 174*fc*
  early recognition of 162
  hypotensive decompensated 175*fc*
  impending 449
  management of 159
  stages of 162*t*
  types of 160*t*
Short stature, idiopathic 425
Sick sinus syndrome 149
Sickle cell disease 71, 217
Simethiconet 389
Sinus rhythm 147
Sinusitis, acute 7
Skeletal muscle relaxant 456, 458
Skin
  and soft tissue infections 3, 35
  lighteners 248
  pinch 100
Sodium
  bicarbonate 258, 462
    administration 183
  cromoglycate 373
  nitrite 252
  polystyrene sulfonate 463
  stibogluconate 317
  thiosulfate 252
  valproate 368
Somatropin 425
Sparfloxacin 48, 294
Spinal cord injury, acute 428
Spiramycin 317
Spironolactone 138, 392, 473
Staphylococcal scalded skin syndrome 5
Staphylococcus
  aureus 3, 28, 31, 33, 63, 66
  epidermidis 63, 66
  saprophyticus 63

Status asthmaticus 113, 375, 425, 428
Status epilepticus 119, 358, 362, 364, 366, 368, 406, 408
   management of 119
   seizures 367
Stavudine 327
Steroids 168
   role of 76
Streptococcal pharyngitis, acute group 293
Streptococcus
   pneumoniae 64, 168
   pyogenes 4, 64
Streptomycin 76, 77
   sulfate 295, 300
Strongyloidiasis 87, 312
Succinylcholine 464
Sucralfate 389
Sulbactam 40, 268, 272
Sulfadiazine 295, 317
Sulfadoxine 309
Sulfamethoxazole 25, 50, 281, 295, 472
Sulfasalazine 464
Sulfonamides 488
Synthetic human growth hormone 425
Syphilis 23
   congenital 36

T

Tachyarrhythmia, supraventricular 351*t*
Tachycardia 258
   atrial 355
   functional ectopic 350
   supraventricular 147, 350, 352, 355
   ventricular 148, 350, 355

Taenia saginata 87, 311, 312
Taenia solium 87
   intermediate stage infection of 87
Tapeworm infections 87
Tazobactam 4, 294, 471
Teicoplanin 51, 68
Telavancin 51
Telithromycin 56
Tenofovir 328
Terbinafine 334
Terbutaline 112, 114
   sulfate 379
Terfenadine 416
Tetanus 28, 36, 236
   antitoxin 28
   immunoglobulin 28, 242
   neonatal 416
   prevention of 236*t*
   prophylaxis 216*t*
   toxoid 214, 215
   treatment of 243
Tetracycline 49, 295, 488
   derivative antibiotic 282
   group antibiotic 282
Tetralogy of Fallot 177, 177*t*, 349, 397
   management 177
   prevention 177
Theophylline 111, 260, 380
   salt 380
      combination preparations 381
Thiabendazole 312
Thiamine 432
Thiazide 130, 138
   diuretic 390, 391
Thiopental sodium 368, 465
Thioridazine 261, 409
Thrombocytopenic purpura 429
Thrombosis 452
Thymidine analogues 93

Thyroidectomy, preoperative 428
Thyrotoxic crisis 428
Thyrotoxicosis 349, 422, 428
   neonatal 428
Thyroxine sodium 430
Tiagabine 368
Ticarcillin 40, 41, 296, 468, 471
   disodium 296
Tigecycline 53, 69
Tinidazole 318
Tobramycin 48, 297, 469, 471
Tolmetin sodium 401
Tonic clonic seizures, generalized 366
Tonsillopharyngitis 5
Tooth extraction 440
Topiramate 124, 368
Toxicity 249
Toxocara, larval infection of 88
Toxocariasis 87
Toxoplasmosis 89
   acquired 316
   congenital 36, 316
Tracheitis bacterial 9
Tramadol 401
Tranexamic acid 465
Tranquilizers 402
Triamcinolone 430
Triamterene 393
Trichinella spiralis 87
Trichinellosis 87
Trichomonas vaginalis 89
Trichomoniasis 22, 89, 314, 318
Trichuriasis 88
Triclofos sodium 410
Trifluoperazine 258, 410
Triflupromazine 420
Trimethoprim 25, 50, 281, 295, 472
Trovafloxacin 48
Tuberculosis 13, 71, 74, 78
   childhood 74
   infection 14
   pulmonary 78
Typhoid
   conjugate vaccine 222
   fever 25
   vaccines 222
Ulcerative colitis 464
Universal Immunization Programme 231

U

Upper respiratory tract infections 5
Ureaplasma urealyticum 34
Uric acid lowering agent 440
Urinary acidification 434
Urinary retention, nonobstructive 382
Urinary tract
   infection 36
      recurrent 71
   obstruction 21
Ursodeoxycholic acid 466
Ursodiol 466

V

Vaccination, dose and schedule of 226
Vaccines 205
Vaginal infections 22
Vaginosis, bacterial 22
Valganciclovir 324
Valparin 369
Valproic acid 368
Valsartan 137, 350
Vancomycin 4, 51, 67, 297, 468, 472
   resistant enterococcus, treatment of 69

Varicella 234
    vaccine 207, 223
    zoster
        immunoglobulin 243
        virus 91
Vasodilator 139, 341t, 345
Vasopressin 339, 431, 466
    analog 423
Ventriculoperitoneal shunt infection 14
Verapamil 251, 260, 355, 473
Vertigo 417
Vibrio cholerae 64
Vigabatrin 369
Viral infection 90
    treatment of 90t
    types of 90, 91
Viral load 92
Visceral larva migrans 88, 310
Visceral leishmaniasis 315
Vitamin 431
    A 432
    B1 432
    B12 434
        deficiency 434
    B2 433
    B6 433
    C 434, 436
    D 434
        analog 431
        preparation 431
    D3 434
    E 435
    K deficiency 436
    K1 259, 436
Vomiting 416, 418-420, 460
    radiotherapy-induced 418
Voriconazole 96, 334
Vulvovaginal candidiasis 22, 96

W

Wernicke encephalopathy 433
Whipworm 88, 311
Whole-cell pertussis 216-218
Wilson disease 459
Wound management 216t
Wuchereria bancrofti 86

X

Xerophthalmia 432

Y

Yersinia enterocolitica 65

Z

Zalcitabine 328
Zanamivir 324
Zidovudine 328
Zinc supplements 439
Zonisamide 369